MEDICAL GEOGRAPHY

MEDICAL GEOGRAPHY

SECOND EDITION

Melinda S. Meade
Robert J. Earickson

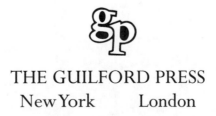

THE GUILFORD PRESS
New York   London

© 2000 The Guilford Press
A Division of Guilford Publications, Inc.
72 Spring Street, New York, NY 10012
www.guilford.com

Printed in the United States of America

This book is printed on acid-free paper.

Last digit is print number: 9 8 7 6 5 4 3 2 1

Library of Congress Cataloging-in-Publication Data

Meade, Melinda S.
    Medical geography / Melinda S. Meade and Robert J.
        Earickson. — 2nd ed.
            p.   cm.
        Includes bibliographical references and index.
        ISBN 1-57230-558-4
        1. Medical geography.   I. Earickson, Robert.   II. Title.

    RA792.M42 2000
    614.4'2—dc21   00-035421

Preface

Much has changed in the world and in the discipline of geography since the first edition of this text was published in 1988. The Soviet Union has fallen apart, and with it the Soviet health care system. The free market economically, politically, and socially has become a global runaway force. AIDS, which in the mid-1980s was a new epidemic of poorly understood etiology, has become a modern pandemic plague of enormous demographic and social impact. Infectious disease in general, newly emerging or now unaffected by our drugs, is renascent. World population has grown by more than 1 billion, has lowered its fertility to three children per family and its growth rate to less than 2%, and has picked up and headed for the city. Health promotion has become the world theme, and biomedicine has been forced off its pedestal. Social science has developed an interdisciplinary theoretical perspective and a new vocabulary for addressing old processes. Geographic information systems, with their ability to manage and portray spatial data, have become the dominant tool in geography and have transformed a variety of health analyses and the structuring of public data. Medical geography as a subdiscipline has become less concerned with the optimization of health service delivery or a dichotomy between health service and disease ecology (etiology). Instead, it has become increasingly concerned with health geography as a behavioral and social construction and disease ecology as an interface between the natural (physical world) and cultural dimensions of existence.

This text still endeavors to provide a broad-based, comprehensive survey of the rich diversity of medical geography for upper-division undergraduates and graduate students while also serving as a sound reference for the complexities of classifications, processes, and systems. Our perspective remains holistic and international. We still hope to provide the necessary biological background for geographers to understand disease processes and the necessary geographical background for health researchers to understand spatial processes. Students who have used the text in the past decade have included medical doctors pursuing a doctorate in epidemiology; graduate students in geography working on their doctorates; graduate students from such public health disciplines as epidemiology, biostatistics, health behavior, nutrition, health administration, and public policy; undergraduate geography majors; and premedical undergraduates with majors in chemistry or biology but little background in the social sciences or geography. It is difficult to meet the needs of such varied students, with their different competencies in statistics, mapping, and geography. Because of this, the current edition has fewer special interest vignettes. Most of the methodological material that was previously presented in vignettes has been incorporated into new chapters, which focus on data and spatial analysis. Because there is such a range of opinion about where this material is best used in a course (given the variety of classes), the two new chapters have simply been placed at the end of the book. Something also needs to be said about references. We have attempted to write a general textbook that reads along without the constant interruption of strings of citations, most of which are publications themselves citing the common source of their idea/term or general knowledge in a field ("It is hot in the tropics [x, 1958]" or "The malaria plasmodia (schistosome, tick, etc.) has several life stages [y, 1999]"). Where possible, we referenced the seminal ideas and influential discussion, not all the most recent applications of those ideas. Our references are not meant to be a comprehensive bibliography of work in medical geography. The approaches, information, or examples we used are listed under "References." Students can usually identify relevant material by its title. "Further Reading" contains related reading, much of it suitable for term papers and further study, which includes excellent, relevant geographic studies written by important geographers but that were not actually included in the chapter. Finally, specific original ideas, quotes, or individual studies reported are specifically referenced in the body of the text. Thus the chapter on diffusion has more references than the others, because so many of the ideas, methodologies, and research findings have been contributed by a few individuals and so little has yet become general knowledge.

Our hope is that this text will be a sound foundation for the future development and practice of medical geography and that it will inspire geographers and others to bring their own special subdisciplinary knowledge to enrich and advance this growing course of study. Finally, we wish to acknowledge and appreciate the many examples and even words in this text that belong to the two former coauthors of the first edition, John W. Florin and Wilbert M. Gesler, who were each too preoccupied at this time with other books they were writing to join in this revision.

Contents

ON AIRS, WATERS, AND PLACES

Whoever wishes to investigate medicine properly, should proceed thus: in the first place to consider the seasons of the year, and what effects each of them produces (for they are not at all alike, but differ much from themselves in regard to their changes). Then the winds, the hot and the cold, especially such as are common to all countries, and then such as are peculiar to each locality. We must also consider the qualities of the waters, for as they differ from one another in taste and weight, so also do they differ much in their qualities. In the same manner, when one comes into a city to which he is a stranger, he ought to consider its situation, how it lies as to the winds and the rising of the sun; for its influence is not the same whether it lies to the north or the south, to the rising or setting sun. These things one ought to consider most attentively, and concerning the waters which the inhabitants use, whether they be marshy and soft, or hard and running from elevated and rocky situations, and then if saltish and unfit for cooking; and the ground, whether it be naked and deficient in water, or wooded and well watered, and whether it lies in a hollow, confined situation, or is elevated and cold; and the mode in which the inhabitants live, and what are their pursuits, whether they are fond of drinking and eating to excess and given to indolence, or are fond of exercise and labor, and not given to excess in eating and drinking.

From these things he must proceed to investigate everything else.

—Hippocrates (c. 400 b.c.)

1

Questions of Medical Geography

Medical geography uses the concepts and techniques of the discipline of geography to investigate health-related topics. Subjects are viewed in holistic terms within a variety of cultural systems and a diverse biosphere. Drawing freely from the facts, concepts, and techniques of other social, physical, and biological sciences, medical geography is an integrative, multistranded subdiscipline that has room within its broad scope for a wide range of specialist contributions. Medical geography is both an ancient perspective and a new specialization. As illustrated by the quote from Hippocrates, he (460?–377? B.C.) was familiar with the importance of cultural–environmental interactions more than 2,000 years ago. This ecological perspective on disease and health continued to be philosophically important, even dominant, until the emergence of germ theory in the second half of the 19th century. Thus, the 18th- to 19th-century physicians who first used the term "medical geography" and who struggled in dozens of works to describe and organize the avalanche of new information about human diseases, cultures, and environments, were continuing the holistic Hippocratic tradition (Finke, 1792–1795; Fuchs, 1853; Hirsch, 1883–1886). Their descriptions are being rediscovered and reevaluated by geographers and other scientists once again concerned with disease ecology (Barrett, 1980). Barrett, especially, has researched 19th-century roots of medical geography, that era's explanation of disease distribution and etiology, and the beginning of disease mapping (Barrett, 1991, 1993, 1996, 1998).

Geographic variation in health has long been studied under such interdisciplinary rubrics as geographic pathology, medical ecology, medical topography, geographical epidemiology, geomedicine, and so forth. The perspective and methodology of geography has now been applied to the study of health, disease, and care for 50 years. The emergence of a systematic interest in medical geography can be dated from the first report of the Commission on Medical Geography (Ecology) of Health and Disease to the International Geographic Union in 1952. Another 15 years passed before the work of pioneering researchers and teachers in a dozen countries resulted in a substantive focus on medical geography in the international community (for the English-speaking world, see especially Stamp, 1964, in the British Commonwealth and May, 1950, 1958, in the United States). The development of medical geography in several countries is described in the first chapters of a festschrift to Andrew Learmonth (McGlashan & Blunden,1983).

After considering some basic definitions and terminology about health and disease, this chapter describes the evolution of medical geography and its relationship to geographic questions, theories, and methodologies. The various approaches and interests it outlines become the subject matter of the chapters of this book.

DEFINITIONS AND TERMINOLOGY

Definitions of Health and Disease

Everyone knows what health is, and yet a precise definition of health is difficult to come by. This problem is shared by researchers who, in studying health, ironically need to measure disease. Health, however, is more than the absence of disease. We know that greater health is usually equated with lower mortality and morbidity rates and that health, of course, is a good thing in itself. The problem remains of how to define health without reference to disease.

The first major definition to present health as a positive entity, a presence to be promoted and not merely an absence to be regretted, occurs in the 1946 charter (preamble to the constitution) of the World Health Organization: "Health is a state of complete physical, mental, and social well-being and not merely the absence of disease or infirmity." This influential statement was important for the philosophical position it stated and for the goals it set for government programs and research funding. It has not proved useful, however, for implementing any standards or research designs that require criteria. It is ideal, utopian.

May's (1961) definition of disease was for many years referred to by geographers. He stated that disease is "that alteration of living cells or tissues, that jeopardizes survival in their environment" (p. xv). There are several important points in this definition of disease. The organism has an environment to which it relates. The idea that disease jeopardizes survival implies that there may be different levels of health without there being disease. An office worker, for example, need not have the physique or eyesight of a hunter. One may be born with a physical handicap and lead a productive life into old age, depending on the society within which one lives and its technology. May, however, was a physician before he did geography, and it shows; present understanding and interest in such dimensions as mental health, mind–body interaction, and sociocultural morbidity context are difficult to reconcile to this more biomedical model.

An influential definition comes from Dubos (1965): "States of health or disease are the expressions of the success or failure experienced by the organism in its efforts to respond adaptively to environmental challenges (p. xvii)." This definition implies a system whose parts can exist in different states of interaction. Health is not necessarily a condition of physical vigor but a condition suited to reaching goals defined by the individual. The most important word is "adaptively." Dinosaurs were highly adapted to their environment but could not cope with environmental changes. There is a dynamic quality to health. Dubos's definition, however, defines what health results from, not what it is.

In this book, we adhere mainly to J. Ralph Audy's (1971) definition: "Health is a continuing property that can be measured by the individual's ability to rally from a wide range and considerable amplitude of insults, the insults being chemical, physical, infectious, psychological, and social" (p. 142). This definition will be elaborated on in Chapter 2, but here it should be noted that health is present until death and is a dynamic quality continually engaged in coping with a changing social and physical environment. Audy says that health can be measured, but this has proved difficult except for such specific aspects as immunological or nutritional health. Researchers have used many indices and surrogate measures over recent years, and they have filled government reports and suggested criteria, but each definition is limited to its narrow purpose and has never become widely accepted. In the end we are still measuring the absence of disease.

Terminology

A familiarity with some terminology is necessary before the availability and limitations of data on health and disease can be appreciated. This section presents some of the most commonly used terms.

Diseases are referred to as *congenital* when they are present at birth. These may be of genetic origin, as is hemophilia; they may be acquired in the womb, as with drug addiction or chemical-induced deformity; or they may be acquired during the process of birth itself, as when severe inflammation of the eyes results from passage through a birth canal infected with the bacteria of gonorrhea. Diseases are referred to as *chronic* when they are present or recur over a long period of time, and as *acute* when their symptoms are severe and their course is short. *Degenerative* diseases are characterized by the deterioration or impairment of an organ or the structure of cells and the tissues of which they are a part. *Infectious* diseases result from the activities of living creatures, usually microorganisms, that invade the body. *Contagion*, transmission of infectious disease agents between people, may be direct through person-to-person contact or indirect through the bites of insect vectors or via fomites (or vehicles) such as contaminated blankets, money, or water.

Figure 1-1 illustrates one way of looking at the continuum of health and disease. The term "clinical" refers to conditions that have symptoms that can

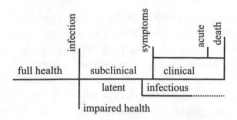

FIGURE 1-1. The health continuum, illustrating terminology and stages of ill health between full health and death.

be presented to a physician for observation and treatment. In a *subclinical* condition, an infectious agent may enter the body, multiply, stimulate the production of antibodies, and be eliminated from the body without the person being consciously aware of any illness. Usually the only way that subclinical infections can be detected is through serology, or the identification of antibodies and other immune reactions in the blood. Quite a few diseases produce acute reactions in only a small proportion of those infected. Other common diseases are mild infections when acquired in childhood and often pass unnoticed. In either case, public health officials are sometimes startled to find from serology that a "rare" disease has in fact infected the majority of the population.

Sometimes an infectious disease has a period of *latency* or *incubation* between the time the infection occurs and the appearance of clinical symptoms. Although the disease is not manifest, people are sometimes infectious. The common cold, for example, usually has an incubation period from 1 to 3 days, but people may be infectious for 24 hours before their own symptoms appear. Measles has an incubation period of about 10 days until onset of fever; people are then infectious for the 3 or 4 days until the rash appears, as well as for several days afterward. Because disease data usually are not produced until clinical symptoms are diagnosed, statistics at any given time usually underestimate the amount of disease in a population. Problems with time lag, apparent health, and time of diagnosis are accentuated when degenerative diseases are studied. The latency period between initial stimulus and the diagnosis of presented symptoms for cancer, for example, is commonly more than 20 years and may vary by several years for individuals, depending at what stage of the disease they are diagnosed.

A disease is *endemic* when it is constantly present in an area. It may occur at low levels, occasionally popping up here or there, as typhoid does in the United States (hypoendemic), or it may occur with intense transmission, as malaria does in parts of Africa (hyperendemic). Sometimes a hypoendemic disease can flare into rapid spread, perhaps in response to the dislocations of warfare or malnutrition from crop failure. Sometimes diseases that are not endemic are introduced and spread rapidly. A disease is said to be *epidemic* when it occurs at levels clearly beyond normal expectation and is derived from a common or propagated source. Epidemic disease may include an outbreak spreading through a population or widespread degenerative diseases, such as lung cancer.

The terms "incidence" and "prevalence" are often confused or used loosely and wrongly. *Incidence* refers to the number of cases of a disease being diagnosed or reported for a population during a defined period of time. It refers to new cases. *Prevalence* refers to the number of people in a population sick with a disease at a particular time, regardless of when the illness began. Thus, the incidence of tuberculosis in Texas in 2000 refers to the number of new cases diagnosed there that year, whereas the prevalence of tuberculosis in Texas in 2000 includes the total number of Texans suffering from the disease that year. The incidence and prevalence rates of chronic diseases, especially, can be very different.

TRADITIONS AND EVOLUTION

Place was important to medicine until the middle of the 19th century. For 2,000 years medicine was concerned with geographic variations in air, water, soil, vegetation, animals and insects, diet, habit and custom, clothing and house type, government, and economy. The 19th century saw a paradigm change, a change in the great overarching idea of how disease occurred and what questions were worth asking. In the last century *germ theory*, or what is known as the "doctrine of specific etiology," has resulted in revolutionary advances. The discovery that microbes invade human bodies and cause alterations that result in disease led to asepsis and sterilization, vaccination, antibiotics, chlorination of water and treatment of sewage, and over 30 more years of life for the average person in a developed country.

Specific etiology, or one cause (germ) that is both necessary and sufficient for each disease, is less relevant to a society in which people die from heart disease, cancer, kidney failure, alcoholism, and violence. These are diseases of multiple, complex causes based as much in culture as in biology. Even for infectious diseases, germs are no longer considered to be the "sufficient" cause. The tubercle bacillus is necessary to cause tuberculosis, but the disease depends on nutrition, genetics, treatment, the presence of disease conditions, crowding and ventilation, spitting, and mental attitude. The etiology and control of strokes or infertility are even more complex. Yet the progress of specific etiology has been paralleled by the progress of specialization and the increasing divorce of body from mind and environment.

As the contradictions between the dominant biomedical orientation and the health needs of people increased, the social sciences became more involved. Besides geography, the last few decades have seen the development of flourishing concentrations in medical anthropology, medical sociology, medical economics, and psychology. Historians are reconsidering the significance of disease for major social and economic changes. They are investigating the role that historical connections between empires and the development of trade has played in the spread of disease or concepts of disease causation. Changes in technology such as glass making and the invention of the internal combustion engine have profoundly altered the disease maintenance and health care systems. Political factors influence government policy and determine the availability of sewerage systems and potable water as well as the mix of medical systems and the distribution of resources. Such organizations as universities, foundations, and insurance companies attract the attention of political scientists by affecting the quantity and goals of foreign aid and the standards and technology of domestic care. Medical economics has demonstrated the great monetary savings of prevention programs. The problems of technological development and ever-rising medical expenses on one hand and an aging population with uneven economic resources on the other demand that that flexible and innovative strategies be developed. Sociologists have demonstrated the importance of class and ethnicity in everything from defining the sick role and choosing a doctor to diet and exercise habits. How far people are willing to travel for care and what care is accessible and acceptable to them are as sociologically relevant as occupational exposures to hazards and lifestyle changes. Anthropologists have illuminated the many cultural belief systems about disease causation and prevention and the pharmaceuticals and therapy strategies of traditional medical systems. Issues of diet and mental health have received special attention.

Medical geography draws on the concepts and uses the techniques of all these disciplines and adds spatial and ecological perspectives. It exemplifies the interdisciplinary nature of geography, bridging the gap between the social and the physical and biological sciences. Cognate disciplines for training a medical geographer include epidemiology, history, sociology, economics, anthropology, psychology, zoology, entymology, botany, parasitology, meteorology, geology, urban planning, health administration, environmental engineering, and biostatistics.

Traditions

Geographers argue endlessly about the nature of their discipline. Some dichotomize geography into the study of physical or human phenomena. They separate, for example, the study of geomorphology or climatology from the study of economic processes or politics. This separation often provides a useful framework for structuring programs of study, but it is simplistic for geographic research purposes, for many geographical subdisciplines pose questions that link physical and cultural dimensions. A more useful organization is defined in terms of the nature of questions posed and the approach to answering them (Amedeo & Golledge, 1975). Before that, however, this section looks at the four traditions Pattison (1964) identified at the heart of geography, and at a little of their history as they have been developed in medical geography.

Pattison's four traditions were spatial, regional, man–land, and earth science. The first of these to develop in American medical geography was the man–land (or "human–environment," as we would term it today). The focus on how humans as cultural beings and the physical environment they live in interact and affect each other, and on the nature of those linkages, is for geographers in this tradition the essence of the discipline. At the beginning of the 20th century, many geographers followed a basic premise called *environmental determinism*. The assumption was that the physical environment caused, or at least had a dominating effect on, human environments, activities, and biology. However, the simplistic methodologies of the time could not handle the complexities to which they were applied. There followed a philosophical progression to the idea that a wide variety of human activity developed within the constraints of the environment: *possibilism*. Eventually, environmental determinism and possibilism were replaced as the dominant paradigm in the discipline by a behavioral approach in the spatial tradition of human geography that treated the environment as totally subservient to the will of humans or ignored it completely. The man–land tradition continued to evolve, especially on the West Coast, into more ecological wholeness. Today, the approach of cultural ecology considers humans to be cultural beings whose existence is inextricably interwoven with the environment.

Medical geography, as a subdiscipline and specialty within the discipline of geography, does not have a long history. Jacques May, the "father" of medical geography in the United States, initiated the subdiscipline (1950, 1954) and wrote *The Ecology of Disease* (1958). This represented the culmination of a long intellectual evolution on May's part. He had begun as a French surgeon in Siam (now Thailand) and spent most of his years at the major French hospital in Hanoi. He started by questioning why his patients in the tropics experienced disease and responded differently under surgery and medical care than did the European patients described in textbooks. He progressed to an interest in their multiple infections and to the conditions of their lives, and then to an understanding of the cultural and environmental conditions that produced and limited their health and disease. British geographers in particular were familiar with tropical conditions in the colonial world and diseases such as malaria. Stamp (1964) and Learmonth (1952, 1972, 1988) described world patterns of infectious disease to the public as well as to geographers. John Hunter (1966, 1974) taught medical geography at Michigan State University from the 1960s until the 1990s, and from that large department seeded American colleges with geographers who had at least that initial exposure to the subject. Fonaroff (1968) introduced the subject to many with his masterful article on the changing ecology of malaria in Trinidad. The curriculum of human ecology at the University of Illinois strongly affected the founding of medical anthropology at Berkeley and influenced J. Ralph Audy (1971), chairing international health at San Francisco Medical School. From that curriculum also came Warwick Armstrong (1965; 1973), the first medical geographer with a master's degree in public health, who established medical geography in Hawaii. Meade (one of the authors) became the first American geographer to do both a master's (Hunter) and a doctorate (Armstrong) in medical geography (as cultural ecology).

The interests of the earth science tradition have been largely included within the cultural ecology of disease. Light, heat/cold and the seasons, electromagnetic waves, and sound relate to biometeorology. Toxic pollution, radiation of various types, and properties and trace elements of soil and water are often related to degenerative diseases. Developing this aspect of disease ecology involves depth in geology, climatology, and biogeography especially.

The spatial tradition, Pattison noted, emphasizes distance, form, direction, position, location, and the distribution over space which most geographers consider essential to the core of the discipline. In medical geography this tradition has developed two components: locational analysis and spatial analysis (Meade, 1980). Geographical theories and techniques for determining optimum location, designing transportation networks, and measuring distribution have been applied to locating medical personnel and facilities. The classic "journey to work" studies of economic geography have become health service demand and market area analyses. This tradition emphasizes spatial organization. It uses analysis of pattern to get at the process that generated it. Given some understanding of the processes that generate locational distributions, some geographers address more applied questions: What is the optimum location for a specific purpose? How can the greatest efficiency in spatial structure (as transportation systems, urban places, communications, or administration) be advanced? In other words, the conceptual and methodological understanding is used and extended in locational decision making. A medical geographer might ask where ambulances should go when transporting different levels of emergency, such as severe burns or common heart attacks; where a birth control clinic should be located for maximum access by a target populations; or how an area of uneven distribution of population, income, and health facility utilization divided under various political units should be optimally regionalized to save costs on expensive new equipment.

There were three main sources of this vigorous strain of medical geography. The first was the studies on locational analysis for the Swedish health system by geographers at the University of Lund (Godlund, 1961). The second was the Chicago Regional Hospital Studies, in which Richard Morrill brought both Pyle (1971) and Earickson (Morrill & Earickson, 1968) into the geography of health service. The third was the first widely read book to introduce a generation of geography graduate students to the subject, Shannon and Dever's (1974) *Health Care Delivery*. Within a few years annual meetings generated hours of papers on health service location and utilization and scores of medical geographers found jobs in planning and marketing. As geographers began to focus on the inequalities of health care provision, it became clear that the way countries organized their health care systrems had a major effect on the dimensions of health care inequality. Concepts of political economy became increasingly important. State practice and public policy and the structure of society moved out of sociology into geographic analysis (Eyles & Woods, 1983) and across the sea to the national Canadian health promotion endeavor. Studies increasingly focused on topics such as territorial injustice and environmental racism and the structural context of why people get sick, rather than simplicities of distance. Jones and Moon's (1987) influential book moved the social context of not only health care but health into the mainstream of geographic study. The deinstitutionalization of the mentally ill in the United States and failure to develop the community service provision and shelter to care for those with mental illness, substance abuse, or victims of domestic violence changed the focus and influenced the methodologies of geographic research and exposition (Dear & Wolch, 1987; Wolch & Dear, 1993).

Spatial analysis is so intrinsic to geographic thinking that many geographers would find it strange to discuss it separately. In medical geography, however, it has found special focus in the study of disease diffusion and the analysis of diseases or disease factors of unknown etiology. When the epidemiological and statistical study of the spread of contagious disease within a population and its subgroups is considered spatially, settlement forms and urban systems and transportation networks and trade flows and global connections and population mobility become the objects of modeling. Pyle (1969) started this with his study of how the changing process of diffusion of cholera in 19th-century United States reflected the maturing infrastructure and urban system of the country. Recent studies of the diffusion of influenza, measles, cholera, and hepatitis have become elaborate and powerful, as reviewed in Cliff and Haggett (1988) and Thomas (1992). A different aspect of spatial analysis has been study of the covariation in space of occurrence of disease and possibly related factors or of environmental and social conditions. These studies are often classified with medical geographic studies of disease ecology, but they emphasize the methodologies of spatial analysis, especially cartography and other systems of geographic information and analysis.

The final tradition, regionalization, has often been regarded as an ultimate goal rarely attained. Regional geography has a long tradition, going back to the Greeks. It focuses on integrating all the variable phenomena in order to characterize the special identity of particular places and areas. True integration of the great complexities of culture and environment, geography as synthesis, is the highest expression of regional geography but is seldom achieved. More often geographers work with limited regions created for particular research purposes. Some regions, *uniform* or *formal* regions, delimit areas that are homogeneous for certain variables. In this way, the Islamic world or Anglo-America is a region, as is the Cajun dialect area or the grassland biome (vegetational region). Other regions, called *functional* regions, delimit areas within which interaction occurs. Areas in which people patronize a certain shopping mall, read a certain newspaper, or root for a certain ball team are functional regions. The epistemological purpose of regionalizing is the reduction of variance through classification. In other words, grouping all an area's "like" things together helps organize the cacophony of variation into patterns that are useful for recognizing the underlying processes.

In medical geography, regionalization may take the form in locational analysis of delimiting an ambulance service area or hospital market area; in cultural ecology, it may determine the limits to the area and living sytem within which a disease agent circulates, and so define the disease *nidus*; in spatial analysis it may involve determining the space in which several factors and conditions of disease co-occur and so suggest an etiological hypothesis. At a national level of regionalization, some of Jacques May's (1958, pp. 30–32) initial descriptions of how the Vietnamese got their diseases are still among the best syntheses. They lacked, however, geographic dimensions such as the larger social and economic structure, transportation and other infrastructure, as well as the location of health services and how well they provided prevention and intervention. The strongest attempt so far to pull such multiple dimensions together into the geography of health and disease place comes from German studies in geomedicine at Heidelberg (Jusatz, 1969–1984).

The special and basic tool of geographers, in service of all its traditions, is the map. Cartography, the construction and interpretation of maps, has held a central place in geography. Most geographers have a profound love affair with maps. An old saying in the field is, "If it can't be mapped, it's not geography." Although a wide variety of statistical techniques are used in geography, as in other social sciences, maps are a unique, powerful, and flexible tool for analysis of geographical phenomena. A map is a model of the world that, through the use of point, line, and area symbols, can integrate many dimensions of reality. The rapid development of the methodologies for spatial data analysis, known as *geographic information systems* (GIS), is revolutionizing the old tool of mapping and the questions that the discipline of geography can answer as well as ask. Such systems hold profound significance for the future work of medical geography.

Questions

The strands of medical geography have evolved from all these traditions in the larger discipline. They have been variously emphasized in Soviet, German, British, Australian, Indian, French, and North American schools. The following six questions, largely paraphrased from Amedeo and Golledge (1975), can be applied to research in medical geography, although they were originally used to emphasize the common perspective of geography regardless of its specializations.

1. *Why is a phenomenon distributed in a particular way?* There is enormous variation in the incidence of diseases on the surface of the earth. Rates for cancer of the esophagus, nasopharynx, stomach, colon, and other sites may

vary 100-fold between countries; 10 babies in 1,000 die in one country, 300 in another; measles, leprosy, tuberculosis, and malaria are mild in one place and deadly in another. There is also enormous variation in the access of people to physicians, hospital beds, medicines, and other health services.

The first step in addressing why phenomena are distributed in certain ways is to accurately describe where they are located. Traditionally, various forms of mapping have fulfilled this purpose. Today, maps are sometimes abstracted into graphs, or their x and y coordinate systems are used to delimit classes for statistical frequency distributions. Regardless of the means of construction or use, accurate maps are a valuable first tool of analysis.

National atlases of mortality have been produced in Great Britain, Japan, and finally, in the United States (by the National Center for Health Statistics, 1997). Atlases of mortality from cancer have had a strong impact in the United States and in China. Indeed, atlases of disease occurrence and diffusion such as the *Welt-Seuchen Atlas* (Rodenwaldt & Jusatz, 1952–1961) have been the most recognized contribution of geography to the health professions. British geographers have been especially vigorous in mapping disease distribution with accuracy and sophistication. The role of statistical mapping and the analytical use of mapping in general are not, however, widely recognized outside the field.

Some geographers have used aggregated, census-derived demographic and socioeconomic data in multivariate statistical analyses to explain the distribution of such phenomena as physician specialists, bronchitis, suicide, and teenage pregnancy. Some geographers have used microscale, interview, and field-mapped data to illuminate connecting paths between environmental, cultural, and demographic patterns and occurrence of disease or of health care practices. Some have generalized distributional patterns of vegetation and topography to delimit regions of landscape within which certain kinds of disease transmission occur. Whatever the scale or approach, accounting for the spatial distribution of health-related phenomena is the dominant purpose of medical geographic inquiry.

2. *Why are facilities and businesses located where they are?* Why are the offices of physicians, public clinics, or research hospitals located in certain places and not in others? How do the locations of different levels of specialization relate to each other? Why, for example, do facilities to handle heart attacks and those to give cancer radiation therapy have different locational distributions? Are health facilities located in the most efficient places, and can knowledge of the processes behind their locational needs be used to optimize location?

These types of questions were first emphasized in the United States but today are attracting international geographic attention. Whatever the political economy of a country's health service system, there is a need to optimize the location of emergency service facilities and to build expensive facilities such as those for dialysis in places that will be accessible to the future distribution of people in need.

3. *Why do people move in certain directions for certain distances?* The movement of people over space has inevitably attracted a lot of geographic attention. Population geography studies human mobility at many scales. Economic geography investigates consumer behavior. Medical geography is concerned with how far people will travel to get different health services, and why they go to one place and not to another. It is concerned with patterns of human mobility and frequency of contact as these affect the diffusion of contagious disease or the exposure of people to places of disease transmission. Medical geographers have studied the transfer of diseases from Europe and Africa to the New World, the exposure of people to the hazard of schistosomiasis in certain bodies of water at certain times of day, and how far a teenager will travel to get contraceptive information. Why people move as they do is a question basic to understanding health service utilization and the transmission of disease.

4. *Why do innovations spread as they do?* Not only people but ideas and material goods diffuse across space through time. A few medical geographers have addressed the diffusion of medical technology, such as changes in diagnosis, procedure, nomenclature, or concepts of disease causation. Most have considered the spread of infectious agents analogous to the spread of other innovations and have studied the relationship to settlement systems and activity patterns. How do changes in the size of cities, the density of populations, or transportation links affect the diffusion of disease? Can one use the spatial pattern that results from the spread of a disease in a neighborhood, within an urban system, or across a region to understand the process? Can one learn enough of barriers to and corridors for diffusion that one can learn to control an epidemic?

5. *Why do people vary in their perception of the environment?* If distance means different things to different people, they will use health care services differently. Indeed, their perception of what causes illness will result in different preventive and curative behavior. When several medical care systems are available, people will choose among them according to their perceptions of efficacy for particular health problems. The occurrence of illness itself will vary, often by ethnic group, according to how the sick role or pain thresholds are defined. Thus, one office worker will be absent to go the the doctor with a sore throat while another will work with terrible congestion and a mild fever, which he or she does not report. Perception of class or ethnic differences in treatment or vocabulary and language can create "social distances" more influential in where people go than the mileage they must transit.

Just as people vary in their perceptions of the hazards of flood, so do they vary in perceptions of the hazards of unboiled water, unbelted automobile accidents, or malaria transmission. Such perceptions affect the material environment as well as human activities and influence the planting of trees, drainage of water, and other alterations of the earth.

6. *How do objects, ideas, processes, and living beings interact to characterize and constitute places?* Some of the medical topographies of the 17th and 19th cen-

turies attempted to answer this question and explain why places were or were not healthy (Chalmers, 1776; Dickson, 1860; Ramsey, 1796). May (1958, pp. 30–32) addressed the problem well in his classic description of how the rice-farming peasants of Vietnam contracted diseases from the way they lived on their land. The regional (country) monographs in medical geography currently being produced by Jusatz and others in Heidelberg systematically consider the dimensions of environment, population, and health care that determine the health status of populations and their subgroups. In general, however, there have been few attempts to understand how the health status of a certain population in a certain place has resulted from the interaction of the people, their environment, and their culture, or with how it might change in the future.

Directions

There are several stimuli to encourage new developments in medical geography. From the dimension of biology comes the prospect of "mapping" the human genome and eventually being able to identify the presence of particular genes for susceptibility or even intervention treatment. From the dimension of cybernetics and information come powerful new computer applications and questions about how information is coded and networked in living systems, including human cultural ones, and how it gets expressed or used. The increased availability of digital spatial data is fueling an increased awareness by government agencies and public health officials of the usefulness for investigation of GIS and spatial analysis. Satellite images and scans of planet earth are exponentially increasing sheer *data* beyond present hope of comprehension or management. Global demographic, economic, social, and political reorganizations are disintegrating conventional wisdom. Science, and especially social science, is becoming internationalized. All these changes and more demand new theoretical developments and ways of understanding.

There are several forms of developing theory in response. New social theories are addressing larger structural issues and ways of considering the context of relationships and events (Cloke, Philo, & Sadler, 1991). A fundamental restructuring of the social sciences is impending. This turns on the elimination of three basic cleavages: that between history and the social sciences over data, bias, and means of knowing; that between studies of developed, "civilized" Western societies and studies "in the field" of the rest of the world (eliminated by the internationalization of the social sciences); and that among the nomothetic social sciences as separate disciplines (stemming from the 19th-century ideological world view of state, market, and society as separate entities) (Wallerstein, 1996). Even the tripartite division of academic thought into humanities, social science, and natural science is being questioned by the recognition in cultural studies that social processes matter even as they condemn Newtonian scientism, and Newtonian scientism is undermined in the natural sciences by indeterminancy and complexity (Gulbenkian Commission, 1996). As partly a social science, geography is part of this ferment. All of human geography is being *reconstructed* (Dear, 1988). *Place* is being reconceptualized (Agnew & Duncan, 1989; Entrikin, 1991).

There has been long-standing tension in medical geography between the study of health services and of the epidemiology of disease. The conversation about this has been transformed somewhat. That part of inquiry that draws its theory and methodology from economic, urban, and social geography is actively participating in the changing perspectives and approaches of postmodern social theory. In social geography the individuality of human perception has become an indeterminacy principle that challenges the basis of knowledge and science (Laudan, 1990). Some argue that medical geography should be "postmedical" and be "relocated" within social geography (Kearns, 1993). Others argue that public health, and even medicine, no longer follow a "biomedical model" any more than science as a whole is Newtonian; that medical geography has always been about public health, not "medicine," and that medical geography needs to incorporate the new approaches of social theory to society and behavior and perception but retain a holistic, inclusive approach to the ecology of health and disease (Mayer & Meade, 1994). Fundamental to the perspective from social geography is that research on population health be "theoretically informed" (i.e., social theory) and be "situated" in the relations of power within society. Research is beginning to be published that accomplishes the linking of cultural perspectives with a political economy analysis that highlights the importance of place and cultural context and is based on empirical field-based case study (Madge, 1998).

Place and landscape have reemerged as concepts central to geography, essentially restating the ancient interest in region. *Place* as a collective experience can be used to analyze the consequences of illness or health service provisions and otherwise relate to recent health philosophies (Kearns, 1993). Within geography there has been a new conceptualization of the meaning and uses of its ancient interest in "landscape." This has been expressed as an interest in healing landscapes, internal landscapes of identity, and landscape in literature and in popular culture which reveals the viewer. This current is drawing on the approaches and methodologies of the humanities as it situates medical geography (Kearns & Gesler, 1998). The new journal, *Health and Place*, has become an important forum for publication in medical geography.

The human–environment tradition also is evolving. New theories in cultural ecology are relating field-level observations to larger organizational relations and phenomenological questions by developing a political ecology analogous to political economy (Price & Lewis, 1993). This approach in the past has addressed mostly agricultural development and change, but Mayer (1996) points out the theoretical possibilities for the ecology of disease and health. Another theoretical approach to the organization of information and status of systems (such as those that result in states of health) is developing out of Prigogine's studies of self-organizing systems (Schieve & Allen, 1982), theorization on information and ecology (Moran, 1990), and the new epistemological apprehensions that have become known as "chaos theory" or "complexity theory" which model indeterminancy (Prigogine & Stengers, 1984; Kellert, 1993). As Greenberg points out, the study of environmental health in stressed neighborhoods requires a holistic view of multiple hazards and varied effects, such as ozone, housing, genetics, segregation, job accessibility, and demography (in Gesler, 2000). It is in the midst of all these new approaches to understanding that the powerful new methodologies of spatial data management and analysis are transforming the ability to address the questions.

THE COURSE OF MEDICAL GEOGRAPHY

After explosive growth in the late 1970s and early 1980s, medical geography has become less exotic as a subdiscipline and more maturely stable and integrated into the profession. As with U.S. geography as a whole, however, there is perceived fragmentation, represented by Paul's (1985) metaphor of a branching tree, and a need to reidentify the core of the discipline and focus on a future.

Instead of the branching tree, Learmonth (1985) inverted the metaphor to that of a stream system. Using this analogy, the headwaters of medical geography lie in the ecology of infectious disease, in the human–environment tradition of geography. Early tributaries added field work, cartography, the study of Third World countries, and the study of development. As the mighty Mississippi is joined by the broad Missouri, analysis of health service delivery, with its own headwaters in the economic and urban geography of developed countries, joins a couple of decades downstream; and in years when federal government funding is plentiful it can rise in flood. Although after their confluence the stream flows continue to be distinguishable for a period of years, their waters increasingly intermingle. The river continually receives new tributaries, from the conceptual sheds of central place, perception, structuralism, ecology, biomedicine, and cognate disciplines in social science. New streams of technologies and techniques join. When the river reaches its sea, human health status, it contributes the flow and deep currents of all of geography to understanding the health of places and their peoples. Reflected in this sea, geography better contemplates and understands itself as a discipline.

The river is whole. Diagnosis and treatment depend on the resources and social structures present, after all, and later diseases result or not from the prevention and treatment of earlier ones. Iatrogenesis (causation by physicians or medical treatment), preventive vaccines, and cardiopulmonary resuscitation are as relevant to the geography of health and disease as are water impoundments, toxic waste, and travel by jet aircraft. But the river has abandoned meanders; it does have backwaters; it even causes localized water-logging and thick muck. In short, as we sail on our mighty river, we need to pay attention to both the macroscale changes in habitat, land use, population, and mobility and the local eddies and sandbars; or to the satellite imagery and the cultural ground truth.

The Challenge of Medical Geography

The development of medical geography has been part of a response to inadequate theory, methodology, and understanding of health and disease in our society. The integrative perspective of geography and the questions and methodologies of geography's various traditions are needed. In the words of John Hunter (1974),

> The application of geographical concepts and techniques to health-related problems places medical geography, so defined, in the very heart or mainstream of the discipline of geography. I would suggest that there is no professional geographer, whatever his or her systematic bent or regional interest, who cannot effectively apply a measure of his or her particular skills or regional insights towards the understanding, or at least partial understanding, of a health problem. This is the essential challenge of medical geography. (pp. 3–4)

REFERENCES

Agnew, J., & Duncan, J. (1989). *The power of place: Bringing together geographical and sociological imaginations.* Boston: Unwin-Hyman.

Amedeo, D., & Golledge, R. G. (1975). *An introduction to scientific reasoning in geography.* New York: Wiley.

Armstrong, R. W. (1965). Medical geography: An emerging specialty? *International Pathology, 6,* 61–63.

Armstrong, R. W. (1973). Tracing exposure to specific environments in medical geography. *Geographical Analysis, 5,* 122–132.

Audy, J. R. (1971). Measurement and diagnosis of health. In P. Shepard & D. McKinley (Eds.), *Environ/mental: Essays on the planet as a home* (pp. 140–162). Boston: Houghton Mifflin.

Barrett, F. A. (1980). Medical geography as a foster child. In M. S. Meade (Ed.), *Conceptual and methodological issues in medical geography* (pp. 1–15). Chapel Hill, NC: University of North Carolina, Department of Geography.

Barrett, F. A. (1991). "Scurvy" Lind's medical geography. *Social Science and Medicine, 33,* 347–354.

Barrett, F. A. (1993). A medical geographical anniversary. *Social Science and Medicine, 37,* 701–710.

Barrett, F. A. (1996). Daniel Drake's medical geography. *Social Science and Medicine, 42,* 791–800.

Barrett, F. A. (1998). Alfred Haviland's nineteenth-century map analysis of the geographical distribution of diseases in England and Wales. *Social Science and Medicine, 46,* 767–781.

Blunden, J. R. (1983). Andrew Learmonth and the evolution of medical geography: A personal memoir of a career. In N. D. McGlashan & J. R. Blunden (Eds.), *Geographical aspects of health* (pp. 15–32). New York: Academic Press.

Chalmers, L. (1776). *An account of the weather and disease of South Carolina.* London: Charles Dilly.

Cliff, A. & Haggett, P. (1988). *Atlas of disease distribution: Analytic approaches to epidemiological data.* New York: Blackwell.

Cloke, P. , Philo, C., & Sadler, D. (1991). *Approaching human geography: An introduction to contemporary theoretical debates.* New York: Guilford Press.

Dear, M. (1988). The postmodern challenge: Reconstructing human geography. *Transactions of the Institute of British Geographers, 13,* 262–274.

Dear, M. J., & Wolch, J. R. (1987). *Landscapes of despair.* Princeton, NJ: Princeton University Press.

Dickson, J. H. (1860). *Report on the medical topography and epidemics of North Carolina.* Philadelphia: Collins.

Dubos, R. (1965). *Man adapting.* New Haven, CT: Yale University Press.

Eyles, J., & Woods, K. (1983). *The social geography of medicine and health.* London: Croom Helm, and New York: St. Martin's Press.

Entrikin, J. N. (1991). *The betweenness of place: Towards a geography of modernity.* Baltimore: Johns Hopkins University Press.

Finke, L. L. (1792–1795). *Versuch einer allgeminen medicinisch-pratkischen geographie* (3 vols.). Leipzig: Weidmannische Buchhandlung.

Fonaroff, L. S. (1968). Man and malaria in Trinidad: Ecological perspectives of a changing health hazard. *Annals of the Association of American Geographers, 58,* 526–556.

Fuchs, C. F. (1853). *Medizinische geographie.* Berlin: Duncker.

Geddes, A. (1978). Report to the Commission on Medical Geography. *Social Science and Medicine, 12D,* 227–237.

Gesler, W. (1999, March). *Medical geography.* Paper presented at the meeting of the Association of American Geographers, Honolulu, HI. Forthcoming in C. G. Willmott, & G. Gaile (Eds.), *Geography in America at the dawn of the 21st century.*

Godlund, S. (1961). *Population, regional hospitals, transportation facilities, and regions: Planning the location of regional hospitals in Sweden* (Lund Studies in Geography Series B: Human Geography No. 21). Lund, Sweden: Department of Geography, Royal University of Lund.

Gulbenkian Commission, (1996). *Open the social sciences.* Report of the Gulbenkian Commission on the Restructuring of the Social Sciences. Stanford, CA: Stanford University Press.

Hippocrates. (1886). *The genuine works of Hippocrates* (F. Adams, Trans.). New York: William Wood.

Hirsch, A. (1883–1886). *Handbook of geographical and historical pathology* (3 vols.; C. Creighton, Trans.). London: New Sydenham Society.

Hunter, J. M. (1966). River blindness in Nangodi, Northern Nigeria: A hypothesis of cyclical advance and retreat. *Geographical Review, 56,* 398–416.

Hunter, J. M. (1974). The challenge of medical geography. In J. M. Hunter (Ed.), *The geography of health and disease* (pp. 1–31). Chapel Hill: University of North Carolina, Department of Geography.

Jones, K., & Moon, G. (1987). *Health, disease and society.* London: Routledge & Kegan Paul.

Jusatz, H. J. (Ed.). (1968–1984). *Medizinische Landerkunde* (Vols. 1–6; Geomedical Monograph Series). Berlin: Springer-Verlag.

Kearns, R. A. (1993). Place and health: Towards a reformed medical geography. *Professional Geographer, 45,* 139–147.

Kearns, R. A., & Gesler, W. M. (1998). *Putting health into place: Landscape, identity, and well-being.* Syracus, NY: Syracuse University Press.

Kellert, S. H. (1993). *In the wake of chaos: Unpredictable order in dynamical systems.* Chicago: University of Chicago Press.

Laudan, L. (1990). *Science and relativism.* Chicago: University of Chicago Press.

Learmonth, A. T. A. (1952). The medical geography of India: an approach to the problem. In K. Kuriyan, (Ed.), *The Indian Geographical Society, the silver jubilee volume* (pp. 201–202). Madras: The Indian Geographical Society.

Learmonth, A. T. A. (1972). Medicine and medical geography. In N. D. McGlashan (Ed.), *Medical geography: Techniques and field studies* (pp. 17–42). London: Methuen.

Learmonth, A. T. A. (1985). Commentary. *Social Science and Medicine, 20,* 407–409.

Learmonth, A. T. A. (1988). *Disease ecology: An introduction.* London: Basil Blackwell.

Madge, C. (1998). Therapeutic landscapes of the Jola, the Gambia, West Africa. *Health and Place, 4,* 293–311.

May, J. M. (1950). Medical geography: Its methods and objectives. *Geographical Review, 40,* 9–41.

May, J. M. (1954). Medical geography. In P. E. James & C. F. Jones (Eds.), *American Geography: Inventory and prospect.* Syracuse, NY: Syracuse University Press.

May, J. M. (1958). *The ecology of human disease.* New York: MD Publications.

May, J. M. (Ed.). (1961). *Studies in disease ecology.* New York: Hafner.

Mayer, J. D. (1996). The political ecology of disease as a new focus for medical geography. *Progress in Human Geography, 20,* 441–456.

Mayer, J. D., & Meade, M. S. (1994). A reformed medical geography reconsidered. *Professional Geographer, 46,* 103–106.

McGlashan, N. D., & Blunden, J. R. (1983). *Geographical aspects of health: Essays in honour of Andrew Learmonth.* New York: Academic Press.

Meade, M. S. (1986). Geographic analysis of disease and care. *Annual Review of Public Health, 7,* 313–335.

Moran, E. F. (1990). *The Ecosystem approach in anthropology.* Ann Arbor: University of Michigan Press.

Morrill, R. L., & Earickson, R. (1968). Variation in the character and use of Chicago area hospitals. *Health Services Research, 3,* 224–238.

National Center for Health Statistics. (1997). *Atlas of U. S. mortality.* Washington, DC: U.S. Government Printing Office.

Pattison, W. D. (1964). The four traditions of geography. *Journal of Geography, 63,* 211–216.

Paul, B. K. (1985). Approaches to medical geography: An historical perspective. *Social Science and Medicine, 20,* 399–407.

Price, M., & Lewis, M. (1993). The revinvention of cultural geography. *Annals of the Association of American Geographers, 83,* 1–17.

Prigogine, I., & Stengers, I. (1984). *Order out of chaos: Man's new dialogue with nature.* New York: Bantam Books.

Pyle, G. F. (1969). The diffusion of cholera in the United States in the nineteenth century. *Geographical Analysis, 1,* 59–75.

Pyle, G. F. (1971). *Heart disease, cancer, and stroke in Chicago: A geographical analysis with facilities, plans for 1980* (Research Paper No. 134). Chicago: University of Chicago, Department of Geography.

Ramsey, D. (1796). *A sketch of the soil, climate, weather, and diseases of South Carolina.* Charleston: W. P. Young.

Rodenwaldt, E. , & Jusatz, H. J. (Eds.). (1952–1961). *Welt-Seuchen Atlas* (Vols. 1–3). Hamburg: Falk.

Schieve, W. C., & Allen, P. M. (1982). *Self-organization and dissipative structures.* Austin: University of Texas Press.

Shannon, G. W., & Dever, G. E. A. (1974). *Health care delivery: Spatial perspectives.* New York: McGraw-Hill.

Shoshin, A. A. (1962). *Principles and methods of medical geography.* Moscow: Academy of Sciences.

Stamp, L. D. (1964). *The geography of life and death.* Ithaca, NY: Cornell University Press.

Thomas, R. W. (1992). *Geomedical systems: Intervention and control.* London: Routledge.

Wallerstein, I. (1996). Open the social sciences. *Items. Social Science Research Council, 50,* 1–7.

Wolch, J. R., & Dear, M. J. (1993). *Malign Neglect.* San Francisco: Jossey-Bass Publishers.

FURTHER READING

Agnew, J., & Duncan, J. (1989). *The power of place: Bringing together geographical and sociological imaginations.* Boston: Unwin Hyman.

Banks, A. L. (1959). The study of the geography of disease. *The Geographical Journal, 125,* 199–216.

Gesler, W. M. (1991) *The cultural geography of health care.* Pittsburgh: University of Pittsburgh Press.

Howe, G. M. (1972). *Man, environment, and disease in Britain.* New York: Barnes & Noble.

Joseph, A. E. , & Phillips, D. R. (1984). *Accessibility and utilization: Geographical perspectives on health care delivery.* New York: Harper & Row.

Kiple, K. F. (Ed.). (1993). *The Cambridge world history of human disease.* Cambridge, UK: Cambridge University Press.

Learmonth, A. T. A. (1975). *Patterns of disease and hunger.* North Pomfret, VT: David & Charles.

Madge, C. (1998). Therapeutic landscapes of the Jola, the Gambia, West Africa. *Health and Place, 4,* 293–311.

Mayer, J. D. (1990). The centrality of medical geography to human geography: the traditions of geographical and medical geographical thought. *Norsk Geografisk Tidsskrift, 44,* 175–187.

Mayer, J. D. (1996). The political ecology of disease as one new focus for medical geography. *Progress in Human Geography, 20,* 441–456.

McGlashan, N. D. (1972). *Medical geography: Techniques and field studies.* London: Methuen.

Phillips, D. R., & Verhasselt, Y. (Eds.). (1994). *Health and development.* London: Routledge.

Pyle, G. F. (1979). *Applied medical geography.* New York: Wiley.

Turshen, M. (1984). *The political ecology of disease in Tanzania.* New Brunswick, NJ: Rutgers University Press.

2

The Human Ecology of Disease*

The *human ecology* of disease is concerned with the ways human behavior, in its cultural and socioeconomic context, interacts with environmental conditions to produce or prevent disease among susceptible people. This constitutes the etiology, or causal evolution, of health and disease. Population genetics, physiology, and immunological and nutritional status are important to disease processes and must be understood as prerequisites to sound research into these process. Geography is also important, as its roots are firmly anchored in the study of cultural and environmental interactions.

Geographers have traditionally studied the creation of landscape, the mobility and composition of population, the determinants of economic activity and its location, and diffusion of things, ideas, and technology. All these are of consequence to medical geography. The landscape is composed of insects, medicinal herbs, and hospitals as well as topography, vegetation, animals, water sources, house types, and clothing. Mobility is important to exposure to and transmission of disease. Elements of population composition include not only age structure, ethnicity, and literacy but also immunological

---

*To avoid confusion, let us state succinctly the difference between "human ecology" and a term we used earlier, "cultural ecology." *Human ecology* is a broad term used in anthropology and epidemiology, as well as in geography, to denote the patterns of human interaction with the physical environment, including not only behavior but genetic adaptation and physiological reaction to environmental stimuli, such as air pressure or trace elements in water, as well. *Cultural ecology* is more specific and refers to behaviors and belief systems within a particular culture, such as those regarding diet, house construction, or hygiene. It is a frequent source of confusion that a great urban sociologist, Amos Hawley, used the term "human ecology" and its holistic view to build on the theoretical traditions of Robert Parke and E. W. Burgess at the University of Chicago in the 1920s on the structure and development of cities. His influential concepts and writing at North Carolina's Institute for Research in the Social Sciences led directly to the development of a separate tradition of social human ecology in the social sciences, one largely without a biophysical environment. The usage of "ecological" to mean multivariate studies of complex systems stems from the sociological tradition.

and nutritional status and genetic susceptibility. Health service delivery relates to economic activity, as do occupational health hazards. Disease agents and medical technology are subject to diffusion.

The main purpose of this chapter is to establish a conceptual framework for understanding why human disease and health vary over the surface of the earth. Health is defined in terms of adaptability and is related to complex systems of interaction among habitat (environment), population, and cultural behavior. These three dimensions form a triangular model of human ecology and underlie disease etiology, consequences, and prevention. Each dimension is considered in turn. A concrete example, ascariasis, and a complex field of study, the ecology of nutrition, illustrate the functioning of the model.

HEALTH

J. Ralph Audy (1971) defined *health* as a "continuing property" that could be measured by the "individual's ability to rally from a wide range and considerable amplitude of insults, the insults being chemical, physical, infectious, psychological, and social" (p. 140). One might prefer the term "stimuli," or "hazards," to "insults." Such stimuli may be either negative or positive: The crucial thing is that the individual must respond to them.

Infectious insults consist of the pathogens—agents that cause disease. Every person is infected at all times with many billions of viruses, bacteria, and protozoa that cause no harm, such as intestinal bacteria. Changes in health status can cause a normally benign relationship to alter and become pathogenic. We also constantly receive nonorganic physical insults, such as from electromagnetic radiation. The trauma of tissue damage and broken bones can result from falls and violence. We live in a chemical soup. Our bodies are chemical systems, quite literally composed of what we eat. Petroleum derivatives and nicotine are now part of our chemistry. The absence of an essential vitamin or an excess in a basic food component, such as cholesterol, can also be a chemical insult. Mental and social insults further influence physiological functioning.

Examples of Insults or Stimuli

Chemical	*Physical*
Carbon monoxide	Trauma
Drugs	Radiation
Benzene	Light
Paint fumes	Noise
Formaldehyde	Electricity
Low dietary calcium	Air pressure

Infectious	*Psychosocial*
Prion	Danger
Virus	Crowds
Rickettsia	Isolation
Bacteria	Anxiety
Protozoa	Community
Helminth	Love

It is possible to map, at a variety of scales, every kind of insult. The areas of a town could be mapped based on noise, people's fear of walking down the street at night, air pollution, visual blight or beauty, mosquito density, or alcohol consumption. Such maps could be overlaid to show regions of health hazards. These regions of insults form the environments to which individuals are exposed at the microscale as they move around.

At the microscale are self-specific environments. Everyone is wrapped in an envelope of heat, humidity, bacteria, fungi, and mites and may host lice and fleas. The driver of a car encounters a set of insults that differs by section of the road and the other vehicles around. The infectious and other insults encountered on a bus are quite different from those in a car. Within buildings, one is insulted by microwaves from the walls, magnetism from electricity, light, changes in humidity, infections from other people, and psychosocial challenges from books, television, and conversation. The exact nature and range of insults to which an individual is exposed during a day is unique. Behavioral roles associated with age, sex, class, and occupation create some groupings of insults, however, and geographical location delimits other groupings. These differences in exposure to various health hazards can be modeled.

The idea that health is a "continuing property" and not a characteristic that is either present or absent involves recognition that health exists at various levels. The only absence of health is death. Health can exist at a threshold, marginally, or it can exist amply with great reserves. Audy points out that an insult has a "training" impact. That is, after the body has successfully rallied from the insult, the body is better able to cope with future insults of that kind. One's first public talk, first date, or first exam in graduate school is more difficult to cope with than the 20th. While a person is reacting to a stimulus, however, the level of health is decreased, and that person becomes less able to cope with another insult. A society's fixation on cleanliness, on the other hand, may result in inadequate training of the immune system and increase the susceptibility of the adult.

The way insults affect the level of health, Audy suggested, can most easily be diagrammed for immunological health. In Figure 2-1, two individuals are conceived and born and experience infectious insults. The first becomes infected with a cold virus, and while she is coughing, sneezing, and slightly feverish her health level declines a little. Soon, however, she is immune to that cold virus, and her health rebounds to a higher level. In this way she proceeds through a succession of infectious episodes. Through time, her level of

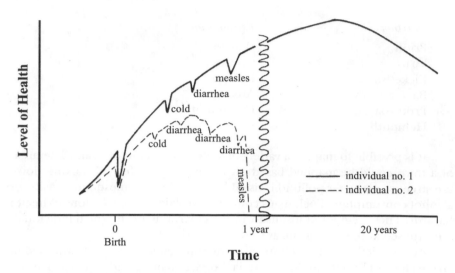

FIGURE 2-1. Health level and insult stress. The discontinuous solid line indicates health level over a lifetime, with a peak of health around age 20. The part before the discontinuity indicates levels of health for two individuals within their first year.

health continues to increase until her early 20s and then gradually declines over the next several decades. The second individual also survives the massive insults that attend birth, but poor maternal nutrition has given her a lower birthweight and level of health. Soon after she rebounds from the cold virus with increased health, she is infected with bacteria that give her diarrhea. She is removed from the food supplements believed to be the cause and even from water, in an effort to stop the diarrhea. Her health level increases slightly as she masters the bacteria, but the episode has precipitated malnutrition because her diet has been marginal. With health lowered by malnutrition, before she can rally and restore herself, she is again assaulted by enteric (intestinal) bacteria. Malnourished, dehydrated, her health level is greatly decreased. As she struggles to rally and grow, she becomes infected with the measles virus. Depleted of health reserves, she cannot rally and she dies. This latter scenario of multiple insults piling up and cumulatively lowering the health level below the vital threshold occurs frequently in Third World countries.

The stress of life events such as marriage and divorce, promotion and being fired, moving, losing a spouse, or having a baby can be scored to predict the likelihood of illness events. It has also been noticed that employee absences due to sickness tend to cluster. Both of these examples of the timing of illness events can be addressed in the terms of the framework that we have developed. Insults require adaptation, and health is lowered during that process, making a person temporarily less able to adapt to the next insult. Around final examination time, for example, many students get sore throats, as the cumulated stresses of little sleep, poor diet, anxiety, and other insults lower levels of health until throat bacteria that have been well controlled suddenly cause clinical illness.

THE TRIANGLE OF HUMAN ECOLOGY

Habitat, population, and behavior form the vertices of a triangle that encloses the state of human health (Figure 2-2). *Habitat* is that part of the environment within which people live, that which directly affects them. Houses and workplaces, settlement patterns, naturally occurring biotic and physical phenomena, health care services, transportation systems, schools, and government are parts of the habitat thus broadly conceived. The following chapters develop other aspects of the habitat; in this chapter the discussion is limited to the constructed part of the habitat, where humans live and work.

Population is concerned with humans as biological organisms, as the potential hosts of disease. The ability of a population to cope with insults of all

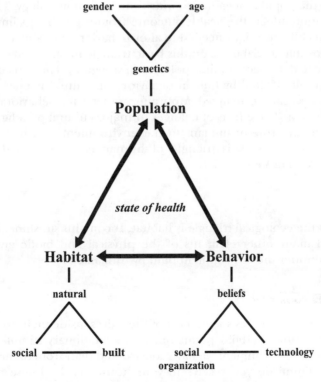

FIGURE 2-2. The triangle of human ecology.

kinds depends on its genetic susceptibility or resistance, its nutritional status, its immunological status, and its immediate physiological status with regard to time of day or year. The effects of age, gender, genetics, and other population components are pervasive but largely implicit in the remainder of this book.

Behavior is the observable aspect of culture. It springs from cultural precepts, economic constraints, social norms, and individual psychology. It includes mobility, roles, cultural practices, and technological interventions. The triangular ecological model differs from sociological models in its separate consideration of behavior and population. Education, for example, is an element of behavior rather than population status. Education involves behavioral exposures to an opportunity in the habitat, an experience that can influence behavior in a way that improves health status by reducing harmful exposures, increasing protective buffering, and inducing alteration of the habitat itself through technology. The social theories of structuration or political/economic/social constructs and perceptions are concerned with this leg of the triangle.

Through their behavior, people create habitat conditions, expose themselves to or protect themselves from habitat conditions, and move elements of the habitat from place to place. The habitat presents opportunities and hazards to the population genetics, nutrition, and immunology. The status of the population affects the health outcome from the habitat stimuli and the energy and collective vigor needed to alter behavior and habitat.

It is possible to elaborate on this basic triangle in many ways. Subsystems can be created for economics, politics, or religion. The effects of global warming (itself affected by human behavior) on natural habitat and behavioral feedbacks can be analyzed. Motivation systems for behavioral alteration can be analyzed. The effects of changes in major cultural paradigms, such as the purpose and role of humans in the environment, can be isolated and spotlighted as insets. This triangle of human ecology is used to discuss women's health in Vignette 7-1.

Habitat

One leg of the ecological triangle is habitat. It contains sunshine, insects, distance, and many other elements of the physical and biotic environment. Here we consider the environment built by humans.

The Built Environment

Asleep or awake, humans spend most of their lives inside their houses or other buildings. Dubos (1965) points out that evolutionary stimuli now come more from the environment we have constructed than from nature.

What stimuli do you receive in your house? Is the house heated and cooled, so that the humidity is also affected? Is it well ventilated? Do any insects live in the woodwork or basement, or do you prefer the vapors of insect nerve poison? Does your dog or cat sleep in the house? Are there windows to let in light? Are there dark corners and rooms? Are there roach droppings or dust bunnies? Is the concentration of dandruff, hair, dust, and allergenic materials higher inside or outside your house? Is there perhaps formaldehyde in the insulation, or lead solder in the pipe joints, or asbestos in the shingles? Do you have radiation sources such as a television or a microwave oven? Or do you have radiation only from electric wiring in the walls? What is the noise level? Do you feel crowded or isolated there?

The type of house, the presence of domestic animals, and the kinds of pens and buildings in which domestic animals are confined are all of consequence to health. It matters to insect ecology (and hence to disease transmission) whether roofs are made out of thatch or corrugated iron and whether windows are screened. It matters for the survival time and contagion of bacteria whether architecture is oriented toward private, shaded, inner courtyards and interior darkness or is open and the interior is almost continuous with the outdoors. It matters whether kitchens are inside or outside the dwellings and whether there are piped water and flush toilets. "Sick buildings" can result from sealing the windows in the interest of energy efficiency but also trapping cleaning fluids and paint fumes.

Details matter in the ecology of disease. A certain kind of chimney can cause a room to be smoky, so that mosquitoes are repelled but eyes are chronically irritated and eventually blinded. Floorboards can be spaced so that food and dirt fall through to be scavenged by pigs and chickens below, or they can be placed tightly together so that one needs to learn to use a dustpan and brush, or they can be carpeted so that fleas can spend their entire life cycle in the living room. Houses can be built out of cold, damp stone and be full of drafts. Alternatively, they can be constructed from mud and straw and provide good nesting cracks for insects. Humans create much of their disease environment.

Changes in the built environment can result in profound alterations of disease conditions. We do not know why some diseases disappeared from Europe and others increased during the last few centuries. Leprosy, for example, used to be common in Europe but no longer is endemic. Dubos (1965) and others argue that changes in the built environment, such as cheaply produced window glass and architectural principles that allowed construction of multiple chimneys, flooded even the houses of the poor with light and warmth, drastically changing the habitat for disease agents. In the cities of industrial Europe the construction of dark, unventilated, and crowded tenements provided an ideal habitat for tuberculosis bacteria. Cropping patterns and food consumption can result in surprising differences in insults. People who grew and consumed rye for bread, for example, suffered much more from ergotism (a toxic condition produced by eating grain infected with ergot fungus) than those who grew or were able to afford to eat wheat.

Settlement patterns, the way people are clustered and distributed on the land, also influence health conditions. On a microscale, geographers look within settlements at the spatial arrangement of residences and land uses. Usually three general settlement forms are distinguished: nuclear, dispersed, and linear. At the macroscale, geographers look at how the settlements are distributed with regard to each other. A settlement system consists of various sizes of settlements, including large cities and the distances, directions, and connections among them which form the structure of a functional region of trade, ideas, and other interactions. The importance of this hierarchical system is discussed in Chapter 10, about disease diffusion.

The most common settlement form is *nuclear.* Most rural people in the world live in houses clustered in a village from which they walk out to the surrounding agricultural fields, with forest and grassland lying beyond. The settlement land use buffers most households from any insect-transmitted diseases from woods and fields, but the nuclear form facilitates the fecal contamination of water sources and the spread of contagious diseases. Houses in a *dispersed* settlement form are located on the farmland of their owners, and neither air nor water provides much focus of contagion for the scattered population. Each household, however, is exposed to diseases originating in the natural surroundings. A *linear* settlement, in which houses are lined up along both sides of a river, canal, or road, has an intermediary position and often is characterized by the worst conditions of the other settlement forms. People are only partially buffered from insect-transmitted diseases because the rear of the dwelling is exposed; and the clustering of houses provides a focus for contagion, especially for those households downstream from other dwellings. In contemporary U.S. terms, the inner city is like a nuclear settlement, exposed to contagion and concentrated pollution, and suburbs, fragmenting the landscapes into which they disperse, reap the hazards of increased tick vectors even as their reduced density retards contagion. Housing sprawled along the highways suffers both the air pollution and vehicular hazards of the city as well as the mosquito and flea pests of the countryside.

Health services are an integral part of the human habitat. Whether a disease is diagnosed and how it is treated depend partly on whether facilities for urine analysis, X rays, brain scans, and various blood tests are available to the physician. Some health facilities lack electricity and in many ways constitute a very different health habitat than that presented by the presence of a university research hospital. Factors as diverse as international economics and roads washed out by monsoon rains can affect the availability of antibiotics or blood for transfusion. The availability and accessibility of health facilities and health personnel comprise a critical part of the health habitat.

The Social Environment

The social environment consists of the groups, relations, and societies within which people live. Audy's conception of health at different levels and depths of reserves and Dubos's (1965) and McKeown's (1988) observations—that

(1) all people exposed to an infection or other risk did not get sick and (2), once sick, people followed varied courses of illness and outcome—had come to seem obvious but were still mysterious. Genetic predisposition, nutritional status, and other population attributes seemed to explain only part. These authors had pointed out that the major declines in mortality resulting from many infectious diseases had occurred prior to effective therapy. Public health improvements in sanitation and changes in year-round availability of good nutrition and such things seemed to explain only part. The ground-breaking studies by Marmot (1986) and others (Marmot, Kogevinas, & Elston, 1987), known as the Whitehall Studies, followed 10,000 British civil servants over two decades and established the importance to health of relative status and not simply economic deprivation to health.

In the study, everyone had abundant food, good shelter, excellent water and sanitation, accessible quality health care, public health information, and general benefits of living in an economically developed country. Yet the clerical/manager civil servants had three and a half times the mortality rates of senior administrator civil servants. The effects of status seemed to work especially through the response to stress. Everyone's blood pressure rose during the workweek, for example, but at home over the weekend the blood pressure of senior administrators fell to healthy levels, whereas that of lower-level civil servants declined only slightly: They seemed to remain continually stressed. Social theorists were quick to realize the implications for race discrimination, gender stereotyping, access to higher education, and social class constructs of many kinds. Addressing the question of how apparently equivalent risks to health became manifested so differently in different people, Robert Evans's (Evans, Barer, & Marmor, 1994) influential studies and writing brought the issue to the forefront of Canadian efforts to promote health as a national priority. Many researchers have confirmed the importance of relative differences in status, and not simply deprivation. The old emphasis on "unhealthy lifestyle choices" and economic deprivation are clearly incomplete and inadequate. There are larger structural and political/economic context and processes involved in determining health.

Even "laboratory" studies at the Duke Primate Center and elsewhere have confirmed that moving a high-status primate to a group where his status is low, and so on, has effects on heart disease, cancer, and the course of infections. But what are the plausible mechanisms? Evans et al. (1994) elucidate the internal biological responses—especially processes of the immune system and endocrine production—which link health status to the perception of the external environment (an interaction of behavior vertex with population vertex to cope with habitat vertex). They point out that many cultural variables affect how distress and disease become manifest in a particular cultural context There are implications for such things as how groups respond to the stress of culture change through coping strategies based on different traditional organization and key values or how epidemiologists conduct community surveys of mental health.

Population

The *nature* of the population, that is, the characteristics, status, and conditions of individuals as organisms, does much to determine the health consequences of any stimulation. Whether the stimulus is a bacterium, light, drug, sound, or thought, the reaction will differ according to the body's biochemical state. This physiology is in part inborn through the genetic code, but it is also influenced by weather, nutrition, previous experience, age, and so on.

Genetics

Genes set the limits of our possible responses to social, biological, and physical experiences. Once it became possible to "read" the DNA (deoxyribonucleic acid) sequence of acids and bases that encodes the structure and processes of life, the sciences of genetics and biochemistry expanded explosively. Our knowledge of how genetic information is stored, transmitted, and activated at the appropriate time is undergoing almost daily revision. The DNA chain can be broken in some places but apparently not in others. Pieces can be switched, overridden, and deleted. Some information has persisted from ancient times, with no known function today. Some is activated to govern the production of enzymes, hormones, or other proteins only at certain times in life and then is "turned off." The functioning of the genetic code is much more complex, and the encoded instructions much more varied, than had been imagined.

The Human Genome Project begun in the early 1990s, is already yielding important medical results. It is an ambitious research undertaking to map the spatial arrangement of chemical functional groups and their interactions on human chromosomes, and so locate the genes and their functions in human heredity. Several genes responsible for serious disease have already been identified: cystic fibrosis, Huntington's chorea, familiar breast cancer susceptibility, familiar early-onset Parkinson's disease. Recombinant genetic technology, using, for example, common viruses to "vector" normal genes into cells to replace damaged and dysfunctional ones, is already leading to new therapies and even promising cures. Even diseases influenced by several genes, like some breast cancer, are yielding to the new technologies, and there is excitement about treatments for diabetes, schizophrenia, and severe forms of obesity, to name a few of the current targets.

Genetically *caused* disease is uncommon, however. Rather than dominant lethal genes, most genetic disease is associated with rare recessive traits which, while terribly important to the individuals and families involved, are not a concern at the population level except under conditions of inbreeding. Hemophilia among the royal families of Europe is the most famous example of such a disease. "Mad King George" may have been a threat to his people, but not from contagion. Harmful traits in a population that is not inbred tend to be eliminated rather than reproduced, and when they are found to occur frequently in a population, one looks for some advantage that they bestow. Most diseases that tend to be transmitted in families or that occur more frequently in particular population groups result from genetic *susceptibility* rather than genetic causation. That is, the disease requires a stimulus, or "cause," to occur, but another person who is not genetically susceptible will not respond to the same stimulus with disease. Some types of cancer and the virulence of diseases such as tuberculosis or measles are thought to be related to genetic susceptibility.

Research in biochemistry and genetics has been overwhelmed by the recent findings on the variability and plasticity of human inheritance. The paired, rod-shaped chromosomes in the nucleus of each body cell contain the paired genes that control heredity. There are specific points, known as structural loci, on the chromosomes for genes governing each characteristic (trait) (what the genome project is mapping). Genes that occupy the same locus on a specific pair of chromosomes and control the heredity of a particular characteristic, such as blood type, are known as *alleles*. When more than one version of the same trait is common, such as blue and brown eyes or Type A, Type B, and Type O blood, the population is said to be *polymorphic* for that trait. Humans have long been recognized to be polymorphic for blood type, skin color, hair texture, stature, and other traits that used to be categorized by the concept of "race." There are, at a conservative estimate, more than 50,000 structural loci, and about one-third of these are polymorphic. Each individual has two different alleles for about one third of these polymorphic structural loci, or about one-tenth of his or her entire genetic inheritance.

One way to illustrate the importance of polymorphism for human health is to consider the histocompatability system (HLA): in short, the genetic control of the body's immune system. "Histo" refers to tissue; "HLA" to human leukocyte antigens, white blood cell substances that induce production of antibodies. The HLA region of the chromosomes has at least four loci. More than 20 alleles may occur at one of these, 40 at another. In total, more than 80 alleles are involved at these four loci, and the possible number of reproductive combinations exceeds 20 million. It has long been known that people have different types of blood, A, B, AB, or O, and that the Rh factor is positive or negative. Currently, more than 160 red blood cell antigens are identifiable. Most have been implicated in blood transfusion reactions and presumably are involved in mother–fetus exchanges. More than 100 variants of human hemoglobin are also known. This is the type of genetic variability involved in acceptance or rejection of organ transplants, defense against cancer, and resistance to diseases such as malaria or measles.

The concept of race has become obsolete insofar as it denotes a classification with concrete existence rather than a convenient categorization for some particular purpose. One can visualize thousands, even millions, of maps of the relative frequencies of genetic traits for antigens and enzymes, hormones, bone structure, skin pigmentation, and other coded instructions for forming human beings. Each mapped surface is continuous over the earth, for almost all of these variants occur everywhere. The frequency of most genetic variations in a population has a spatial gradient (slope), however. The gradients for types of blood antigens, for example, run east–west in Europe, with Type A and Rh factor decreasing to the east. Skin pigmentation and body shape, however, have a north–south gradient in Europe. If people were "racially" grouped by their fingerprints, western Europeans, sub-Saharan Africans, and east Asians would be grouped together because they have "loops" whereas Mongolians and Australian aborigines have "whorls," and Khoisan and central Europeans "arches." If people were grouped by body hair or size of buttocks yet different "races" would be classified.

Studies of identical twins who have identical DNA but may be raised together under the same social influences or separately in different families and circumstances allow genetic effects and shared-environment effects to be separated. Twin studies have identified an astonishing amount of genetic propensity. The range of influences includes things such as color preference and favorite foods, occupational choice and form of exercise, alcohol and tobacco usage, and personality type and risk of cardiovascular disease. Genetic effects extend, apparently, to biological reproduction, as predicted by evolutionary theory. Udry (1996) has argued that under conditions of behavioral choice and opportunity, biological differences in behavioral dispositions will increasingly explain variations in behavior. "Application of this principle to demographic research suggests that, increasingly, gendered behavior, fertility, contraception, abortion, nuptiality, occupational choice, and other behaviors of interest to demographers will be influenced by biological choice" (p. 335). Researchers have used the Danish national register of twins to follow cohorts of twins through the demographic transition (Chapter 4, this volume). Kohler, Rodgers, and Christensen (1999) find that the heritability of fertility changes in systematic ways: Shared environment effects are strong in pretransitional cohorts and under constant social conditions, but when changing social norms and economic conditions allow a broad range of life-course alternatives and deliberate choice, the heritability of female fertility is high and environmental effects become almost irrelevant. This is especially true at the onset of fertility decline, and especially strong for the timing of transition from zero to one child.

The manner in which each genetic distribution compares with environmental, cultural, or disease patterns is of interest. Physical environmental factors such as solar radiation and cultural factors such as method of maintaining livelihood, perceptions of beauty, marriage ideals, and migration histories have all affected genetic patterns. Geographers have joined the search for associations between blood type and disease susceptibility and between metabolic differences and cultural evolution, such as cropping system. Any effort to categorize all distributions, however, has to involve rather arbitrary criteria and great simplification. Biologically the concept of race is still used occasionally as a convenient categorization for the relative frequencies of many alleles, in full recognition that group boundaries and the traits included are arbitrary. When race is used as a grouping of alleles to indicate the overall genetic distance or closeness of populations, it sometimes establishes a useful research framework. The Japanese, for example, have different health problems than do Europeans and Americans also living in industrialized countries at the same latitudes. The disease experience of successive generations of Japanese in the United States has been studied to help untangle genetic, cultural, and environmental factors in cancer etiology. In most scientific usage, race has generally been replaced by the categorization of "ethnicity," for it has been many decades since behavioral, linguistic, or mental characteristics were scientifically associated with the genetic inheritance of physical traits. Anyone doing or reading about research that involves a racial classification needs always to question closely the nature, purpose, and appropriateness of the characteristic used, or whether, for example, careless and lazy usage is neglecting socioeconomic or cultural causal associations. "Race" has, of course, become a social construction, a category experienced or studied as a reality with real consequences for social marginalization, group perception, and health care.

Genetically Based Differences in Metabolism

There is considerable interest today in investigating the genetic base of differences in human metabolism (energy and material transformation within cells) as these differences interact with culture and health. Lactose intolerance and alcoholism are briefly discussed here.

Lactose intolerance is a classic geographic puzzle in human ecology. Lactose is the only carbohydrate in milk. The enzyme lactase splits lactose into glucose and galactose, which are absorbed into the blood stream as nutrients. Lactase appears in the human fetus in the third trimester of pregnancy, reaches a peak at birth, and falls gradually in childhood. The condition of lactose intolerance, or being unable fully to digest milk because of an inability to produce lactase, is the usual condition of most adult mammals, including human beings. Among some populations, notably Europeans, the gene for producing lactase does not shut off, and so most adults are able to digest dairy products. Scientists and others of European descent used to consider this the normal human condition.

Simoons (1969; 1970) has proposed a geographical hypothesis of biological and cultural interaction to explain the distribution of lactose intolerance around the world. He estimates that among Asians, about 90% of the population is lactose intolerant. Among Africans the prevalence of lactose intolerance shifts from tribe to tribe, even from village to village, but in general, intolerance prevails. The question raised by his research is whether, for example, the Chinese lost their ability to digest lactose because they defined cattle keeping as barbaric and consequently excluded from their diet milk and the meat of herd animals (eating the meat of only door yard scavengers such as chickens and pigs), or whether they developed their cuisine because they were unable to digest milk. Similarly, did Caucasians develop a high frequency of lactose tolerance because they became herders of cattle and goats, with mixed farming systems to support their draft animals, or did they take to dairy foods and raise the animals that produced milk because they could digest lactose? In Africa the ethnic groups that herd cattle generally are much more lactose tolerant than the farming groups that do not, but the genetic pattern is complex as a result of invasions, migrations, and intermarriage. Lactose intolerance has important ramifications for worldwide emergency relief (usually involving powdered milk) and protein supplementation, agricultural extension, and development aid of all kinds, as well as vitamin D and calcium supplementation.

Studies involving the metabolism of alcohol have shown that the Chinese, even when acculturated to U.S. drinking habits, tend to metabolize alcohol differently than European ethnic groups. A single glass of wine may produce the dizziness, flushing, and nausea that usually characterize much higher levels of alcohol consumption among Europeans. Some ethnic groups, such as Jews, have low levels of alcoholism while others, such as Russians, have rather high levels. Most such differences have been explained in sociocultural terms, as alcohol plays different roles in different societies. But the question arises: Is the different role of alcohol in European and Chinese cultures a result of or a cause of differences in metabolism of alcohol? As the study of alcoholism progresses, it is being found that upbringing, life stress, familiarity, and social custom are important, but alcoholism also clusters in families. Even when adopted in infancy the children of alcoholic fathers are more likely to become alcoholic, and identical twins reared apart and brought up differently seem to show similar susceptibility (studies have involved small numbers). Alcohol has been produced for millennia in some cultures to store excess grain and to provide an alternative to polluted water; in other societies it has been little used in these ways. As in the case of lactose intolerance, geographical associations of culture, alcohol, and population may help establish patterns and promote understanding of a serious human health problem.

Other Influences on Population Status

Beyond genetics there are many other inputs into the functioning of the human biochemical system. A most important geographical influence is weather. Humans adjust to differences of temperature and humidity, air pressure, altitude and oxygen level, and hours of daylight by altering their body chemistry, physiology, and metabolism. These changes create different nutritional needs and different internal conditions for infectious agents or for drugs (see Chapter 5).

Age is also a critical factor for health status. Those who study geriatrics (diseases of old age) are just beginning to understand the aging process, but many of the biochemical changes are obvious. Metabolism changes in response to different energy requirements when behavioral roles change with age and growth, maturation, and reproduction are completed. Hormone and enzyme production, organ function, and deposition and storage of fats and chemicals in the bones, liver, and blood vessels all change with age. Experience accumulates, and the immune system recognizes and copes with a greater variety of infectious agents—and is sometimes more sensitized from long exposure to a variety of allergenic substances. The regulation of some homeostatic systems, such as temperature control, tends to become less efficient with age; other systems gain in efficiency, from practice.

The age structure of a population in large part determines consequences as diverse as the spread of an infectious agent and the severity of the illnesses it causes, the effects of changes in the weather or of an air pollution episode, the expression of carcinogenic agents in clinical disease, and the need for health services. Because age affects so many dimensions of health status, it needs to be accounted for in virtually every study of disease etiology (see Chapter 6).

Behavior

Human beings are animals which are cultural beings. Culture creates social organization, structuring relationships of power, status, and control of resources. Culture creates belief systems, values, perceptions. Culture develops technology. The study of this vertex comprehends most of social science and the humanities. Cultural behavior interacts with the triangle of human ecology in four ways:

1. Humans create many habitat conditions.
2. Behavior exposes individuals and populations to some hazards and protects them from others.
3 People move not only themselves from place to place but also other elements of disease systems.
4. Behavior affects the health of the population by controlling genetics through marriage customs, nutritional status through food customs, and immunologic status through the technology of vaccination and customs of deliberate childhood exposure.

Each of these aspects of behavior is discussed.

Very little of the earth's surface is unaltered by human activity. Vegetation has been burned, removed, and planted. Water has been withdrawn from below the earth's surface and stored and distributed over hundreds of miles on the surface. The chemical composition of the air and water has been altered. The kind of buildings people construct, the kind of industries they work in, the kind of vehicles and roads they build, and the kind and scale of the settlement systems they live in all form the hazards to which they are exposed. This cultural creation of disease is as true for malaria as for lung cancer. For example, in the northeastern United States people cleared most of the forest for agriculture and growing cities. They thereby eliminated many of the animals. Land has in recent decades reverted to old fields and new forests and presently is being fragmented by expanding suburban settlement and abandonment of industrial sites. With the restoration of habitat and now without large predators to control them, the deer population has rebounded to the highest level in two centuries. This has promoted the spread of Lyme disease and established it as a major public health concern throughout the region.

Besides creating hazards, cultural practices also function to protect people. Many protective customs have been developed. In the Chinese culture realm people habitually drink tea rather than unboiled water. Many of the Jewish and Moslem dietary practices are protective, and the burial of feces is prescribed in the Old Testament. The European custom of using a handkerchief for blowing the nose is as protective as the Chinese custom of blowing the nose onto and spitting upon the street is endangering. Wearing shoes provides almost total protection against hookworm. Frequent washing of hands, especially after defecation or before handling food, is effective protection from diseases as diverse as the common cold and hydatidosis (invasion of tissue by tapeworms; see Table 3-5).

We have learned to construct *buffers* against disease deliberately: Consider the chlorination of water supplies, the use of seat belts, and the prevalence of the water-sealed toilet. There are cultural origins and diffusion paths for protective buffers, and sometimes diffusion and adoption take time. There are also economic and social class barriers to their occurrence. For example, diarrhea is one of the greatest causes of death in the world. Millions of children die of diarrhea because, although it is known how to protect them, the appropriate knowledge and means never reach them.

Behavioral roles, varying by age and sex and often by ethnicity or class, largely determine who is exposed to what. There is great cultural variation in social norms. In one culture men are exposed to the infections of the crowded marketplace because women are thought not to understand money, whereas in another culture women are exposed because men are considered far too unreliable to handle the family money and women are judged superior at bargaining. Who herds animals in pastures and gets hookworm? Who handles dangerous industrial chemicals and gets cancer? Who washes laundry in the morning when *Mansonia* mosquitoes are biting and gets filariasis (a worm infestation; see Table 3-2)? Who tends the orchard in the evening when *Aedes* mosquitoes are biting and gets dengue fever? Who goes to school and gets mumps? Who drives a vehicle and suffers a concussion? Who fights a war and is maimed? Who goes to the city for wage labor and contracts AIDS while separated from home? Who leaves the home village for marriage and faces abuse or depression without social support?

Mobility patterns are of critical importance for the diffusion and incidence of disease, and they are discussed at some length in Chapter 4. Medicinal plants as well as insects that transmit disease have been spread around the world by humans. When people migrate, they carry customs, adaptive in the place of origin, that are often inappropriate in the new place, such as building in Hawaii a house with a steeply pitched roof to shed snow. Such "cultural baggage" may include ideas about poisonous or nutritious plants. Formerly protective behavior may even be harmful in the new place. A good example is geophagy, the practice of earth eating. In parts of Africa pregnant women eat earth formed into molds and sold in market. The earth comes from special sites and is often high in calcium, iron, and other minerals. It is believed to provide critical nutrients missing in the diet. The practice persists in the United States among a few people of African descent. An old woman in rural Georgia may keep a jar of her favorite clay from a local stream bed in her pantry, although she does not need its minerals (inappropriate behavior); and her daughter who has migrated to a northern city may consume laundry starch as a substitute for earth (harmful behavior). With mobility, custom often becomes disassociated from purpose.

It is easy to understand how behavior can affect the genetics of a population. Marriage customs have evolved partly to control genetics. All societies appear to forbid incest, although it is defined in different ways. Some societies prohibit racial intermarriage, whereas others are far more concerned with class status. Technology can affect the genetics of the population. In one society people with poor vision make poor hunters and providers; in another, eyeglasses have rendered eyesight an irrelevant criterion for marriage. Health services and technology enable people with genetic traits for diabetes, hemophilia, or deficient immune systems to live and reproduce. The immunological status of a population used to depend almost entirely on its age structure, because experience with infectious agents accumulates over time. Now technology allows even newborns to be vaccinated for diphtheria, whooping cough, and other frequently fatal diseases. The degree of disease resistance of the population thus has become a cultural construct.

The Cultural Ecology of Ascariasis

Hundreds of millions of people are unaware that they have ascariasis. The disease agent is the intestinal roundworm that is adapted to humans, *Ascaris lumbricoides*. The adult worm in the intestine passes eggs into the feces. The eggs embryonate in the soil for about 3 weeks before they are infective. They are eaten by people, perhaps through soil contamination of vegetables, dust contamination of eating utensils, or a child's eating of dirt. The eggs hatch, and the larvae penetrate the gut wall and make their way to the lungs, where they develop in the rich oxygenated tissue for more than a week. They break through into the lung and are coughed up into the mouth and swallowed once again. This time, as adults, they dwell in the small intestine and pass eggs into the feces. A light infection is usually asymptomatic. The first awareness of an infection may come when live adult worms are seen in the stool or perhaps are passed through the mouth. Heavier infection causes digestive disturbances, abdominal pain, and loss of sleep. Death can (rarely) result from intestinal obstruction.

This life cycle and transmission chain is complex but well-known and medically straightforward. Epidemiologically, small children have the highest rates of infection, followed by mothers who tend small children. It is a disease acquired in the home and its environs. Those who work in the fields or herd livestock may get hookworm but seldom roundworm.

The cultural and environmental interactions involved in ascariasis are actually quite complex, as Figure 2-3 illustrates. A person infected with the roundworm can be treated with antihelminthic drugs. There may be side effects, but unlike the case with other helminthic (worm) infections of the lungs, liver, or blood vessels, the killed intestinal worms are easily eliminated from the body. Sanitary disposal of the eggs prevents humans from ever contacting them. In some cultures, however, even if the adults construct and use latrines or are wealthy enough to have a flush toilet, the home compound may be contaminated by toddlers because they are not diapered. Although embryonated eggs may remain viable for years, the eggs often encounter adverse environmental conditions in the soil. Temperature affects the time they take to embryonate. Physical conditions such as sun or shade, moisture, acid-

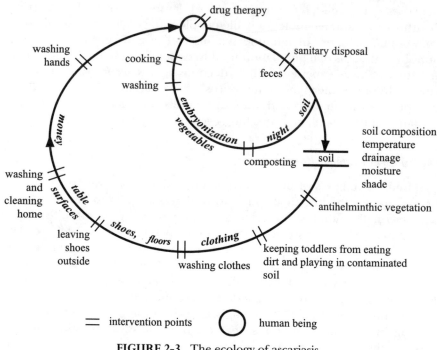

FIGURE 2-3. The ecology of ascariasis.

ity or alkalinity affect whether the embryos can develop and how long they survive. Predators eat the eggs, and plants that produce chemicals to protect themselves from helminths sometimes affect the human parasites as well. Customs regarding defecation habits are very important. A certain stream bank may be used by everyone, or people may seek privacy in their own orchard or woodlot. Customs differ about how far from the house one must go, and about where small children can play. In the Chinese culture realm human waste has been collected and used as fertilizer for millennia. The Chinese were once said to be the most heavily parasitized people in the world because of this practice. Composting at high temperatures sterilizes the eggs, and during the Mao Zedong era it was claimed that this technology had eliminated the problem. Apparently it was not applied universally with equal care, however, as in 1995 the overall prevalence of ascaris in the Chinese population was 47%, or more than 500 million people infected.

The embryonated eggs get into the human mouth through a variety of paths that involve dust as well as direct contamination. Money or dusty fruit may carry the eggs. The eggs often enter the house on dirty feet and contaminate counters, dishes, and hands. All the customs about not wearing shoes into the house, frequency of washing clothes, floors, and furniture, and habitual washing of hands become important. Sometimes these habits depend not only on custom but on the physical availability of abundant water for hygiene. When the nearest well in the dry season is more than a mile distant, when the stream used for water is 5,000 feet down the mountainside, or when water must be melted from snow or obtained by hacking through thick ice, floors tend not to be washed very often.

EVOLUTION, ADAPTATION, AND EMERGENCE

It is an adage that diseases represent evolution in progress. Health is adaptability, Dubos says. Natural selection works on the microbes and it works on the humans. In his classic, Thomas (1974) described the components of our own cells, the mitochondria which perform our respiration and the other foreign bodies, each with their own DNA that is not ours, which are so symbiotic with us that our form of life cannot exist without their presence. Their aging may be our aging. Other forms of DNA strands, prions and plasmids, and stray protein molecules of many kinds pass through generations and across species of pig, duck, dog, and among humans alike. Geography is not much interested in intracellular structures, but this ecological continuum of struggle and cooperation and adaptation and mobility and information is life itself. Whatever we do with our politics and our technology, the microbes will continue their struggles to adapt, evolve, and survive. Just 30 years ago we thought we could eradicate malaria and tuberculosis and perhaps even eliminate infectious disease altogether. Now we know better.

When a disease agent either produces immunity or kills, there must be a

population large enough to support its continuous circulation among susceptible people. Otherwise the disease cannot be maintained, as can be seen
when infectious diseases such as colds or influenza are introduced to small island populations today. A few diseases, such as chicken pox (whose viral
agent, herpes, can lie dormant in an immune person for decades before being shed during the illness known as "shingles" to infect a new generation),
have evolved special strategies for surviving in small human groups. Most human infectious diseases could not have existed before domestication of
plants and animals led to agricultural systems that supported enormously increased human populations with food surplus. These people then created
cities in settlement systems and transformed the nature of human interaction. Disease agents that mutated from animal diseases, as must have happened many times previously in isolated dead ends, now found with urbanization a large enough interacting population to support their continuing
circulation. The measles virus, for example, is closely related to the virus that
causes rinderpest in cattle and the one that causes distemper in dogs. As people domesticated these animals and herded them together, the microbe
could spread more intensely among them. It must have infected people many
times before it managed a strain that survived long enough to be passed to
another person. A settlement system of several hundred thousand interacting
people is necessary to maintain the circulation of measles, which kills or
leaves permanent immunity, and so infectious people must have contact with
new susceptible people. The domestication of animals and their herding together created conditions optimum for an animal virus crossing to people.
Not only measles but smallpox and tuberculosis, for example, have their closest microbe relations in cattle disease agents (it was not accidental that cow-
pox could be used as a vaccine for smallpox).

The ecological information feedback in relationships is important to
both microbe and host. If the infected host does not survive long enough
for the disease agent to get to another host, both will die. A virulent agent,
which multiplies so quickly it overwhelms its host and kills quickly, will not
spread as widely as an agent which becomes attenuated and lets its host carry it around for awhile. The English sweating sickness terrified Europe from
1485 to 1552, for example, but the microbe was so efficient at killing its
hosts that it became extinct. Human hosts, on the other hand, are selected
for resistance to the agent and, less directly, for developing successful cultural buffers. The most common model is that disease agents newly transferred to people are most virulent, become less severe through passage and
over human generations, and eventually become "mild childhood diseases."
In the human gut, bacteria may cause massive tissue destruction and fatal
fluid loss or become intestinal fauna that produce symptoms only under
physiological stress, or commensal residents unknown in their billions, or
even symbiotic agents that help produce vitamins for the human gut to absorb. The general rule is that the more virulent and less adapted the agent,
the newer the disease. There are other strategies, however. Disease agents

vectored by insects in particular (discussed in Chapter 3) may benefit from concentrating great numbers to increase their chance of being taken up by a flea or mosquito and inoculated into another person. Their host does not have to be mobile to infect insects, and how long he needs to survive depends on how many insects there are to feed on him and pick up the infectious agent. Similarly, when many people, or animals, crowd together, they increase the ease of contacting another susceptible host and so the agent can increase its numbers (and hence virulence) to maximize transmission of infection rather than keep its host active to maximize contact with others. Most microbes mutate or combine with passing bits of DNA to create new strains that constantly probe for the best survival strategy. For excellent discussion of the evolution of *Yersinia pestis,* the bubonic plague bacteria, see Wills (1996); for the evolution of genetic strains of HIV and their selection by human behavior, see Ewald (1994).

Various infectious diseases evolved in separate population settlement systems, within which over centuries hosts and microbes had begun to adapt to each other. Diseases remained regionalized for long periods because people infected with a disease agent either died on the journey or became immune before they could reach another region. Even if a few people made contact, ecological relations usually work against successful biological invasion. When the yellow fever virus was introduced to the mosquitoes and monkeys of South America, for example, it found a new place to relocate; when—if—it was introduced to the mosquitoes and monkeys of tropical Asia, however, it found its niche already occupied by the virus of dengue fever, which induced resistance to it. The protozoa that causes African sleeping sickness must have cross the Atlantic with the slave trade, but it never found a fly like the tsetse, which exists only in Africa, to transfer it to a new host. Even though most disease agents are species-specific—that is, the dog round worm does not cause ascariasis in people; human measles does not give a dog distemper—if enough contact is made adaptation will begin.

Throughout history, the progressive development of transportation and mobility has resulted in exchange of disease agents between formerly separated populations (see, e.g., Crosby, 1972; McNeill, 1976). The contact of the Roman and Chinese empires brought a deadly exchange of disease agents, as did the later contact of Europeans and Native Americans. "The Columbian Exchange" brought to the New World the disease agents that had evolved in the domesticated animal herds and crossed to people in the cities of the Old World. It also brought a few disease systems, such as malaria and river blindness, that found equivalent insects to vector them and successfully relocated into parallel ecological niches. Syphilis probably spread with Columbus from the Caribbean to Europe. From Spain to the New World, however, came smallpox, measles, whooping cough, typhoid, diphtheria, influenza, malaria, yellow fever, onchocerciasis, probably tuberculosis, and more. When a new disease agent spreads in a "virgin population," in which there is no immunity from age or experience, it strikes down everyone. When everyone is sick, there is no one to gather firewood, or cook, or even fetch water for the feverish. Epidemic after epidemic spread through the Amer-Indian population, spreading on indigenous trade routes through even North America decades before any English settlers appeared. There is a range of estimates, but probably an 80–90% reduction of population, the loss of 50–80 million people in the greatest holocaust of human existence, resulted. Two centuries later, the people of Hawaii and other Pacific islands did not fare much better.

Today disease agents can easily cross the ocean on a jet airplane. Chapter 4 discusses the accelerating mobility of the human population. Because people can travel and arrive at their destination long before they develop any symptoms, traditional buffers such as quarantine have been rendered moot. Any virus from any place in the world can be anywhere else within a week. The new conditions in an urbanizing world are also creating optimum conditions for the emergence of virulence and crossing of species through the sheer intensity of transmission that has been made possible (see, e.g., dengue hemorrhagic fever in Chapter 3). Finally, old diseases are reemerging as the agents learn to cope with cultural buffers. One of the greatest threats to public health today is the emergence of multiple-drug-resistant tuberculosis, some strains of which are now untreatable with any antibiotics. Streptococcus and other hospital infections are becoming very resistant, as are the salmonellas and shigellas of livestock and people. The resistance of the malaria protozoa to chloroquine and related chemicals has spread around the world, while those on the Thai–Cambodian border today are resistant to every known antimalarial drug except *artemisia,* which has just been introduced from China. Resistance to it has already been induced in a laboratory. We may soon be more helpless before malaria than in the 19th century, when at least quinine worked for those who had it. The threat of emerging diseases is producing major conferences, book perspectives, and new journals.

NUTRITION AND HEALTH

The interaction between nutrition and disease is two way. In themselves, deficiencies of minerals and vitamins constitute diseases, but malnutrition also makes the body more susceptible to disease. Antibodies are not produced quickly or abundantly, tissues heal slowly, bones are more easily broken, membranes become permeable. A malnourished person is more likely to get sick, and the course of the sickness is more likely to be severe and drawn out; the level of health is lowered by the malnutrition, and the person is less able to rally from new insults. Sickness may cause malnutrition. The body commonly responds to fever and nausea with a loss appetite. Feverish people tend to sleep for long periods and not eat regular meals. If diarrhea or vomiting occurs, the body's absorption of nutrients is hindered. Prolonged diarrhea drains the body of salts and disturbs the electrolyte balance. When the body copes with infection, high levels of nitrogen are eliminated in the urine. Even the mild reaction resulting from vaccination will cause nitrogen to be eliminated, so that the body requires protein supplementation for recovery. It is easy to understand how a newly weaned child with borderline nutrition can develop kwashiorkor (a form of severe protein deficiency) after measles, or pneumonia after malnutrition.

Dietary excess can also result in disease conditions. Sugar consumption, for example, is related to the occurrence of diabetes and dental caries. Cholesterol, an animal fat, is related to atherosclerosis. Several salts can cause hypertension.

Regionalization of Diet and Deficiencies

Nutritional hazards can often be associated with cropping pattern, season, or culture realm. Jacques May devoted the last 20 years of his life to studying the ecology of malnutrition and left us a voluminous literature on the subject (1977; see "Further Reading"). He showed appreciation of both the environmental and the cultural side of nutritional patterns.

Environmental parameters of rainfall and evapotranspiration potentials, freezing, heat, soil, evolution, and topography put limits on what can be cultivated. Where droughts are frequent and soils tend to be saline, the various kinds of millets are reliable and yield good protein. Where water is abundant and temperatures warm, rice returns the highest number of calories per acre and provides good nutrition. Winter wheat yields more than spring wheat, but winter wheat usually cannot be grown in Siberia, Manchuria, and much of Canada. Many of our grains evolved in places with long hours of sunlight during the growing season. They either fail to ripen or yield poorly under tropical conditions of an unvarying 12 hours of sunlight. The agricultural patterns of the world formed within these parameters. These are generalizations; rice is grown even in northern Japan, using specially adapted strains. For most of human history 20 inches of rainfall marked the geographical limit of cultivation and the beginning of pastoralism, but in recent years irrigation from tube wells has greatly extended the amount of arable land.

To these physical parameters must be added the cultural patterns that have formed broad dietary regions. Food crops were domesticated in specific cultural hearths and then spread over paths of cultural contact. The natives of Middle America domesticated corn, squash, beans, tomatoes, chili peppers, and numerous vegetables. They did not domesticate many animals and had no equivalent for the cow, but the collective amino acids in corn, squash, and beans are well balanced and provide complete protein. In the Middle East wheat was domesticated and became the staff of life. It was balanced by the domestication of cattle, sheep, goats, and other dairy and meat sources. In Southeast Asia rice was domesticated, and the fish cultivated in the rice fields provided the balancing protein. In West Africa the cocoyam and oil palm were domesticated and combined with millet.

The original domesticates continue to constitute the core regional diets. Each diet is balanced and potentially sufficient for people who can afford to get enough of it. Only the domesticated starch roots, especially manioc (otherwise known as tapioca or cassava), are so deficient in anything but calories that they constitute a poor diet. For most people the cereal grains and legume vegetables such as soybeans or chickpeas are the major sources of protein, although medieval Europeans and their Mediterranean predecessors developed a mixed farming system that used grain cultivation and animal husbandry to mutually support each other. Diversity and variety in diet, however, are everywhere necessary to provide the full range of nutrients. A diet limited to staple foods is often the lot of the poor, and so regional diets are often associated with specific nutritional deficiencies. Table 2-1 lists human nutritional needs, sources of nutrients, and deficiency diseases.

The first and perhaps greatest deficiency association is that of beriberi with rice. It was certainly a great mystery. *Beriberi,* a disease involving weakness, paralysis, and eventual heart failure, results from the lack of thiamine, vitamin B1, which is needed for carbohydrate metabolism. Rice has thiamine in its husk. When rice is milled at home with mortar and pestle, some husk and thiamine remain in the finished product. Milling rice by hand is arduous and time-consuming, and the pretty, white, polished mill rice is greatly preferred. The white polished rice also stores better. Beriberi historically was concentrated in Tokyo and parts of northern China which were at the end of a long transportation of rice from southern regions of the country. The rice was thoroughly milled prior to shipment by canal boat or wagon. To help protect it from weevils, talcum powder was commonly added. This, in turn, led to the cooking custom of thoroughly washing the rice and even throwing out excess cooking water, customs which further diminished the thiamine, which is water soluble. In contrast, in the southern part of India where medical researchers had puzzled over the absence of beriberi despite dependence on rice, the customary treatment was to partially cook the rice before storage and before milling; this parboiling preserved the thiamine. By the end of the 19th century it was known that beriberi befell institutionally crowded populations, such as monks and soldiers and especially sailors and prisoners; that it was most common on the coasts whereas people in the interior of countries seemed immune; that commonly people newly arrived took several months before they developed the disease; that people such as scholars who led sedentary lives, poor laborers eating rice, and soldiers fed on meat and eggs were all prone to develop beriberi; that it was epidemic at the beginning of the rainy season, when plowing was done, but was unrelated to climate because it had spread and climate had not changed; that it occurred from Brazil to Argentina and in the American South but was responsible for up to half the hospitalizations in Kuala Lumpur, Manila, and Tokyo. Researchers looked for a toxin in bad food, for a chemical contaminant, and especially for the newly discovered germs. The Dutch discovered that by feeding their prisoners in Java brown rice they could stop the deaths, but world

TABLE 2-1. Human Nutritional Needs, Sources, and Deficiencies

Nutrient	Major body function	Major sources	Deficiency disease
Balanced amino acids	Precursors of structural protein, enzymes, antibodies, hormones	Good sources: meat, fish, dairy products, legumes Adequate sources: rice, corn, wheat Poor sources: cassava, yams	Kwashiorkor
Fatty acids	Cell membrane function, regulation of digestion and hormones	Vegetable oils	Skin lesions

Water-soluble vitamins

Nutrient	Major body function	Major sources	Deficiency disease
B1 (thiamine)	Removal of carbon dioxide	Organ meats, whole grains, legumes	Beriberi (nerve changes, weakness, heart failure)
B2 (riboflavin)	Energy metabolism	Widely available	Lip cracks, eye lesions
Niacin	Oxidation-reduction reactions	Liver, lean meats legumes (can be formed from amino tryptophan)	Pellagra (skin rash, nerve and mental disorders)
B6 (pyridoxine)	Amino acid metabolism	Meats, vegetables whole grains	Irritability, convulsions, kidney stones
Pantothenic acid	Energy metabolism	Widely available	Fatigue, sleep disturbances
Folacin	Nucleic acid and amino acid metabolism	Legumes, green vegetables, whole grains	Anemia, diarrhea
B12	Nucleic acid metabolism	Muscle meats, eggs, dairy products (not in plant foods)	Pernicious anemia, nerve disorder
Biotin	Fat synthesis, amino acid metabolism	Legumes, vegetables, meats	Fatigue, depression
Choline	Precursor of neurotransmitter	Yolk, liver, grains, legumes	Not known
C (ascorbic acid)	Maintains cartilage, bone, dentine; collagen synthesis (= about 30% of body protein)	Citrus fruits, tomatoes, green vegetables	Scurvy (degeneration of skin, teeth, blood vessels)

(*continued*)

TABLE 2-1. *(cont.)*

Nutrient	Major body function	Major sources	Deficiency disease
Fat-soluble vitamins			
A (retinol)	Constituent of visual pigment; maintenance of epithelial tissue	A or pro-A (beta-carotenes) in green vegetables, dairy products	Xerophthalmia, night blindness, blindness
D	Growth and mineralization of bone, absorption of calcium	Cod-liver oil, eggs, fortified dairy products	Rickets (bone deformity), osteomalacia in adults
E	Antioxidant to prevent cell membrane change	Green leafy vegetables, seeds, shortenings	Anemia
K	Blood clotting	Green leafy vegetables	Internal hemorrhages, severe bleeding
Major minerals			
Calcium	Bones and teeth, blood clotting, nerve transmission	Dairy products, dark green vegetables, legumes	Stunted growth, rickets, osteoporosis, convulsions
Phosphorus	Bones and teeth, body pH balance	Dairy products, meat, poultry, grains	Weakness, demineralization of bones
Potassium	Body pH balance, water balance, nerve function	Meats, milk, fruits	Muscular weakness, paralysis
Chlorine and sodium	pH balance, water balance, formation of gastric juices	Common salt	Muscle cramps, apathy
Magnesium	Activates enzymes, protein synthesis and nerve transmission	Whole grains, green leafy vegetables	Growth failure, weakness, spasms behavioral disturbances
Iron	Constituent of hemoglobin and enzymes in energy metabolism	Eggs, organ meat, meats, legumes, whole grains, green leafy vegetables	Iron-deficiency anemia
Fluorine	Bony structure and teeth	Water, seafood	Higher frequency of tooth decay
Zinc	Constituent of many enzymes, tissue healing, digestion	Widely distributed	Growth failure, small sex glands, slow healing
Copper	Constituent of enzymes of iron metabolism	Meats, water	Anemia

TABLE 2-1. *(cont.)*

Nutrient	Major body function	Major sources	Deficiency disease
Trace minerals			
Iodine	Constituent of thyroid hormones	Marine fish, dairy products, vegetables (depending on soil)	Goiter
Selenium	Association with vitamin E	Seafood, meat, grains	Anemia, cardiovascular disease
Chromium	Glucose and energy metabolism	Fats, oils	Impaired ability to metabolize glucose
Manganese, molybdenum, cobalt, silicon, vanadium, tin, nickel	Constituents of enzymes; functions poorly known in humans; essential to animal nutrition	Organ meats, fats; some widely available	Not reported in humans

Note. Adapted from Scrimshaw and Young (1976, pp. 62–64). Copyright 1976 by *Scientific American.* Adapted by permission.

medical scientists did not read Dutch. Finally Robert R. Williams, working with the military in the U.S. colony of the Philippines, discovered that he could cure the disease with rice-bran water, that beriberi was due to a deficiency, a lack, and not a positive toxin. He later identified and synthesized the missing life chemical, the first vitamin, B_1.

The distribution pattern of the disease was explained by industrial milling of rice and its shipment and storage, along coasts and to cities and institutions. As part of economic development, power mills in the 1960s and 1970s spread along new railroad lines and roads into formerly rural and isolated areas in tropical Asia. The milling, or "polishing," almost completely removes the thiamine, so that without compensating changes in the population's diet, in recent decades development spread beriberi in almost epidemic form. Just at plowing time, when the need for carbohydrate energy is high, beriberi appeared to paralyze the farmer. Enrichment of rice at the mills has proved to be an answer to the deterioration of nutritional ecology, but this did not happen easily. Because of international opposition to companies making money from poor farmers by selling their "quick fix" (supplementary vitamin) instead of improving overall diet by reduction of poverty, it took decades and thousands of lives before the bread-enrichment model of the United States was followed.

The best known of the staple-associated deficiency diseases in the United States is *pellagra*. The disease is first characterized by a distinctive butterfly-shaped rash on the back, which is easily reversed by consuming the vitamin niacin. At advanced stages it results in nerve damage and insanity. Maize, or corn, has little niacin. The way the Native Americans prepared maize (grits) made the most of its niacin, but it needs to be supplemented with niacin-rich foods. In the South, settlers' contact with the Cherokees was prolonged. Maize came to have a very important role in the immigrants' diet. By the end of winter there was often little left for the poor to eat except corn-meal, a situation that became more common in the late 19th century when "King Cotton" became even more important than vegetables in the home garden. A niacin-deficient diet resulted. The majority of patients in southern mental institutions in the 1930s were pellagra victims. As poor people in parts of Africa, South America, and Asia turned to maize for most of their calories, pellagra became a problem.

Pastoralists tend to have ample protein but inadequate B vitamins. The pastoralist who eats few green leafy or yellow vegetables and no butterfat is of-ten short on vitamin A. For children one common result of vitamin A defi-ciency is blindness, because the cornea becomes softened (keratomalacia). Historically, African pastoralists traded meat and milk for vitamin B-rich grains from sedentary farmers and for vitamin A-rich palm oil from the in-habitants of chronically protein-deficient rain forest areas. New national bor-ders and trading systems oriented toward Europe have changed the structure of such nutritional exchanges.

Kwashiorkor, an African word for a protein deficiency disease, is most common in the wet tropics. There are many reasons for this, including the leaching and low nitrogen content of soils and the dietary importance of starchy root crops such as cassava and taro. Although some dwarf, resistant breeds of cattle have been developed and there are vigorous internationally supported breeding programs, over the centuries trypanosomiasis (sleeping sickness) made it impossible to raise livestock in large areas of Tropical Africa. This has meant loss of animal protein from milk (for those who are not lactose intolerant) and meat. In some tropical regions fish are an impor-tant source of protein, especially for places near the sea. In tropical Asia, dried fish made into a sauce is a high-protein condiment universally used on rice and traded far inland. It is no longer clear, however, that protein defi-ciency alone results in kwashiorkor while lack of calories results in the wast-ing of marasmus. They may both be different physiological responses to the absolute insufficiency of food. Deficiency of food overall would suggest that international programs need to focus on increasing agricultural production for small farmers overall rather than importing and popularizing such com-mercial protein enhancers as soy drinks, so continuing research and develop-ment of nutritional understanding will have serious international policy con-sequences.

Rickets, a bone-deformity disease, used to be common in high-latitude countries. The sun's ultraviolet radiation stimulates the human body to pro-duce vitamin D, which is necessary for calcium metabolism. Wrapped in heavy clothing when outdoors and spending most of the low-light winter pe-riod indoors, growing children did not get enough sunlight. The situation became worse in the tenements of the early industrial revolution, with its coal-polluted, dark industrial cities. Fish liver is one of the few dietary sources of vitamin D, and so through processes of cultural ecology cod liver oil became a common tonic. The vitamin is fat soluble, and eventually the happy solution (for lactose-tolerant populations) of adding the vitamin to milk, where it could be ingested with the calcium that needed metabolizing, was found. This has not proved such a simple solution at the same latitudes in China, which does not have a dairy cuisine.

A similar cultural buffer, iodized salt, can solve another metabolic disease that is strongly regionalized in China. Deficiency of iodine, an element needed by the thyroid to make the important metabolic control hormone, thyroxin, results commonly in the gross thyroid enlargement known as goiter and more severely in cretinism, when the growth and development of young brains and bodies are impeded. As recently as 1996 more than 10 million mentally retarded people and tens of thousands of cretins were regionalized within China, a generation lost by the destruction of public health iodized salt proposals as Mao's Cultural Revolution ravaged China. Some current American–Chinese efforts involve adding iodine to irrigation water and seeking other pathways. These people and many others through history live in a place of glaciated soils far from the sea and its fish or salt. In Nepal, for example, the problem has varied historically with whether Nepal traded in friendly relations with India (sea salt) or China. There are other regional concentrations, such as those in upland but tropical central Java, where causation is more complicated and involves goitrogenic plants in the diet that prevent the absorption of what iodine is consumed.

Famine also has its regional patterns. Starvation can claim the poor even in well-fed lands. Crop failure, flood, earthquake, and hurricane can strike anywhere. Hundreds of local famines have been recorded in Europe in the last few centuries. Repeatedly during the 20th century China's Sorrow, the Huang (Yellow) River, escaped its levees to spread across the North China plain and bring famine to tens of millions. The Indian monsoons can fail (to produce an adequate period of rain) several years in a row. Famines tend to occur in areas of unreliable and highly variable annual rainfall. The grasslands and marginal agricultural lands of the African savanna (see Vignette 3-1), as well as land that is under the rain shadow of the Western Ghats and margins of monsoon penetration in India, and the degraded scrublands of northeastern Brazil are all famine-prone. Famines are commonly the result of warfare, as guerrillas or soldiers and bombers make cultivating fields and storing seed grain impossible and armies of refugees are displaced. There is actually little outright starvation on earth today, despite the problems of population growth. There is mass malnutrition of various kinds, and most of that is due to the lack of means or right to get the food that does exist. The political/economic structures of power are seldom more starkly revealed.

There is also the power of cultural preference, prescription, and prohibition. Swine would fit in well with Middle Eastern agriculture, but there are religious injunctions against eating pork. Valuable though cattle are for draft power, milk, dung, and hides in India, the herds would be better fed and stronger if they were culled for meat, but religion proscribes it. The poor and homeless in the United States could get quality protein from the excess dogs killed daily by the animal pounds. The majority of the human race eats tasty dog meat, but in Western civilization it is taboo. Some people have vitamin A and iron deficiencies simply because they culturally do not want to grow vegetables, not because of inadequate land. Some people culturally refuse their children eggs, the best protein available to them, because they are believed to cause worms. Most cultures have strict rules about what pregnant women, sick people, or infants can and cannot eat. Sometimes these prescriptions promote good nutrition, and sometimes they hinder it. There is the widest possible range of opinions about what constitutes good food supplementation for a nursing infant and what children should eat after being weaned. Some infant mortality and kwashiorkor are caused by the lack of income to purchase anything but the local starchy staple; but much of it is caused by ignorance of what an infant needs for nourishment.

World dietary patterns are undergoing many changes. In the last few centuries, crops and animals have spread from their hearths to be incorporated into other dietary regimes. Potatoes have gone from South America to Europe, wheat and soybeans to the Americas, maize to China. Food storage and processing, transportation and finance, and types of ovens and cooking fuels have changed. Local famines resulting from isolated valley floods, hurricanes, or insect outbreaks have largely been eliminated by regional and national economic and political cooperation as new scales of organization have developed. International trade, refrigeration, veterinary science, and the development of new protein drinks, vitamin supplements, and enrichment targets have changed world nutrition. All these nutritional changes affect the health status of populations: because of radical changes in diet, the Japanese have grown taller, and as people in the United States change their diet, they die less frequently from heart disease. Human nutrition around the world is generally better than in past centuries. One result of this improvement is earlier age of menarche and its consequences. The issues of food distribution can be studied and dealt with at a wide range of scales. The purchasing power of the Netherlands or Japan allows them to buy the food they need in the international market, whereas countries such as Bangladesh, which are far more self-sufficient in food, are considered to have a population problem. Issues of social equity have become important worldwide at the national scale as countries struggle with globalization of trade, resources, capital, pollution, and occupational restructuring. For example, the United States exports food to earn a large part of its foreign exchange yet has its own malnourished people. At the family scale, a household may have adequate food, but if it is customary for the male head of the family to eat first and get his choice of any eggs, fish, or special foods, then the dietary intake of pregnant women and small children may be inadequate.

Measurement of the availability of nutrients and diets is difficult. Methods used include 24-hour recall, maintenance of food diaries, the weighing and sampling of foods as they are cooked, and the less intrusive feeding of a "ghost" visitor—an additional plate at table, which can be emptied daily by an investigator. All methods have their drawbacks and deficiencies. Individual and household studies are expensive. One result is that small-area data for nutrition are almost nonexistent. For some purposes state-level marketing data may be adequate, but few data of value are available for medical geographical research in nutrition.

CONCLUSION

Morbidity and mortality vary greatly around the world, not only in quantity but also in the particular diseases involved. Women in Ghana die of malaria, women in the United States die of breast cancer; children in Bolivia die of diarrhea and pneumonia, children in Italy die of automobile accidents. It is more valuable to understand disease processes however, than to construct great mental catalogues and memorize disease patterns as though they were so many imports and exports.

The customs, beliefs, and behavior that characterize each global culture realm and local ethnic group create the environmental conditions and exposure patterns that result in geographic distribution of health and disease. Genetics, to be sure, often underlies susceptibility and resistance, but the distribution of genes is also a result of adaptation to environment, population mobility, and cultural selection. Influences of the physical environment, such as radiation and trace elements and insect and animal communities and their habitat are critical, but they are buffered and even formed by human agency. Entirely natural landscapes scarcely exist.

Medical geography explains the distribution of health and disease and identifies efficient ways to intervene and distribute trained personnel and technology. Every disease has its cultural ecology, its geographic regionalization, and its patterns of diffusion and change.

REFERENCES

Alland, A., Jr. (1970). *Adaptation in cultural evolution: An approach to medical anthropology*. New York: Columbia University Press.

Allison, A. C. (1954). Protection afforded by sickle-cell trait against subtertian malarial infection. *British Medical Journal, 1*, 290–294.

Audy, J. R. (1971). Measurement and diagnosis of health. In P. Shepard & D. McKinley (Eds.), *Environmental: Essays on the planet as a home* (pp. 140–162). Boston: Houghton Mifflin.

Bias, W. B. (1981). Genetic polymorphisms and human disease. In H. Rothschild (Ed.), *Biocultural aspects of disease* (pp. 95–131). New York: Academic Press.

Crosby, A. (1972). *The Columbian Exchange: Biological consequences of 1492*. Westport, CT: Greenwood.

Diamond, J. (1997). *Guns, germs, and steel*. New York: Norton.

Dubos, R. (1965). *Man adapting*. New Haven, CT: Yale University Press.

Evans, R. G., Barer, M. L., & Marmor, T. R. (1994). *Why are some people healthy and others not? The determinants of health of populations*. New York: Aldine de Gruyter.

Ewald, P. W. (1993). The evolution of virulence. *Scientific American, 268*, 86–93.

Ewald, P. W. (1994). *The evolution of infectious disease*. New York: Oxford University Press.

Hunter, J. M. (1973). Geophagy in Africa and in the United States. *Geographical Review, 63*, 170–195.

Kohler, H., Rodgers, J. L., & Christensen, K. (1999). Is fertility behavior in our genes? Findings from a Danish twin study. *Population and Development Review, 25*, 253–288.

Lederberg, J., Shope, R. E., Stanley, C., & Oaks, J. (1992). *Emerging infections*. Washington, DC: National Academy Press.

Marmot, M. G. (1986). Social inequalities in mortality: The social environment. In R. G. Wilkinson (Ed.), *Class and health: Research and longitudinal data*. London: Tavistock.

Marmot, M. G., Kogevinas, M., & Elston, M. A. (1987). Social/economic status and disease. *Annual Review of Public Health, 8*, 111–135.

May, J. M. (1958). *The ecology of human disease*. New York: MD Publications.

May, J. M. (1977). Deficiency diseases. In G. M. Howe (Ed.), *A world geography of human diseases* (pp. 535–575). London: Academic Press.

McKeown, T. (1988). *The origins of human disease*. Oxford: Basil Blackwell.

McNeill, W. H. (1976). *Plagues and peoples*. New York: Doubleday.

Morse, S. (Ed.). (1993). *Emerging viruses*. New York: Oxford University Press.

Newman, J. L. (1995). From definition, to geography, to action, to reaction: The case of protein-energy malnutrition. *Annals of the Association of American Geographers, 85*, 233–245.

Race, R. R., & Sanger, R. (1975) *Blood groups in man* (6th ed.). Oxford: Blackwell.

Scrimshaw, N. S., & Young, V. R. (1976). The requirements of human nutrition. *Scientific American, 235*, 50–64.

Simoons, F. J. (1969). Primary adult lactose intake and the milking habit: A problem in biological and cultural interrelations. *American Journal of Digestive Diseases, 14*, 819–836.

Simoons, F. J. (1970). Primary adult lactose intolerance and the milking habit: Part 2. A cultural historical hypothesis. *American Journal of Digestive Diseases, 15*, 695–710.

Simoons, F. J. (1974). Rejection of fish as human food in Africa: A problem in history and ecology. *Ecology of Food and Nutrition, 3*, 89–105.

Simoons, F. J. (1976). Geographic perspective on man's food quest. In D. Walcher, N. Kretchmer, & H. Barnett (Eds.), *Food, man, and society* (pp. 31–53). New York: Plenum.

Smith, C. J., & Hanham, R. Q. (1982). *Alcohol abuse: Geographical perspectives* (Resource Publications in Geography). Washington, DC: Association of American Geographers.

Thomas, L. (1974). *The lives of a cell*. New York: Viking Press.

Udry, J. R. (1996). Biosocial models of low-fertility societies. *Population and Development Review, 22* (Suppl.), 325–336.

Vermeer, D. E. (1966). Geophagy among the Tiv of Nigeria. *Annals of the Association of American Geographers, 56,* 197–204.

Watterlond, M. (1983). The telltale metabolism of alcoholics. *Science, 83,* 72–76.

Watts, E. (1981). The biological race concept and diseases of modern man. In H. Rothschild (Ed.), *Biocultural aspects of disease* (pp. 1–25). New York: Academic Press.

Whitmore, T. M. (1992). *Disease and death in early colonial Mexico.* Boulder, CO: Westview Press.

Wills, C. (1996). *Yellow fever, black goddess: The coevolution of people and plagues.* New York: Addison-Wesley.

Xu, Long-Qi, Yu, Sen-hai, Jiang, Ze-Xiao, Yang, Jia-Lun, Lai, Chang-Qin, Zhang, Xiang-Jun, & Zheng, Chang-Qian. (1995). Soil-transmitted helminthiasies: national survey in China. *Bulletin of the World Health Organization, 73,* 507–513.

FURTHER READING

Abrahams, P. W., & Parsons, J. A. (1996). Geophagy in the tropics: A literature review. *Geographical Journal, 162,* 63–72.

American Association for the Advancement of Science (1994). Genes and behavior issue. *Science, 264,* 1637–1816.

American Association for the Advancement of Science (1994). Genome issue. *Science, 265,* 1981–2144.

Black, F. L. (1975, February 14). Infectious diseases in primitive societies. *Science, 187,* 515–518.

Boyden, S. V. (Ed.). (1970). *The impact of civilisation on the biology of man.* Toronto: University of Toronto Press.

Cockburn, A. (1967). *Infectious diseases: Their evolution and eradication.* Springfield, IL: Thomas.

Dando, W. A. (1976a). Man-made famines: Some geographical insights from an exploratory study of a millennium of Russian famines. *Ecology of Food and Nutrition, 4,* 219–234.

Dando, W. A. (1976b). Six millennia of famine: Map and model. *Proceedings of the Association of American Geographers, 8,* 29–32.

Emch, M. (1999). Diarrheal disease risk in Matlab, Bangladesh. *Social Science and Medicine, 49,* 519–530.

Garrett, L. (1994). *The coming plague: Newly emerging diseases in a world out of balance.* New York: Farrar, Straus & Giroux; Penguin Books.

Gary, L. E. (1977). Sickle-cell controversy. In A. S. Baer (Ed.), *Heredity and society: Readings in social genetics* (2nd ed., pp. 361–373). New York: Macmillan.

Gopalan, C. (1992). *Nutrition in developmental transition in South-East Asia.* New Delhi: World Health Organization.

Howe, G. M. (1972). *Man, environment, and disease in Britain.* New York: Barnes & Noble.

Learmonth, A. (1988). *Disease ecology.* London: Basil Blackwell.

Logan, M. H., & Hunt, E. E., Jr. (Eds.). (1978). *Health and the human condition: Perspectives on medical anthropology.* North Scituate, MA: Duxbury Press.

Matossian, M. K. (1989). *Poisons of the past: Molds, epidemics, and history.* New Haven, CT: Yale University Press.

May, J. M. (1961). *The ecology of malnutrition in the Far and near East.* New York: Hafner.

May, J. M. (1963). *The ecology of malnutrition in five countries of eastern and central Europe.* New York: Hafner.

May, J. M. (1965). *The ecology of malnutrition in middle Africa.* New York: Hafner.

May, J. M. (1966). *The ecology of malnutrition in central and south-eastern Europe.* New York: Hafner.

May, J. M. (1967). *The ecology of malnutrition in northern Africa.* New York: Hafner.

May, J. M. (1968). *The ecology of malnutrition in French-speaking countries of West Africa and Madagascar.* New York: Hafner.

May, J. M., & McLellan, D. L. (1970). *The ecology of malnutrition in eastern Africa and four countries of western Africa.* New York: Hafner.

May, J. M., & McLellan, D. L. (1971). *The ecology of malnutrition in seven countries of southern Africa and in Portuguese Guinea.* New York: Hafner.

May, J. M., & McLellan, D. L. (1972). *The ecology of malnutrition in Mexico and Central America.* New York: Hafner.

May, J. M., & McLellan, D. L. (1973). *The ecology of malnutrition in the Caribbean.* New York: Hafner.

May, J. M., & McLellan, D. L. (1974). *The ecology of malnutrition in eastern South America.* New York: Hafner.

May, J. M., & McLellan, D. L. (1974). *The ecology of malnutrition in western South America.* New York: Hafner.

Miller, L. H. & Carter, R. (1978). Innate resistance in malaria: A review. *Experimental Parasitology, 40,* 132–146.

Schofield, C. J., Briceno-Leon, R., Kolstrup, N., Webb, D. J. T., & White, G. B. (1990). The role of house design in limiting vector-borne disease. In S. Cairncross, J. E. Hardoy, & D. Satterthwaite (Eds.), *The poor die young* (pp. 189–212). London: Earthscan.

Stannard, D. (1989). *Before the horror: The population of Hawaii on the eve of Western Contact.* Honolulu: University of Hawaii Press.

Stearns, S. C. (1999). *Evolution in health and disease.* New York: Oxford University Press.

VIGNETTE 2-1.   Biological Classifications of Importance to Health

Medical and biological terminology can be very intimidating. The first stop on the way to read something in a medical journal is often the reference shelves to find a medical dictionary. It can still be confusing when a single parasite is referred to in two or three ways in different sources. This introduction to the classification system may be a useful reference.

An infectious disease's causative organism, variously known as a germ, microbe, pathogen, or parasite, is the *agent* of the disease. It may be a virus, a rickettsia, a bacterium, a protozoan, or a worm. The type of disease agent is important for understanding the possibilities of intervention in the disease cycle. At the smallest and simplest end of the infectious agent continuum are various bits and strings of protein, tiny short loops of DNA, and similar mysterious molecules called prions, plasmids, and new things every year. They do not seem to meet the historic definitions of "life."They have no nucleus of control, no container of their being, seemingly no being to contain as they drift among individual animals and species of animals and even between animals and plants. But they can be replicated. They can change the behavior of DNA and, for example, make a strain of bacteria more virulent, or cause the destruction of brain cells. Next are the viruses, simple loops of information which did not used to be considered living, either. Outside living tissue, viruses cannot reproduce. Pharmaceutical drugs have little effect on them—except for the potential of some of the new pharmacopeia developed through research on AIDS. The best weapon against viruses is a vaccine. Rickettsias cannot live outside cells, but in other respects they are similar to bacteria and have been regarded as degenerated bacteria that have lost their containers. They live very well within arthropods and get introduced to people during "blood meals." Rickettsias and bacteria both are sensitive to antibiotics, which means that infected people can be treated. Mass treatment programs based on a single injection are sometimes possible. The more complicated organisms, protozoa and especially helminths (flukes, filaria, and intestinal worms), are difficult to treat on a mass basis because powerful drugs that have many adverse side effects must be used. Hospitalizing half the population to treat schistosomiasis, for example, is not only too costly in agricultural work time and medical care but can seem useless when people return home to be reinfected. Treatment of individuals, such as returned United States tourists, is usually possible. Worms of various body organs are especially difficult to treat, especially when they exist in heavy loads of hundreds, because only intestinal worms have a ready mode of egress from the body; the others, dead and unable to disguise themselves, become masses of internal foreign matter for the body to attack. Currently, there

VIGNETTE 2-1, TABLE 1. Some Medically Important Taxonomy

Phylum	Order	Family	Genus	Species	Disease Caused or Vectored
Arthropoda	Acarina (class Arachnida)	Trombiculidae	*Trombicula* (mites)	*T. akamushi*	scrub typhus
		Ixodidae	*Dermacentor* (ticks)	*D. andersoni*	RMSF, tularemia, etc.
				D. variabilis	RMSF
			Ixodes	*I. dammini*	Lyme disease
	Siphonaptera	Sarcoptidea	*Sarcoptes* (mites)	*S. scabie*	scabies
		Pulicidae (fleas)	*Xenopsylla*	*X. cheopis*	plague
			Pulex	*P. irritans*	tapeworm
	Diptera	Pediculidae (lice)	*Pediculus*	*P. humanus*	typhus, relapsing fever
		Psychodidae	*Phlebotomus* (sandflies)	*P. various*	leishmaniasis
		Simuliidae	*Simulium* (blackflies)	*S. damnosum*	river blindness
		Tipulidae	*Glossina* (tsetse flies)	*G. palpalis*	African sleeping sickness
		Tabanidae	*Chrysops* (deer flies)	*C. discalis*	tularemia
		Culicidae (mosquitoes)	*Culex*	*C. fatigans*	filariasis
				C. pipiens	encephalitis
			Aedes	*Ae. aegypti*	yellow fever, dengue fever
			Anopheles	various, any	malaria
Platyhelminthes (flatworms)	Trematoda		*Schistosoma* (blood fluke)	*S. hematobium*	schistosomiasis
				S. japonicum	schistosomiasis
				S. mansoni	schistosomiasis
			Fasciolopsis	*F. buski*	intestinal fluke
		Digenea	*Gastrodiscoides*	*G. hominus*	intestinal fluke
			Clonorchis	*C. sinensis*	liver fluke
			Fascida	*F. hepatica*	liver fluke
			Opisthrochis	*O. felineus*	liver fluke
			Paragonimus	*P. uestermani*	lung fluke
	Cestoda		*Taenia*	*T. solium*	pork tapeworm
				T. saginata	beef tapeworm
			Echinococcus	*E. granulosus*	hydatidosis (dog tapeworm)
Nemathelminthes (roundworms)	Nematoda	Ascaridoidea	*Ascaris*	*A. lumbricoides*	ascariasis (roundworm)
		Trichurata	*Trichinella*	*T. spiralis*	trichinosis
		Strongylata	*Ancylostoma*	*A. duodenale*	hookworm
			Necator	*N. americanus*	hookworm
			Strongyloides	*S. intestinalis*	strongyloides

Group	Subgroup	Genus	Species	Disease
Protozoa	Filarioidea	*Wuchereria*	*W. bancrofti*	bancroftian filariasis (elephantiasis)
		Onchocerca	*O. volvulus*	river blindness
		Dracunculus	*D. medinensis*	dracunculiasis (guinea worm)
	Mastigophora (flagella)	*Leishmania*	*L. donovani*	Kala-Azar
			L. braziliensis	American leishmaniasis
	Trypanosomatidae	*Trichomonas*	*T. vaginalis*	vaginitis
		Trypanosoma	*T. gambiense*	African sleeping sickness
			T. rhodesience	African sleeping sickness
			T. cruzi	Chagas Disease (American trypanosomiasis)
Sarcodina (pseudopods)	Entamoeba	*Giardia*	*G. lamblia*	diarrhea
		Entamoeba	*E. histolytica*	amebic dysentery
Sporozoa (no adult locomotion)		*Plasmodium*	*P. falciparum*	falciparum malaria
			P. vivax	benign tertian malaria
			P. malariae	quartan malaria
Bacteria	Spirillaceae	*Vibrio*	*V. cholerae*	cholera
	Bacillaceae	*Bacillus*	*B. anthracis*	anthrax
		Clostridium	*C. tetani*	tetanus
		Yersinia	*Y. pestis*	plague
	Mycobacteriaceae	*Mycobacterium*	*M. tuberculosis*	tuberculosis
			M. leprae	leprosy
	Spirochaetales	*Borrelia*	*B. recurrentis*	relapsing fever
			B. burgdorferi	Lyme disease
		Treponema	*T. pallidum*	syphilis
Rickettsiae		*Rickettsia*	*R. rickettsii*	Rocky Mountain spotted fever
			R. prowazekii	typhus
		Coxiella	*C. burneti*	Q fever
Virus	RNA viruses	*Picornavirus*		enteric viruses, rhinoviruses (intestinal, respiratory)
		Arbovirus	arthropod-borne	encephalitis, hemorrhagic fevers (various, numerous)
		Myxovirus		influenza, mumps, measles
		Retrovirus	HIV	AIDS
	DNA viruses	*Adenovirus*		respiratory
		Herpesvirus	varicella-zoster	chickenpox-zoster (shingles)

are no successful vaccines for any of the complicated organisms. and indeed they have enough genetic material that they seem able to adapt and prevent complete immunity to them by their hosts.

Multiple terminology is often used to refer to a specific insect or parasite. Usually this draws on genus or family classification to invoke known characteristics of breeding, attaching, eating, and so on which separate the groups. For example, an article might use the terms "trombiculid mite," "the trematode," and, in the same paragraph, "the fluke" or "the schistosome."People commonly say "insect bite" when they mean "arthropod bite" (i.e., ticks are not insects). A "filarial" worm is a long, thread-like worm that may live in lymph glands or under the skin but which reproduces and disseminates itself by producing "microfilaria" (microscopic larvae) that arthropods can take up with a blood meal. Elephantiasis and river blindness are "filarial diseases" vectored by arthropods; roundworm and tapeworm are not. To refer to a bacteria as a spirochete, or a vibrio, or a bacillus, is to comment on the bacteria's mobility, its ability to survive in the soil or water, its contagion. Vignette 2-1, Table 1 shows the relationships of different scales of classification for some of the most important agents and vectors.

3

Landscape Epidemiology

The landscape that distinguishes a place is a complex expression of physical, biotic, and cultural processes. When one knows how to analyze its elements and patterns, one can usually determine what diseases can occur. This is true at every scale, from the microecology of a house and its backyard to the transcontinental migratory paths of birds and the viruses they disseminate. As world population grows and the world economy changes, landscapes are being altered in ways that increase risk of disease or enhance protection from it.

This chapter is about the cultural ecology of transmissible disease, or the ways in which regions impart pattern to disease distribution. The broad term, "communicable disease," as used by the Centers for Disease Control and Prevention includes all diseases due to a specific infectious agent which is transmitted from an infected host to a susceptible host, whether directly or indirectly through an intermediary vector. We treat the directly transmitted agents, contagious ones, mainly in Chapter 8 (this volume), on diffusion. This chapter is about vectored diseases, which parasitologists and entomologists call transmissible. The cultural ecology of vectored diseases needs to address the biogeography of the arthropod vectors and their animal hosts. The Russian parasitologist/geographer Pavlovsky called this biotic regionalization of vectored diseases landscape epidemiology. Today, studies of the regionalization of vectored diseases, often using GIS and sometimes satellite imagery, are increasing internationally. Most of them use the following concepts; but few of them apply the Russian name, landscape epidemiology.

Before we take up the elaboration of disease systems and their regionalization, however, basic terminology and system parameters must be established. Then the cultural ecology of several diseases—yellow fever, bubonic plague, malaria, dengue hemorrhagic fever, schistosomiasis, and Lyme/Rocky Mountain spotted fever—are discussed at length. The latest available data on the prevalence of these diseases and more, complete with detailed epidemiologies and often maps, are available on the World Health

Organization website (Vignette 12-1). Each of these diseases is of major importance not only to human health but also to the advance of scientific understanding about the nature and occurrence of different types of transmission systems. Finally, the use of landscape epidemiology to regionalize the occurrence of, and locate points of intervention in, vector-borne disease systems is summarized.

REGIONS

There are four types of regions involved in the study of landscape epidemiology. The first is biotic. Climate, altitude, and latitude combine to create broad biotic regions, *biomes,* with predictable locations (see Vignette 3-1). These include not only plants and animals but also particular types of insects and microbes. If the biome's natural fauna and flora are displaced through land development, their replacements tend to be crops and domestic animals also distinctive to that biome.

The second type of region is also biotic: *realms of evolution.* Because oceans, deserts, and great mountain ranges formed barriers to the exchange of genetic information as the continents drifted apart, complexes of plants and animals followed separate paths of evolution in South America, Africa south of the Sahara, Asia south of the Himalayas and Yangzi (Yangtze) River, Australia, and in the remainder of Eurasia (Palearctic) and North America (Nearctic). These realms of evolution include microbes and insects as well as the more visible mammals and birds that popularly demarcate the regions. As trade and political empires established contacts beyond their culture realms, the biotas of the evolutionary realms were exchanged (see Vignette 2-1). Deliberately, in the case of food crops, and unintentionally, in the case of disease agents, sweeping processes of global readaptation were set in motion. Historians have only relatively recently paid attention to the health consequences that followed upon connection of these realms (McNeill, 1977). When the maritime and land-based transportation and trade networks of the Roman empire connected with those of the Chinese empire, for example, terrible epidemics swept the Mediterranean world. The best studied connection of evolutionary realms is that between the Old World of Eurasia and Africa and the New World of the Americas. The Columbian Exchange involved the exchange of scores of crops and animals and the introduction to the New World of malaria, yellow fever, typhus, bubonic plague, cholera, typhoid, smallpox, scarlet fever, schistosomiasis, river blindness, and other pestilence with catastrophic consequences for the Native Americans.

The third type of region, *culture realm,* is a broad cultural area delimited by the extent of particular cultural practices and beliefs that largely originated in the primary culture hearths. China and the United States, for example, occupy vast territories with the same latitude and often similar climatic patterns, but because their inhabitants use the land differently and have different settlement forms, house types, and technology, their landscapes are distinctive. The use of human waste for fertilizer in the Chinese culture realm (which includes Korea, Japan, and Vietnam) and the use of dogs for herding sheep in the Euro-American cultural spheres are examples of regional patterns associated with health consequences: intestinal parasites and dysentery in the former, and hydatid disease (see Table 3-5, later in this chatper), tapeworm, and numerous flea- and tick-transmitted diseases in the latter.

The fourth type of region, *natural nidus* (focus or cluster), has been defined by Soviet and German geographers. A natural nidus is a microscale region constituted of a living community, among the members of which a disease agent continually circulates, and the habitat conditions necessary to maintain that circulation in the disease system. The more familiar term, "focus," is frequently used instead, but it does not carry the connotation of microecology of soil and bugs and vegetation and animal movement as well. The life cycles and transmission chains of nidal diseases are complex. This chapter describes several examples of different types of systems.

TRANSMISSIBLE DISEASE SYSTEMS

The biological agent of a disease is the infectious information that is necessary (but seldom sufficient) to cause it. It is commonly known as the germ or parasite. The organism infected by a disease agent is called the *host*. When animals are the ordinary hosts, the disease is known as a *zoonosis*. A disease that often infects both people and animals is an *anthropo-zoonosis*. When animal hosts serve as a continuing source of possible infection for human beings, our anthropocentric name for them is a *reservoir* and we regard ourselves as the host (although the animals are actually the primary host). A disease always present, or *endemic,* to an animal population is said to be *enzootic,* and one epidemic among animals is said to be *epizootic.* Some diseases are transmitted directly by contact or inhalation. Others are transmitted through contaminated food or water. This chapter is mainy concerned with disease agents that are transmitted by an arthropod.

The arthropod that transmits the disease agent between hosts, and in which the agent multiplies and often goes through life-cycle changes in form, is known as a biological *vector. Biological* distinguishes the vectors from flies or inanimate objects that may merely transport the agents mechanically (as vehicles or fomites). Many people speak of vectors as "insects," but ticks and mites are not, strictly speaking, insects. The more inclusive category is the phylum, Arthropoda (Vignette 2-1). *Arbovirus* includes all arthropod-borne viruses. The major vectors are mosquitoes, biting blackflies, ticks, mites, sand flies, fleas, and lice; but gnats, midges, and other arthropods are sometimes involved. Most disease agents are strictly limited to transmission by a single species, or at most a genus, of vector. This establishes limits to their distribution because vectors have specific habitat requirements.

Intermediate hosts are organisms that are necessary to some stage of the agent's life cycle. Hosts in which the agent attains maturity or its sexual life stage are the *primary* or *definitive* hosts; hosts for the agent's asexual or larval stage are intermediate hosts. The fluke that causes schistosomiasis, for example, must alternately infect people and snails. The snails do not transmit the agent to people; they are not vectors but intermediate hosts. Nevertheless, it is often convenient to treat intermediate hosts as though they were vectors, because the same kinds of population dynamics and intervention strategies are involved. Sometimes this concept is even further enlarged, as when dogs are treated as "vectors" of rabies to people. Such careless usage may be helpful for mathematical modeling of a disease system from our anthropocentric viewpoint.

Transmission Chains

The first chain of transmission diagrammed in Figure 3-1 involves direct communication of the agent by contact between people. Animals also communicate contagion (chain 2). It is possible for people to get a zoonotic infection, for example, through contact with skin fungi or consumption of raw milk.

Chain 3 illustrates a vectored human disease having no animal reservoir. The absence of a reservoir raises a possibility that does not exist for most anthropo-zoonoses, disease eradication. Although birds, reptiles, and monkeys have their own forms of malaria, for example, human malaria is solely a human disease transmitted by *Anopheles* mosquitoes. There was therefore some hope in the 1950s that it could be eradicated. We shall consider later some of the reasons that it could not.

Most vectored diseases involve transmission of agents among animals (chain 4). Many of these cycles are so ancient that agent and host have mutually adapted and no disease symptoms appear in the infected hosts. Sometimes people are accidentally infected when they intrude on the animal habitat. Usually they develop no disease at all, as they are not a compatible host. Occasionally they are so susceptible to the rare infection that case mortality rates are high. People are usually dead-end hosts, meaning that they cannot give the agent to a vector for transmission to another host. For example, the amount of virus circulating in the blood is known as *viremia*. When people are incidentally infected with viral encephalitis by a mosquito that had previously fed on an infectious horse or chicken, they do not develop viremia sufficient to serve as a source of infection for another mosquito imbibing a little of their blood. Encephalitis cannot, therefore, be spread among people by mosquitoes. Even when clusters of cases occur, they result from exposure to the zoonotic chain.

The final chain in the diagram represents the main focus of this chapter, anthropo-zoonoses, which can be transmitted between animals or between

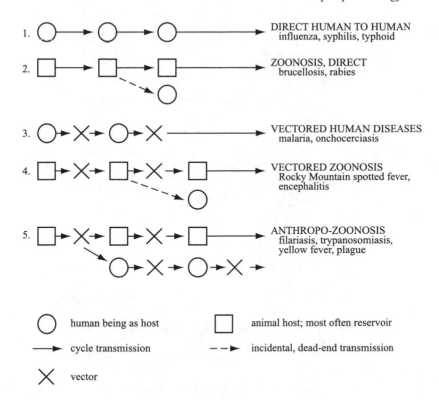

1. DIRECT HUMAN TO HUMAN
influenza, syphilis, typhoid

2. ZOONOSIS, DIRECT
brucellosis, rabies

3. VECTORED HUMAN DISEASES
malaria, onchocerciasis

4. VECTORED ZOONOSIS
Rocky Mountain spotted fever,
encephalitis

5. ANTHROPO-ZOONOSIS
filariasis, trypanosomiasis,
yellow fever, plague

○ human being as host   □ animal host; most often reservoir

⟶ cycle transmission   – –▶ incidental, dead-end transmission

✕ vector

FIGURE 3-1. Chains of disease transmission.

people by vectors and which sometimes cross between the two systems. The first disease for which this complicated system was discovered was yellow fever.

Yellow Fever

Until the 20th century, yellow fever was one of the most feared diseases in the Western Hemisphere. The step-by-step discovery of its transmission chain, with the subsequent recognition of the implications for many other diseases, ranks as one of the milestones of medical science (Figure 3-2).

Pandemics (international epidemics) of yellow fever swept the Americas in the 18th century. The pandemic of 1793–1804, for example, started in Grenada and spread through the Lesser Antilles and Venezuela, finally striking ports from New Orleans to Boston. During this Napoleonic period, the French suffered losses of more than 30,000 men in their garrisons in Guadaloupe, Martinique, and Santo Domingo. By the late 19th century, yellow fever was endemic from Brazil to Yucatan and throughout the Caribbean; it was seasonally epidemic along the Atlantic seaboard. Then the United

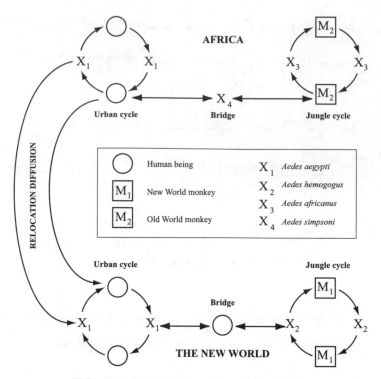

FIGURE 3-2. Yellow fever transmission chain.

States Yellow Fever Commission determined that the infectious agent (a virus, now known to be a group B togavirus) was transmitted by the mosquito *Aedes aegypti.* Using this first proof of arthropod transmission of human disease agents, General Gorgas attacked the mosquito in Cuba, thereby suppressing the endemic focus. Soon after, suppression of yellow fever allowed construction of the Panama Canal. After the 1905 pandemic was stopped in New Orleans by anti-*Ae. aegypti* operations, the newly established Rockefeller Foundation undertook the task of eradicating *Ae. aegypti* throughout the Caribbean. Partly because the mosquito was an introduced species that was only superficially established, the operation was a success. Yellow fever appeared to have been eliminated.

Then came isolated reports of yellow fever—not epidemics—and investigation discovered that the agent was transmitted among monkeys by mosquitoes, especially *Ae. hemogogus* (see Figure 3-2). This astonishing finding was dubbed the "jungle cycle." Woodcutters and settlers, exposed by their behavior to the monkey-biting jungle mosquito, occasionaly contracted the disease, but as long as *Ae. aegypti* was absent there was no urban cycle and no epidemic.

In West Africa, whites had been dying of yellow fever in "the white man's graveyard" for centuries. It was thought, however, that Africans did not get the disease, which was epidemic only in coastal European settlements. Further study revealed that Africans had greater resistance (lower case mortality) to the disease but that in many parts of Africa the infection was almost universal. That is, studies of blood (serology) showed that antibodies to the virus were very common. The mosquito *Ae. aegypti*, which evolved in Africa, was demonstrated to be transmitting the virus among people in the African towns and villages (so that the "urban cycle" was also the "village cycle"). Further search demonstrated that there was also a jungle cycle: *Ae. africanus* and related mosquitoes were transmitting the virus among monkeys. That yellow fever originated in Africa is indicated by the resistance of human population, the ubiquity of *Ae. aegypti* there, and by a further complication to the system. There is a mosquito, *Ae. simpsoni*, which breeds in the curled leaves of banana plants and other vegetation on the fringe of human settlements. It bites people in the villages and monkeys in the forest. Because *Ae. aegypti* is indigenous and exists in many forms fully adapted to various niches (e.g., breeding in tree holes), its eradication seems impossible. Because of *Ae. simpsoni*, which does not have an equivalent in the New World system, the infection that is enzootic in the monkeys (which serve as a reservoir for the disease) can be easily reintroduced to the villages and towns even when the urban transmission chain is broken. The jungle cycle is intimately linked to the village cycle, and yellow fever continues to occur.

The major defense in Africa is the potent vaccine for yellow fever. In tropical America, however, vaccine is used mainly for those occupationally exposed to the jungle cycle. Efforts to prevent the disease have been concentrated on preventing *Ae. aegypti* from becoming reestablished in the cities, which recently seems again to be a losing battle. Because yellow fever does not occur today in the United States, there is little incentive for this country to spend billions of dollars and massive efforts to eradicate *Ae. aegypti*, which is widespread and deeply ensconced. As a consequence, the mosquito is repeatedly exported, via shipped goods, from the United States to Venezuela and other places in Latin America, where it has been repeatedly eradicated.

Once the intricacies of this vectored disease were understood, the puzzles of many other vectored diseases became solvable. Scientists looked for other arthropods capable of transmitting agents and for other animal reservoirs.

Vector Ecology

Most disease agents require specific hosts in which they live and are even more restrictive about the cold-blooded arthropods in which they reproduce. Because the agent usually goes through changes in life stages and multiplies within the vector, most arthropods cannot be biological vectors. An inappropriate arthropod finds its throat blocked, its abdomen too heavy for flight, and its life expectancy so shortened that death occurs to the arthropod and agent before transmission. A vector poorly adapted to an agent implies that the relationship is of recent origin. For example, part of the evidence that ty-phus is a relatively recent disease in humans is that the human louse itself dies from the infection. Transmission comes through a bite or another abra-sion contaminated with louse feces or crushed-louse fluids, instead of from repeated blood meals, which would occur in a well-adapted system. (Fleas sometimes die, too, from ingesting large amounts of bacteria such as *Yersinia pestis*, which multiply and cause the blood to clot; clot chunks then enter the wound with the next desperate blood meal of the haplesss flea. It is not clear whether this occurs with species in the natural nidus.)

A full range of arthropods is involved in disease transmission almost everywhere, but one may identify broad patterns that generally coincide with biomes (see Vignette 3-1). At high altitudes and latitudes, the tick is an espe-cially important vector (Table 3-1). This is because it is capable of transmit-ting rickettsias and viruses transovarially (into its eggs), so that all the thou-sands of ticks that hatch from an infected tick's eggs are equally infected, through generations. In this way the disease agent is transmitted despite freezing temperatures, which stop transmission by killing adult mosquitoes and the agent they carry.

Mosquito-transmitted diseases are most important in warm, humid lands where the insect can live long and reproduce frequently (Table 3-2). Repro-duction in mosquitoes is temperature dependent and occurs more quickly when the temperature is warm. The female mosquito takes blood to get pro-tein to lay its eggs (male mosquitoes do not bite people). A mosquito trans-mitting malaria in Georgia, if it were to become infected from its first blood meal after emerging as an adult, might infect 11 to 13 people in its life. The same species in New York would be unlikely to infect more than 4 or 5. As temperatures get colder, the metabolism of mosquitoes slows down. Below freezing it stops entirely, and death follows. A few mosquitoes, such as the vector of La Crosse encephalitis, sometimes pass the infection *transovarially*, but this is rare (see Table 3-2). Thus the disease cycle is interrupted annually in cold climates. A disease such as yellow fever can be introduced only as an epidemic in the middle latitudes and does not become endemic there, as it was in the Caribbean. In the wet–dry tropics, some mosquitoes have the abili-ty to *estivate*, or to hide and dehydrate during the dry season, and survive. The adult, infected mosquitoes can renew the transmission chain when the rains come. There is growing appreciation of yet another biological strategy. Many viruses transmitted by mosquitoes, including several kinds of encephalitis found in the United States, are actually zoonoses of birds. They are annually reintroduced along the great bird flyways during avian migration and arrive just in time for the new spring mosquitoes to become infected. The virus sim-ply winters in warmer climes.

Flies inhabit a wide range of biomes (see Table 3-3). In general, they are most important in arid places. The flies of Australia, of the wet–dry tropics, and of arid grazing lands are infamous. A few types of these flies are blood-sucking vectors of human disease. The most notorious of these is the tsetse

TABLE 3-1. Some Diseases Vectored by Ticks and Mites

Disease	Agent	Major vector	Endemic locale	Reservoir/comments
Viral				
Encephalitis, Central European	Togavirus, group B	Tick: Ixodes spp.	Europe	R: rodents
Encephalitis, Russian Spring—Summer	Togavirus, group B	Tick	Europe, North Asia	R: rodent; tick transovarial transmission
Louping ill	Togavirus, group B	Tick	Great Britain	R: sheep
Rickettsial				
Rocky Mountain spotted fever (similar to boutonneuse fever, South African tick typhus, India tick typhus, etc.)	*Rickettsia ricketsii*	Tick: *Ixodes* spp.	North America, especially southeast Piedmont	R: small mammals; tick transovarial transmission
Scrub typhus (tsutsugamushi disease)	*Rickettsia tsutsugamushi*	Larval trombiculid mites: *Leptotrombidum akamushi* and *deliens*	Asia: Siberia to Indonesia	R: rodents; mite transovarial transmission
Bacterial				
Tularemia	*Francisella tularensis*	Ticks: dog, rabbit, Lone Star	North America, continental Europe	Zoonosis of rabbits and rodents
Relapsing fever (endemic)	*Borrelia recurrentis*	Ticks: *Ornithrodoros* spp.	Tropical Africa, Mediterranean, Asia Minor, Americas	R: rodents; tick transovarial transmission
Protozoan				
Babesiosis	*Babesia microti*	Tick	Nantucket Island, United States	R: rodents; rare in humans

fly, which transmits trypanosomiasis (African sleeping sickness). This disease mainly affects animals. In one form, *Trypanosoma rhodesiense,* it is an anthro-po-zoonosis that has a reservoir in African wildlife and is virulent in humans. In another form, *Tr. gambiense,* it is milder, is slower to kill, and has its reservoir mainly among people, with animals being incidental. There are still other forms that affect only animals. The disease has had a major impact on human population distribution and nutrition by making the raising of animals

TABLE 3-2. Some Diseases Vectored by Mosquitoes

Disease	Agent	Major vector	Endemic locale	Reservoir/ comments
Viral				
Chikungunya	Togavirus, group A	*Aedes* spp.	Africa, Southeast Asia	R: monkeys
Encephalitis, eastern equine	Togavirus, group A	*Aedes* spp.	Americas	R: birds
Encephalitis, western equine	Togavirus, group A	*Culex tarsalis*	Americas	R: small mammals, reptiles?
Encephalitis, Japanese B	Togavirus, group B	*Culex tritaenio-rhynchus, C. gelidus*	East Asia, Pacific Islands	Pig amplifying host
Encephalitis, St. Louis	Togavirus, group B	*Culex* spp.	Americas	R: birds
Encephalitis, Murray Valley	Togavirus, group B	*Culex annulirostris*	Australia, New Guinea	R: birds
Encephalitis, La Crosse	Bunyavirus, group C	*Anopheles triseriatus*	Central United States	Transovarial transmission
fever	Togavirus, group B	*Aedes aegypti*	World tropics; hemorrhagic form, Southeast Asia	R: monkeys, Southeast Asia
Yellow fever	Togavirus, group B	*Aedes aegypti*	Tropical Africa, tropical forest South America	R: monkeys
Protozoan				
Malaria	Plasmodium: vivax (tertian) falciparum (malignant) malariae (quartan) ovale (W. African)	*Anopheles* spp.	Tropics and subtropics	Humans are source
Helminthic				
Filariasis (elephantiasis)	Nematode: *Wuchereria bancrofti*	*Culex fatigans, Aedes* spp.	Tropics and subtropics	No reservoir: infective mircofilaria, night or day periodic, depending on local vector; zoonosis of wild and domestic animals in Malaysia
Filariasis (elephantiasis), Malayan	Nematode: *Brugia malayi*	*Mansonia* spp.	Southeast Asia, India, China	

TABLE 3-3. Some Diseases Vectored by Flies and Reduviid Bugs

Disease	Agent	Major vector	Endemic locale	Reservoir/ comments
Viral				
Sandfly fever	Bunyavirus, group C	Midge: sand fly *Phlebotomus papatasii*	Mediterranean climate areas, Asia Minor, Central and South America	Human–fly complex crucial
Bacterial				
Tularemia	*Francisella tularensis*	Deer fly	North America, Europe, Japan	Zoonosis of rabbits and rodents
Bartonellosis (Oroya fever, Carrion's disease)	*Bartonella bacilliformis*	Sand fly: *Phlebotomus* spp.	Andean valleys in Peru, Ecuador, Columbia	People are source
Protozoan African trypanosomiasis (sleeping sickness)	*Trypanosoma gambiense, Trypanosoma rhodesiense*	Tsetse fly: *Glossina* spp.	Tropical Africa	Humans are source for *gambiense* R: wild game and cattle for *rhodesiense*
American trypanosomiasis	*Trypanosoma cruzi*	Reduviid bugs	Tropical America	R: wild and domestic animals
Leishmaniasis, visceral (Kalaazar)	*Leishmania donovani*	Sand fly: *Phlebotomus* spp.	Tropics and subtropics, Mediterranean	R: dogs, cats, rodents in different places Fatal untreated
Leishmaniasis, cutaneous (Oriental sore espundia, uta)	*Leishmania tropica, L. brasiliensis, L. mexicana*	Sand fly: *Phlebotomus* spp.	Arid margins of Asia, Africa, Mediterranean, South and Central America	R: dogs, rodents
Helminthic				
Onchocerciasis	Nematode: *Onchocerca volvulus*	Blackfly: *Simulium* spp.	Tropical Africa, Central America to Amazon	Humans are source
Loaiasis	Nematode: *Loa loa*	Mangrove fly: *Chrysops* spp.	West and Central Africa	Humans are source

for protein and draft power virtually impossible across large areas of Africa. Even this fly, however, needs water to breed and becomes less active when humidity is very low. The biting blackfly, *Simulium damnosum,* which is the major vector of onchocerciasis (river blindness), lays its eggs in oxygenated, fast-flowing water by anchoring them to underwater stones. Exposure to the disease cycle, as the name suggests, is associated with use of the fertile soils near the streams and rivers or with use of the rivers for laundry, fording, or fishing. Hunter (1980) has described the complexity of the disease system and the multisided, integrated attack that is needed to control it. The various forms of leishmaniasis transmitted by sand flies are characteristic of rather arid terrains, but the fly requires some humidity and is often found only at specific altitudes where the relative humidity is high enough. It finds shelter from the sun and low humidity in the plaster and adobe walls of human dwellings and the burrows of rodents.

Analyzing the efficacy of a vector requires detailed knowledge of its particular biology. The following characteristics, for example, affect mosquitoes' usefulness as vectors: flight range, altitude range, sex ratio, breeding habits, preferred breeding sites, life expectancy, alternative (nonblood) food, activity time, host preference, resting habits, biting habits, and tolerance for specific virus, microfilaria, protozoan, and other agents.

Some mosquitoes require fresh water with no pollution; others need organic pollution such as sewage. Some breed in containers, tree holes, or leaf tendrils; others need open water. A few like brackish conditions. Some mate for life when they emerge as adults from the water; others hover around blood sources, hoping to find a mate. Some are weak fliers, others are easily carried long distances by wind, and others are stong fliers, even upwind. Most mosquitoes prefer to bite other animals, including snakes, frogs, and birds, rather than humans, but a few species prefer people, and others tolerate them when hungry enough. Some mosquitoes readily enter human dwellings and after feeding rest on the walls; others never enter dwellings and bite only outside. Some are active during morning or evening; others are active only at night. The detailed ecological requirements for specific mosquitoes are inherent in the landscape, and the distribution of relevant species determines where various disease agents can be spread.

Aedes aegypti is an especially dangerous vector, as is evident from its ecology. It prefers to bite people; it is active during times of day when people are active; it breeds in containers and has adapted well to opportunities offered by human dwellings, such as rain gutters, flower pots, jars of bath water, toilet bowls, and backyard trash containers. It has readily spread around the world with human help, much as the rat has. This is due to its habit of laying eggs just above the water line in containers. The eggs can thus sail across the ocean and hatch when the water jars are filled in the new port. Aside from the human louse, *Ae. aegypti* is probably our most commensal (domiciliated) arthropod. It transmits several of the most dangerous viruses (see Table 3-2).

THE LANDSCAPE EPIDEMIOLOGY APPROACH

Landscape epidemiology is a geographic delimitation of the territory of a transmitted disease in order to identify cultural pathways for disease control. In Europe, several holistic approaches to the study of arthropod-borne or naturally occurring diseases have been developed. In Germany, for example, a holistic ecological approach was developed under the leadership of Helmut J. Jusatz. He produced the first world atlas of epidemic diseases (Rodenwaldt & Jusatz, 1952–1961) which not only portrayed disease distribution but also analyzed its association with climate, topography, hydrology, and flora and fauna. This work was expanded into a series of monographs on the medical geography of such countries as Kenya, Kuwait, and Korea (Jusatz, 1968–1980). This holistic approach and focus on ecological associations, *landschaftokologische*, includes settlement and cultural patterns. In U.S. medical geography, by contrast, the study of the natural ecology of disease has been weak. Instead, the cultural ecology approach of Jacques May has been very influential. May's disease-mapping project with the American Geographical Society first introduced disease as a geographical subject in North America. His influence was established through this project and decades of writing and editing books about the ecology of disease and nutrition. The physical and cultural processes elucidated by May and Jusatz need to be integrated into an understanding or transmissible diseases in varying cultures and environments. The modeling approach of Pavlovsky provides a framework to do this.

Landscape epidemiology was developed by a Russian parasitologist/geographer, Eugene N. Pavlovsky. One of the leading parasitologists of the former Soviet Union, he was director of the Zoological Institute of the Academy of Sciences and president of the Geographical and Entomological Societies of the USSR. Because of the importance of the landscape epidemiology approach, the Institute of Medical Geography became a separate entity in the Soviet Academy of Sciences. Pavlovsky (1966) developed the *doctrine of natural nidality*, or the natural focus of disease. In a *natural nidus*, infection is maintained among wild animals and arthropod vectors. These zoonoses, which Pavlovsky determined and established by fieldwork, occur in particular kinds of terrain. There is a biogeography to the life cycles of the arthropods and various animals involved. Their food sources, soil, climate, slope, exposure, and other ecological parameters determine local distribution and possible occurrence of the disease cycle. By knowing the conditions necessary for specific diseases, scientists can use the landscape to identify disease hazards. Landscape modification can create, or be used to prevent, the establishment of disease cycles. Perhaps the easiest way to understand the concepts of landscape epidemiology is to consider one of Pavlovsky's best know examples, bubonic plague.

Bubonic Plague

"*Ring around the rosy*" (the rash around the flea bite), "*a pocket full of posey*" (posey was used as an amulet to ward off evil spirits and disease), "*ashes, ashes*" or "*achoo, achoo*" (for the sign of the cross made on the foreheads and house doors of sick people; in the German variety, the sneeze as lethal harbinger producing the response, Gesundheit), "*we all fall down*" (and die). So deep is the apocolyptic experience of the bubonic plague in the European soul that 600 years after the Black Death, their cultural descendents still teach their children the bubonic plague song.

Bubonic plague is a natural nidal disease which has spread to parallel ecologic nidi in many parts of the world, and created new resident urban ecologies as well. The infection drains from the flea bite into the lymph nodes, which become swollen buboes. When they rupture, infection of the blood (septicemia) spreads the bacteria throughout the body. Endotoxins cause shock, blood coagulation, and hemorrhaging into the skin vessels, often turning the body black. Untreated bubonic plague today has a case mortality rate of 50–60% (Benenson, 1995). A second form of plague occurs under certain circumstances of climate and crowding and intensity of infection. Secondary infection of the lungs then causes contagion to other people as a pneumonic plague and infects them through the respiratory system. Untreated septicemic plague and pneumonic plague are fatal. The great plagues of massive deaths have involved the highly contagious, lethal pneumonic form. Wills (1996) gives an excellent discussion of the evolution and natural history of bubonic plague.

The bacteria that are the agents of bubonic plague may have been cycling among rodents in the grasslands of Central Asia since prehistory (although McNeill thought the original focus was in the Indian Himalayan foothills and the infection spread to Eurasian steppes in the second millenium). There is also an ancient focus of plague among rodents in the Great Lakes area of Africa, and it is not clear whether the bubonic plague that was the Plague of Justinian (A.D. 542–543) and came to Constantinople from Egypt originated in India or Africa. The tropical black rat, *Rattus rattus,* had managed to cross from the Indian Ocean to the Meditteranean Sea ports. Newly introduced to Europe, it did not yet occur in northern Europe, and thus that devastating epidemic remained limited to the eastern Meditterranean. In 1346, bubonic plague did spread out of the steppes to the coastal ports and across to Europe. By the time of the Black Death, 1348, the black rat had spread throughout the cities of Europe. Population pressure was also severe. Europe was primed for a pandemic which would reduce its population by more than a third.

Bubonic plague is a rodent zoonosis transmitted by fleas (Table 3-4). The rodents in the Central Asian grasslands, the natural nidus of plague, show no symptoms; that is, they are quite resistant to their ancient infection. Consider for a moment what makes up the living community in which the agent of bubonic plague, the bacterium *Yersinia pestis,* circulates continually (Figure 3-3). The rodents live in burrows deep enough to provide insulation from the severe heat and cold of Central Asia. Under the grass, the horizon of organic soil is deep. The soil is drained well enough that the burrows are unlikely to be flooded, even when the snow melts in spring. The degree of flooding or drainage depends on local slope, as do the amount of rainfall

TABLE 3-4. Some Diseases Vectored by Fleas and Lice

Disease	Agent	Major vector	Endemic locale	Reservoir/ comments
Rickettsial				
Typhus fever, epidemic	*Rickettsia prowazekii*	Fluids of body louse, *Pediculus humanus*	Cold climes, especially mountains South America, Himalayas, Balkans	Source is people
Typhus fever, murine, endemic	*Rickettsia typhi*	Flea, especially *Xenopsylla cheopis*	Worldwide	Rats
Bacterial				
Plague, bubonic	*Yersinia pestis*	Flea, especially *Xenopsylla cheopis*	Widespread natural foci; western United States, Vietnam, South Africa, South America, Central Asia	R: rodents
Relapsing fever (epidemic)	*Borrelia recurrentis*	Louse, *Pediculus humanus*	Local areas in Asia Minor, North and East Africa, South America	Source is people; in outbreaks from nidal tick-borne

and the solar radiation received. In the burrow are nesting materials of organic nature, grass roots, and variety of flies, roaches, and other arthropods that take shelter there. Among the worms and arthropods, which might be predators, flea eggs hatch into larvae, which live off the organic matter. Because rats breed frequently and have large litters, there are susceptible baby rats for adult flea vectors to infect when they eat. Therefore, actively infected young rats are often present to feed the rat fleas when they first emerge from the larval stage. In vacated burrows, adult fleas can maintain infection for months while waiting for new hosts.

The landscape must also have the right kind of vegetation for the rats to eat and a certain mix of predators and competitors to regulate the population. There are also micrometeorological limits to this vegetation and fauna. Sometimes fire serves to scatter the rodents and introduce infected fleas to new burrows. At the margins of the territory, where winter cold or summer droughts are so severe that the rat population is unstable, it is difficult for the bacteria to continually circulate to new hosts. Experts in the former Soviet Union became quite precise in identifying the slope, exposure, soil type, acid/base balance, vegetation associations, and so forth that mark areas where the transmission chain is most likely to be established. They concen-

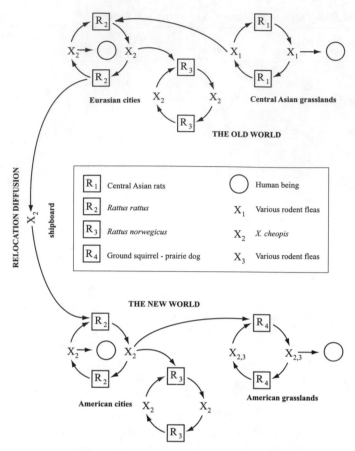

FIGURE 3-3. Bubonic plague transmission.

trated on fumigating burrows in that landscape and managed to reduce greatly the natural focus of bubonic plague in Central Asia.

Occasionally nomads and hunters must have camped in this natural nidus of the disease, and individuals must have been bitten by fleas and died, perhaps scores of miles away. When infected fleas were carried by caravan in bedding or on bodies from this natural nidus to a city such as Constantinople (today's Istanbul), a transference, or relocation diffusion, of disease cycle occurred. The hungry fleas bit urban rats, which were quite susceptible to this new infection and died in droves. As the urban rats died and turned cold, their fleas sought new hosts and spread the epizootic. Urban rat populations were, and are, enormous. As the rodents died in the millions, many millions of fleas looking for hosts encountered human beings. One type of flea, *Xenopsylla cheopis,* made an especially dangerous vector because of its willingness to bite humans, who are avoided by most flea species.

The cultural ecology of European medieval cities was ideal for epidemics of plague. Housing was very crowded; water was of limited availability, especially in the quarters of the poor; hygiene was terrible. Soap was a luxury; hot water was virtually unknown; food was stored in and near dwellings, which rats knew. The 13th-century population boom had led to massive deforestation and overexpansion of areas of agricultural development, which caused erosion and pushed beyond its limits the transportation system's ability to supply foodstuffs to the growing cities. The climate had worsened and grown colder and wetter (causing more ergotism, too), and crop failure was more frequent. There was inflation, common malnutrition, and even starvation, filth, and disruption. Europe was primed for "the Plague." As people fled the epidemic, or as goods were transported with their stowaway fleas and rodents, the disease agent reached new towns and even the new rat populations of northern Europe. Bubonic plague swept from east to west across Europe, and then returned from west to east through a new generation of susceptible children. Some people developed a terminal pneumonia that enabled the bacteria to spread by direct means also (through respiratory contagion). The first wave of the Black Death killed a third of the population of Europe. In some places more than half died. Each successive wave, however, had lower case mortality rates, which dropped from nearly 90% to 60% and perhaps less in places.

As the brown rat, *Rattus norwegicus*, spread into Europe in succeeding centuries and outclimbed, outfought, and displaced the black rat, *R. rattus*, the ecology of the disease changed. The brown rat was not as sociable. The black rat was originally a wild, tropical rat before it became domicilitated, preferring to hang around people's houses and storehouses and barns where it was warm. *Rattus norwegicus* was from the temperate latitudes of Asia. It preferred to live in sewers and other places where it could avoid people and some of its own kind. The parameters of contact between dead rats, fleas, and people changed. Many of the housing and nutritional conditions changed, too, under new population and economic conditions. The great pandemics abated. Bubonic plague has continued, however, to break out when war or other severe disturbances have destroyed the ecological balance.

Meanwhile, plague had been carried by ship to the cities of the New World. In the late 19th century, for example, an epidemic in San Francisco led white citizens there to burn down crowded Chinatown. This conflagration effectively dispersed the rats. From the urban rat epizootics, wild rodents must have become infected. Today, bubonic plague is enzootic in the rodents of the Southwest. In the grasslands of the southwestern United States, prairie dogs and ground squirrels live in burrows in which most of the nidal conditions of Central Asia are duplicated.

A few people die every year in the southwestern United States from bubonic plague. Frequently, later investigation determines that a cat brought home an infected ground squirrel or that some similar event occurred (cats are so susceptible to bubonic plague they even develop buboes; perhaps there was more than superstition to their association with witchcraft). From time to time an epizootic will become evident among ground squirrels in a national park, and the park will have to be closed. A public health threat exists that campers or other travelers in the southwestern arid grasslands will pick up some infected fleas in their baggage (like Asian travelers before them) and transport them to a city where there is a large rat population that has become quite tolerant of our worst rat poisons. Rats infected with the plague have been caught in monitoring traps in Golden Gate Park in San Francisco. Most U.S. geographers, however, understand little about the biogeography of the natural nidus of bubonic plague in their country and, unlike their (former) Soviet counterparts, have not been involved in any effort at control or eradication.

Plague outbreaks have occurred in most of the world's great ports, and plague has become enzootic among the gerbils of South Africa, field rats of India and of Java, and marmots of Manchuria. Worldwide, more than 220 species of rodents have been shown to harbor plague, although the incidence of plague has been declining. The war in Vietnam showed again, however, that when the cultural–biological interface is disturbed, plague can flare into epidemics quickly. Tens of thousands of cases of bubonic plague occurred in refugee-swollen Saigon and the disturbed countryside of South Vietnam. Outbreaks of the deadly pneumonic form followed but were contained in the cities by antibiotic therapy and a short-lived vaccine. In 1994, in Surat, India, plague broke out in the squatter slums and panicked the nation. Monsoon failures had compounded the rural–urban migration to bring rural migrants into the crowded housing; food had been imported to the region and stored; rats had been observed dying in nearby villages. Government officials were initially afraid of inciting panic, but later, although hundreds of people died, a major epidemic was prevented from spreading by meeting travelers at train, bus, and airplane stations. Some countries quarantined passengers arriving from India. It is not certain whether the containment strategy worked or the infection was in fact some other *Yersinia* infection and not true plague. What is clear is that the underlying ecology has not been addressed.

Natural nidality involves defining the micrometeorological, geomorphological, and biogiographical limits of a biological community. May (1958a) described these concepts in a different way. He wrote of multifactor diseases: Each factor had its own spatial distribution, and all factors had to coincide to create the disease conditions. In the example of plague, the bacterium (agent) is one factor. The rat host (reservoir) is a second. The flea vector is a third. The human host is a fourth. May called a place where the three factors of agent, vector, and reservoir coincide, but disease is not known because no humans are present, a "silent zone" of disease. When people, such as pastoralists in the grasslands or woodcutters in the forests, penetrate into the silent zone, disease can result. In the former Soviet Union, Pavlovsky's hypothesis that the potential for disease could be identified from the simple existence of certain environmental conditions was important in developing mining or industrial towns in Siberia. Planners working with landscape epidemiology could design housing, protective clothing, or work scheduling to shield the human population from exposure to the zoonosis. In the United States, there has been limited work on the biogeography of zoonoses. Instead, the silent zone concept is being extended to nonbiotic environmental hazards, such as toxic land.

THE CULTURAL DIMENSION OF WATER-DEPENDENT DISEASE TRANSMISSION

The importance of the human role in habitat modification, of cultural buffering systems, and of human mobility for disease systems was discussed in Chapter 2. These factors are illustrated here with three diseases: malaria, dengue hemorrhagic fever, and schistosomiasis. These three diseases are chosen not only because of their importance but also because they are water-based in different ways. They also serve as examples of how activities that promote economic development, especially in the tropics, can modify nidal conditions and affect disease patterns.

Malaria

Malaria is by far the most serious vectored disease in the world. In the 1950s it was possible to dream about eradicating malaria because it has no reservoir. In the 1960s eradication or control over large areas of Asia and South America was achieved. In the 1990s, it again infects more than half a billion people. Malaria kills 1–2 million people a year (over 900,000 in tropical Africa), totally incapacitates tens of millions, and causes hundreds of millions to struggle in exhaustion with chronically severe anemia. About 40% of the world's population, in more than 100 countries, live in regions where malaria is endemic today. Malaria was known to kill millions of people each year, but even so, the health improvement in the 1960s in countries in which malaria was almost eradicated was eye-opening. Infant mortality rates plummeted. Fertility rates increased as those miscarriages and cases of infertility that were due to malaria disappeared. The terrible pressure malaria has exerted on the human population over the ages is demonstrated by the presence of high-mortality genetic diseases, most famously sickle-cell anemia, that were selected by evolutionary processes because they offered some protection against the greater mortality costs of malaria. Yet the case mortality rate for malaria is low compared to that of most serious diseases. Malaria is generally, depending on type, a chronic, debilitating disease. Despite decades in which scientific armament has been marshaled against malaria, it is resurgent in many countries where only two decades ago it was virtually eradicated. Cases in Sri Lanka, for example, went from 1 million a year in the 1950s to less than 10, to 38,500 cases in 1982 (4% falciparum) to 676,000 cases in 1987 (27% falciparum) to 1 million a year in the 1990s. It is still estimated that about 80% of all clinical cases and 90% of parasite carriers live in tropical Africa. More than 1.7 billion people live in once-endemic areas in which transmission had been greatly reduced but is now reinstated, and in which the ecology is unstable and the situation is deteriorating. The mosquito vectors are resistant to all the major insecticides, the agent is resistant to all the major drugs, and the ancient scourge is upon us again.

The disease cycle consists of direct transmission of the agent between humans by various species of *Anopheles* mosquitoes. There is no animal reservoir, although monkeys, birds, and other animals have their own forms of malaria. The agent is a protozoan, of a form called a plasmodium, occurring in four types. *Plasmodium vivax* causes benign tertian malaria, historically prevalent in Europe. It has a liver-dormant stage (hypnozoites) that allows it to survive even long winters and to reactivate in time to infect the spring mosquitoes. Its case mortality is low enough for it to have been nicknamed "benign tertian." It does not occur in West Africa where people genetically lack Duffy antigens in their blood cells and seem immune to it. *P. ovale,* the least common malaria, occurs only in West Africa—perhaps as a niche replacement. *P. malariae* causes quartan malaria. It is so old and adapted a human parasite that science has yet to discover how it hides and relapses in the blood. The most dangerous form of malaria is caused by *P. falciparum.* It has more than a 10% case mortality rate and often has unusual symptoms of disorientation, coma, shock, and renal failure. Apparently it has most recently transferred from birds. It spreads slowly because it has not yet fully adapted to *Anopheles,* which are not bird feeders. It lacks the ability to go dormant in the human liver and so must reproduce in enormous numbers—which so block, explode, and shatter the circulatory system that it can kill in hours—in order to infect mosquitoes and stay in hypercirculation and continual reinfection.

All the forms of malaria have a complicated life cycle within the body although they differ in detail. The protozoa have much more genetic information, are much more complex and adaptable and cagy, than the comparatively stupid bacteria. The sexual form, gametocytes, emerge from hiding inside the red blood cells within the gut of the *Anopheles* mosquito, mate in its gut wall, and reproduce large numbers of sporozoites which migrate to the salivary glands and get inoculated into people. They swim to the liver, within which they grow and mature over a week or two into the blood forms, merozoites, which enter red blood cells and commence gobbling hemoglobin and multiplying by factors of 10. They consume the red blood cells and break out of the empty husks in a synchronized manner (hence the alternation of fever and chills). The merozoites inside the cells produce the male and female gametocytes, which do not circulate in the blood (and so are not killed by drugs) but do not reproduce, either, until they are taken up by a mosquito to complete the cycle, in about 2 weeks. The complexity of this cycle is such that the hematozoites dormant in the liver were not discovered until 1980, after a century of intense microscopic observation. Each stage has different surface proteins, different antigens, different nutritional needs, different behavior. The multiple, changing symptoms, forms of hiding, and details of human immunological response are still of such baffling complexity and mystery that malaria has defied decades of intense effort to make a vaccine.

The cultural ecology of malaria is also one of the most studied. May (1958a) described a village in the highlands of Vietnam, which had low-grade, endemic malaria. It was a drain on the population's energy, but it was not the worst of these highland villagers' problems. The people lived in houses on stilts and tied their water buffalo and cattle under their houses. They cooked in the houses. These customs were quite different from those of the lowland Vietnamese who moved into the highland area one year. The lowlanders built their houses on the ground and kept their animals in proper barns. They also had cooking sheds separate from the houses. They were rapidly driven out of the highlands by epidemic malaria. The local species of *Anopheles* that transmitted the agent was not a strong flier. The height of a house on stilts deterred her. She preferred to bite animals and seldom went past the tethered animals under the house. She, like all *Anopheles*, was active at night and especially in the evening, when the house was full of smoke. The cultural practices of the upland people thus constituted a rather successful protective buffer. Changing nothing in the system except the cultural behavior of the people was enough to render the land uninhabitable.

The experience of the United States illustrates some of the complex forms of cultural interaction with the biotic disease system. Originally malaria was an Old World disease. The British brought *P. vivax* to North America, and the slaves they imported brought *P. falciparum* from Africa. The early, glowing reports of how healthy the colonies were faded as malaria spread. The nuclear settlements of the plantations were especially good foci of disease transmission. The coastal plantations became so deadly that the owners spent their summers in resorts (the foundation of several beach and mountain resort towns) and cities such as Savannah. The greater resistance of Africans to the disease became a common explanation of why the institution of slavery was "that which is necessary."

People did not know the cause of the disease, but they were keen observers. They knew that as the forest around Savannah was removed and land was converted into rice fields, malaria increased. They thought it was the miasma ("mal aria" means bad air) that the trees had protected them from. In what was probably the first environmental legislation for the public health, the city demanded that all land within a mile of the city be used only for dry agriculture. It compensated farmers out of tax revenues for the loss they incurred by not being able to grow rice or indigo. Malaria decreased in Savannah for a few decades, until the disturbances of the Civil War.

Malaria was *the* American disease of the late 19th century. The confluence of the Ohio and Mississippi was so deadly that many would travel there only in winter. The census of 1890 undertook a survey of cause of death (Figure 3-4). Although not up to today's statistical standards of reporting, the rates it recorded for malaria, over 7,000 deaths per 100,000 people across the South and more than 1,000 in such states as Michigan, Illinois, and California, are impressive. An average case mortality rate of 5% means that almost the entire population was infected over large areas. Yet by 1930 malaria had disappeared from the North and West, and caused fewer than 25 deaths per 100,000 peole in the South except for a few counties. What had happened?

The United States has one important malaria vector, *Anopheles quadrimaculatus.* It breeds in water where it can anchor its eggs on vegetation that intersects the surface in open sunlight and where the currents are not too strong. When the forest was removed across the country, sunlight was let in to marshes and to the poorly drained glaciated land of northern states. Rice plantations planted lots of intersecting vegetation, and much occurred naturally elsewhere. Slow travel by rafts and barges turned canals and rivers into linear transmission channels. Susceptible migrants picked up the infection along the waterways, and travelers who were infected spread it to new places. Houses were of poor quality, and their glassless windows and slatted walls offered little obstruction to mosquitoes. People commonly had poor nutrition and had few animals to divert the mosquitoes. At the turn of the century, the poorly drained land of the glacial till country was deliberately drained for agriculture. Houses were more often constructed of brick or other good ma-

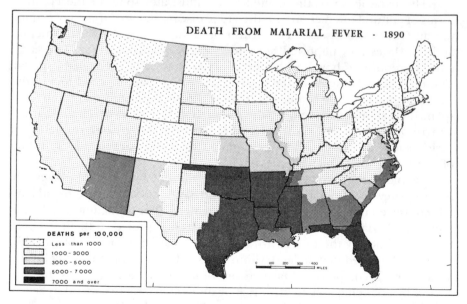

FIGURE 3-4. Malarial deaths in the United States, 1890. Adapted from U.S. Census Bureau (1890, map 17).

terial and had glass windows and screens (mainly to keep flies out). Transportation shifted from the rivers and canals to the railroads, and settlements as well as travelers shifted to the dry upland. The numbers of animals increased. The nutrition of the people improved. Quinine, an antimalarial drug, was available at a more reasonable price when the tariff against its importation (from Java, mainly) was finally dropped. The slower breeding of the mosquito in the cold climate of the North led to the disappearance of northern malaria. In the South the incidence was greatly reduced as the population became more settled (and therefore less mobile), but some counties near sinkholes or the oxbow lakes of the Mississippi remained highly malarious.

Eradication Campaigns

In the late 19th century, Laveran discovered the agent of malaria, and Ross proved its transmission by *Anopoheles* mosquito. In the United States, a public health official named Carter (1919) was amazed at how little use had been made of this knowledge to prevent malaria. The disease was so common in the South as to be taken for granted, and he had to demonstrate to state and other officials the tremendous economic costs of lost workdays and debilitated farmers. The new Rockefeller Foundation became interested. It supported the training and staffing of entomologists and other experts and the creation of public health departments at the county level. Carter himself determined the flight range of the U.S. vector (one mile), its water preferences, and the effects of the water impoundment for mills. Commonly mills were closed on Sunday, and on Monday the elevated mill ponds were drawn down. He determined that this was good, because it stranded the flotage that anchored larvae.

Carter's findings became relevant when the Tennessee Valley Authority (TVA) proposed to construct dams that would impound large bodies of water in the malarious South. The economic value of developing cheap electricity was obvious, but what was the cost to the public health if malaria again became epidemic? The Army Corps of Engineers worked closely with health officials. All people near the proposed reservoirs were checked for malaria and treated, and all dwellings within a mile of the reservoir were screened. All vegetation was cleared within 10 feet above maximum and below minimum water levels to prevent intersecting vegetation. The water level had to be fluctuated, in spite of navigational needs, at fixed times of the year in order to strand flotage. It all worked, and malaria almost disappeared from the TVA area, instead of becoming epidemic.

Similar measures were adopted elsewhere, and levels of malaria were reduced. When threatened by a resurgence of malaria brought by soldiers returning after World War II from fighting in malarious countries, the United States mobilized for eradication of the disease. The military office that had tried to eradicate malaria around military bases where soldiers were training was located in Georgia. It was transformed to head the mobilization against malaria. The weapon was the new insecticide, DDT, which could be sprayed on houses and would for months afterward kill the mosquito vector when it rested on the walls after taking its blood meal. In a massive effort workers sprayed millions of houses across the South and detected and treated thousands of cases. Malaria was eradicated in the United States. The institution that had coordinated the attack became the Centers for Disease Control, located in Atlanta, Georgia (the previously malarial South), rather than Washington, DC.

When soldiers returning decades later from the war in Vietnam brought in relapsing malaria cases by the thousands, public health concerns were again raised. The plasmodia, however, found the environment so modified that they could no longer get established in the United States. Few people now sleep where mosquitoes can fly into their bedrooms and bite them, and detection is swift and treatment intensive. The control of malaria in the United States has been so complete that many people forget why reservoir landscapes have exposed banks and fluctuating water levels. Uses for recreation, livestock, and fish cultivation are coming into conflict with water-management laws that were enacted in every state in the South for control of malaria. Public health workers have grown complacent and government officials ignorant. Yet today, because of population mobility, more than 1,000 cases of malaria a year occur. Some cases have been fatal when physicians failed to recognize the disease. There has, after a gap of 30 years, been indigenous transmission in Texas, California, Michigan, Florida, New Jersey, and even New York City.

Beginning in the late 1950s, the World Health Organization attempted to eradicate malaria worldwide. The effort achieved notable successes, especially in Southeast Asia and Central America. By the 1970s, however, health officials talked about control instead of eradication, and in the 1980s they lost control. In most places the eradication campaign had made little progress at all, especially in tropical Africa where falciparum predominates and prevalence remains at traditional levels that induced a lethal genetic adaptation. Many reasons for the failure of eradication have been offered by authorities. In some cases maintenance and surveillance failed when, for budgetary reasons, the special malaria teams were combined with multipurpose health programs. The international availability and costs of insecticides have changes. Some (Farid, 1980) believe that when the reduction in malaria led to faster population growth, the capitalist countries cut back their financial support; some even suggest that support was intentionally withdrawn from the eradication effort because of a desire to keep Third World countries poor, sick, and dependent. Whatever faults there were in administration and in financing, however, the original hopes of eradication were probably unrealistic because they failed to appreciate the complexities of tropical ecosystems.

In temperate countries, such as the United States, there are few vector species. Sheets of open, fresh water with intersecting vegetation were the breeding area. Spraying walls of houses with a residual insecticide interrupted transmission because the vector bit at night in the houses and then rested on the wall. Figure 3-5 illustrates the contrasting, very complex vector ecology in tropical Malaysia. *Anopheles sundaicus* breeds in brackish water, such as mangrove swamps along the coast. *A. campestris* breeds in rice fields, while *A. letifer* likes coconut, rubber, and swamp trees at low elevations. *A. umbrosus* is the vector of the forest. *A. balabacensis* will breed in the shaded streams of the natural forest or of the rubber tree replacement forests. All these vectors must compete with many other species of mosquito. Each of the vector species occurs in relatively small numbers and prefers to bite animals. Some species bite people only outdoors in the early evening and never enter houses. Others enter houses but fly out the window afterward and rest under vegetation. Most of the *Anopheles* species in Figure 3-5 are normally the vectors of endemic, chronic malaria at low levels. *A. maculatus*, however, breeds in streams exposed to sunlight and readily bites humans. It rapidly increases to very large numbers when given the simple, open habitat it prefers. Thus, when the forest is cut down for land development schemes or plantations and the forest streams are exposed to sunlight, *A. maculatus* rapidly increases in numbers and as a vector of epidemic malaria is one of the most dangerous in the world.

The objective of the eradication campaigns was to interrupt transmission, using some of the known intervention points (Figure 3-6). Residual insecticides sprayed on houses were used to kill the adults after they have taken a blood meal. Humans were examined, and often chloroquine was given as a general prophylaxis to the entire population, to kill the plasmodia in their blood. It was recognized that the mosquitoes could not be suppressed forever. The hope was that when they came back, the agent of the disease would

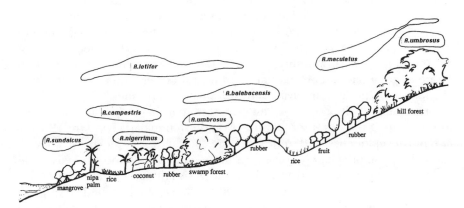

FIGURE 3-5. Malaria vectors in Malaya. The size of the "clouds" indicates the relative importance in each habitat, or land-use zone, of various species of *Anopheles* mosquitoes in peninsular Malaysia. Adapted from Sandosham (1970). Copyright 1970 by Medical Association of Malaya. Reprinted by permission.

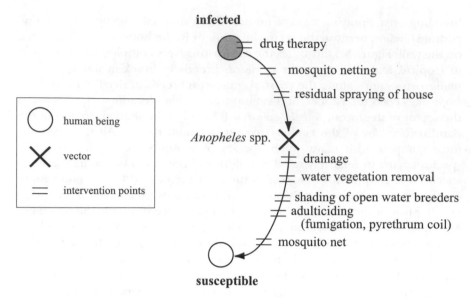

FIGURE 3-6. Malaria intervention. Malaria is vectored by various species of *Anopheles* mosquitoes, but human malaria only infects humans.

no longer exist in that place. This strategy had worked in temperate lands, but the complex ecology of the tropics was frustrating. Although some vectors bit people in their bedrooms at night, rested on the wall, and died, others bit people only outdoors or flew out the window after biting people and never touched the insecticide. Broader attempts to interrupt breeding did not work. Oiling water bodies or stocking them with tilapia fish, which eat mosquite larvae, did not affect mosquitoes breeding in tree holes or hoof prints. People cutting firewood in the mangrove swamps continued to be bitten by *A. sundaicus*. For many such reasons, when the wall-resting, common vector became resistant to the insecticides and rebounded, some malaria was still present in the community, and the transmission chain resumed. Often the population had lost any partial immunity, however, and epidemics, higher infant mortality, and intensified health problems resulted.

Human mobility also played an important part in eradication failure. Laborers clearing the forest for planting would catch malaria from the *A. maculatus*-borne epidemics and return to their villages. People from areas in which the plasmodia had become resistant to cholorquine prophylaxis would migrate to other areas and introduce the resistant strain. Prothero (1961) had earlier demonstrated in Africa the importance of labor-shed (a vast area within which people migrate to work) and pastoral mobility patterns for reintroducing an infection to cleared areas. There was international failure to analyze the problem and coordinate efforts at the appropriate scale. Refugee movements confounded what efforts were made.

In some places there is recurrent interest in permanently altering the environment, through drainage and housing, for example, to defeat in detail the ecology of the local disease system rather than relying on the magic bullets of chemistry. New efforts to develop a DNA-vaccine, a totally new technology, go on apace. A new drug, *Artemisia annua* (qinghaosu) from traditional Chinese pharmacopoeia is proving useful for multiple-resistant strains of plasmodia, but no one doubts that it is already being too commonly (mis)used on the Thai–Cambodia border and resistance will soon develop. No one now even dreams of eradication of this ancient scourge.

Dengue Hemorrhagic Fever

In the 1950s, a dangerous new disease began spreading in Southeast Asia. It was first noticed in Manila, but within a few years it was occurring in Thailand. At first it primarily struck Asian children and had a case mortality of over 10%, although that has fallen to around 3% with better therapy. Investigators considered many factors, including diet, racial susceptibility, and complications from other diseases, without finding the disease agent. Virologists finally isolated the agent, which is identical to the virus that causes dengue fever. Like many arboviruses, it is classed as a togavirus (wearing a covering). Like the virus that causes yellow fever, it is also antigenically identified as a Group B virus (by tests of hemaglutination). It occurs in four types, simply called 1, 2, 3, 4.

Dengue fever is a monkey zoonosis transmitted by *Aedes albopictus* in the forests of Southeast Asia. All four serotypes occur in that jungle cycle, where dengue probably evolved. *Ae. albopictus*, alias "the tiger mosquito" because of its striped legs, will bite people and does breed in containers around human habitation, but it likes vegetation and generally prefers other animals. Dengue fever has been a ubiquitous childhood disease among the rural population of Southeast Asia. With urbanization during the last century, the disease at first disappeared from the urban population, because the vector was not common in towns. With the arrival of *Ae. aegypti* from Africa, however, dengue became epidemic in the cities, where people had not developed the usual adult immunity. *Ae. aegypti* is a super vector. In Southeast Asia it breeds in clear water in containers ranging from empty tin cans to large urns that store bathwater for the dry season. Dengue became endemic in the urban population, affecting mainly children. It was in this milieu that dengue hemorrhagic fever first emerged.

Dengue fever had been notorious for the aches (its alias is breakbone fever) and rash it causes, but it had never been a killing disease. What is probably its first pandemic spread appears in Benjamin Rush's description of it in Philadelphia in 1780, undoubtedly a visitor from the triangular slave–rum–sugar trade of the Caribbean. There were sporadic epidemics in the 19th and early 20th centuries until mosquito control and the eradication of *Ae. aegypti* from the Caribbean and South America brought decades of repose (even as it ended epidemics of yellow fever). In recent decades *Ae. aegypti* has again recolonized the Caribbean and much of South America (Gubler & Trent, 1993).

The new hemorrhagic form of dengue kills more than 15,000 people a year, most of them children, 10,000 of them in India. It usually puts infected people in the hospital when abdominal pain and high fever occur, 2 or 3 days after infection. There is bleeding into the mucous membranes of the abdomen and into the skin, as well as vomiting. This stage may be followed by a shock syndrome, which was responsible for most of the early deaths but is better treated today. Intense research has focused on dengue hemorrhagic fever/dengue shock syndrome (DHF/DSS), and some aspects of the mystery are now clear.

There are several hypotheses about the etiology of DHF. One is that while thousands of rhesus monkeys were caged on the docks of Singapore, en route to U.S. laboratories for development of the poliomyelitis vaccine, jungle strains were introduced to the city. Another hypothesis was that the virus had mutated. All four types of the virus were isolated from dying patients, however, and it seemed unlikely that all four types would mutate at the same time. The modified hypothesis is that *Ae. aegypti* is such a supervector that all types of dengue have been able to become more virulent: Transmission opportunities are so excellent they can chance endangering their hosts more (see Chapter 2). The new disease is indubitably associated with *Ae. aegypti.* As the mosquito has spread among coastal towns and along the railroads and roads, DHF has spread with it. In the urban systems of Southeast Asia, squatter slums and people living on boats have greatly increased the supervector's breeding habitat. As rain gutters, storage jars for rain from roof runoff, ant traps around table legs, flowerpots, and garbage heaps have proliferated, so has the mosquito.

The most widely supported hypothesis today is that DHF is caused by the immune system overresponding to repetitive infection with dengue. The troop movements of World War II in the Pacific, amidst all armies, refugees, and prisoners, moved strains vigorously among Australia, New Guinea, the Philippines, Japan, Indonesia, and Thailand and ensured that all four serotypes were widespread. As people have migrated to the city from different regions, they have brought all four types of dengue fever into simultaneous circulation. Population mobility and the supervector have combined to increase the chance that a child will be infected with two different types of dengue virus within a relatively short span of time. Some researchers (Halstead, 1980) believe that the immune system of some children reacts so strongly to a second infection by a related, but different, dengue virus that the hemorrhagic-shock syndrome results.

Dengue hemorrhagic fever continues to increase and to spread. The initial biennial frequency of the disease has largely disappeared. It occurs throughout the year but increases during the peak mosquito-bite periods associated with the monsoon. Better treatment has brought down the death rate, but tens of thousands of children continue to be hospitalized each year in all the countries of tropical Asia. Following the reestablishment of *Ae. aegypti* in the Caribbean in the 1970s, in the 1980s dengue virus spread epidemically and in the 1990s DHF/DSS became endemic from Cuba to Venezuela and Brazil. At first the syndrome was not common, but since the arrival of a Southeast Asian biotype of dengue it has emerged. One thing not yet understood is the difference between dengue viruses that cause DHF/DSS in the presence of preexisting dengue antibody and those that do not. *Ae. aegypti* is common in the United States. There is public health concern that dengue will not only launch some epidemics but become established in Texas or Florida. The introduction of *Ae. albopictus* to Texas in 1985 from a boatload of tires has heightened concern. *Ae. aegypti* is a much more dangerous, anthropophilic vector, but *Ae. albopictus* poses a new threat because it survives winter better. In Asia it occurs through China and Japan. In the United States, the tiger mosquito has already spread from Texas to Virginia. It is not as happy in paved cities as *Ae. aegypti*, but it seems to love the suburbs.

Dengue fever has been closely tied to international population mobility from tourism and business. Travelers' information for dengue as well as malaria prophylactis and other health information is kept current on the website of the Centers for Disease Control and Prevention.

Schistosomiasis

Schistosomiasis, endemic in at least 73 countries, is the most rapidly spreading serious infectious disease in the world. More than 200 million people are infected by the schistosome, and perhaps a quarter milllion die each year from its depradations (World Health Organization, 1999). Schistosomiasis (sometimes called bilharzia in Africa) is not ordinarily fatal, just debilitating. It is not, strictly speaking, a vectored disease, but it is definitely natural nidal.

The parasite is a schistosome, a kind of blood fluke that lives in the veins (see Table 3-5 and Vignette Table 2-1). Although there are five species, three account for most human disease. *Schistosoma japonicum* and *S. mansoni* inhabit the veins around the intestine; *S. hematobium* inhabits the veins around the bladder. *S. mansoni* occurs in Africa, the Arabian peninsula, and Latin America from the Caribbean to northeastern Brazil. *S. hematobium* occurs in Africa, the Middle East, and small foci in India. There is no significant reservoir for these transmissible diseases except people. The rarer *S. intercalatum* is limited to parts of West Africa where it mainly affects sheep, goats, and other nonhuman mammals. Schistosomiasis has been found in several pockets along the Mekong River (to which it was introduced by Japanese soldiers) in mainland Southeast Asia and has recently been associated with a new species, *S. mekongi*. *S. japonicum* occurs in East Asia and limited areas in the Philippines and Sulawesi. In addition to humans, dogs, cats, pigs, water buffalo, field mice, and rats host the agent and comprise a persistent reservoir.

Schistosomiasis is a chronic disease that, in cases of intense infection,

TABLE 3-5. Some Semivectored Diseases with Intermediate Hosts

Disease	Agent	Main intermediate host(s)	Endemic locale	Comments
Viral				
Rabies	Rhabdovirus	Canidae (foxes, dogs, coyotes, jackals)	Worldwide, except some islands	Also bites of skunks, bats, raccoons: wildlife rabies increasing in United States
Helminthic				
Clonorchiasis (liver fluke)	Fluke: *Clonorchis sinensis*	Freshwater fish, snails: Amnicolidae	East and Southeast Asia	Human infection from larvae in cysts in raw fish, eggs passed in feces
Hydatidosis	*Echinococcus granulosus* (dog tapeworm)	Definitive hosts dogs, wolves; intermediate hosts herbivores, dog—sheep—dog cycle most important; also dog—kangaroo—dog, wolf—moose—wolf, dog—cattle—dog	Where dogs are used for herding: Middle East, Australia, Argentia; also Kenya	Human infection from ingestion of eggs from dog fecal contamination
Schistosomiasis (bilharzia)	Fluke: *Schistosoma mansoni, S. haematobium, S. japonicum*	Snails: *Biomphalaria* spp. for mansonian, *Bulinus* for other types	*S. japonica* in East and Southeast Asia; *S. mansoni* in Africa, Northeast South America and Caribbean; *S. haematobium* in Africa, Middle East to India; *S. intercalatum* West Africa	Humans are main source; domestic animals involved with *S. japonicum;* infection by skin contact with water
Trichinosis	Intestinal roundworm, *Trichinella spiralis*	Swine; bears, dog, cats	Variable worldwide, depending on pork habits	Human infection from eating raw or undercooked meat

can be disabling. It weakens people and causes them to die from other things. In places where it occurs, such as the Nile valley, it fequently infects more than half of the population. The symptoms of the chronic infection result mostly from passage of enormous numbers of eggs. Common symptoms include fever, headache, pain, and bleeding into the urinary tract or intestine. Millions of eggs may block blood vessels. Worms wander from the veins they normally inhabit and go astray into other organs. In cases of heavy infection, the passage of the infesting parasite through the liver can injure the tissue. Individual worms produce eggs for several years and have been known to do so for more than 20 years.

From the veins around the intestines, eggs are passed in the feces; from those around the bladder they are passed in the urine. Hooks on the eggs tear holes to get out of blood vessels and result in bloody urine and other blood loss. Most human waste is deposited into or washed into water. When the schistosome eggs enter water, a form called miracidium hatches and swims downward searching for a snail of the proper genus. The presence of suitable snails has allowed schistosomes to spread to Central and South America; they failed to find suitable snails in the United States. In China, the usual amphibious nature of the intermediate host snails, which support *S. japonica*, allowed a type of intervention (burying and drowning snails) not possible for the aquatic snails in Africa.

After the parasite multiplies in the snail, it breaks out in a microscopic form called cercaria and swims to the surface looking for people. When it encounters bathers, it penetrates their skin and follows a complicated internal path through metamorphosis in the liver to its eventual home in a blood vessel as a sexually reproducing adult trematode. The temperature of the water, the speed of the current, and the hours of sunshine all become critical factors in how long the cercaria survives in the water without a host.

The cultural side of the equation is the water-contact behavior of the population. To contract schistosomiasis, people do not need to eat or drink anything contaminated. They merely need to walk, swim, bathe, or do their laundry. In semiarid lands or in dry times of the year, human activity often centers on water sources. If the appropriate snail is present and its habitat is favorable, a traveler or immigrant can introduce the schistosome eggs and begin a cycle. The more clustered the population is, the more intense the cycle of infection can become. As the floods of the great rivers are controlled, as irrigation is extended into arid lands or converted from seasonal basin irrigation systems to perennial systems, and as fertilizer and fish ponds enrich the water, so the habitat of the snails that are intermediate hosts is increased, and the disease spreads in Africa and in South America.

The age structure and activity patterns of the population affect the disease's epidemiology. Farmers in the field do not use latrines. Children cannot be kept from swimming in the canals. Women must do laundry. The time of day and the place of contact in the river or canal expose people to different activity levels of the cercariae and to different levels of snail and water contamination foci. Deep wells with hand pumps to provide water for laundry and bathing have often reduced incidence in women and children. The expansion of irrigated agriculture has increased occupational exposure. Incidental foci of exposure may be things such as the water basins used for ablutions by Moslems before prayers at a mosque.

Figure 3-7 illustrates intervention points in the life cycle of schistosomia-

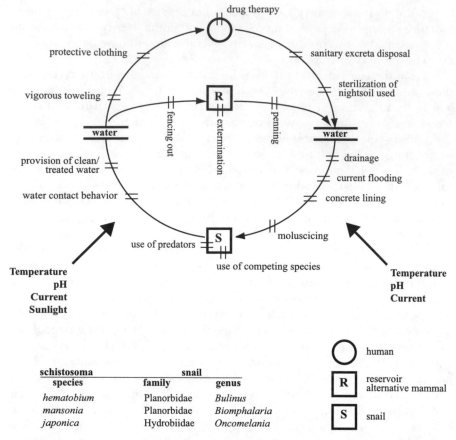

FIGURE 3-7. Schistosomiasis intervention. Each kind of schistosomiasis has a different genus of snail for intermediate host. Environmental characteristics of bodies of water are important at two points in the schistosome's life.

sis. Chemoprophylaxis of the population can kill the adult worms. The drugs are powerful, however, and have many side effects. Usually hospitalization is necessary and few peasants can afford the time and lost work. The few U.S. tourists who get infected can be successfully treated and cured at home, but where a large local population is infected and subject to reinfection, there is no feasible treatment. If all urine and feces were disposed of in a safe manner, contamination of the water could not occur; but given the nature of agricultural work and the activities of rural children, complete sanitary disposal is often not feasible. In some places, such as lower Egypt, the water table is so high that latrines provide little separation of waste and water. Fast water, drainage, and concrete linings of ditches that are regularly cleaned can decimate a snail population. Molluscicides have been used to protect certain settlements or urban populations. They are expensive, as they continually wash away downstream, where they may accumulate and result in fish kills and other harmful effects. There is considerable interest in biological controls. Many animals have forms of schistosomiasis that are not infectious for humans (such as those resulting in "swimmer's itch" in the United States) but that may infect suitable snails and outcompete the human parasite. Some success with biological competition has been achieved in the laboratory, but dominance seems to be temperature dependent and transfers poorly to the field. Clean, safe water can be supplied for domestic use. The water-contact behavior of a population can be modified to some extent if enough is known about the disease hazards. For example, the time of day when certain contact activities occur, such as washing the laundry, might be altered so as to take place when cercariae are less active.

The spread and increase in schistosomiasis are so serious that many kinds of international research are focused on it. Scientists are working on vaccines, on new drug therapies, and on biological competition and predation. Health educators and social scientists are working on modification of population behavior and the design of protective systems. The complex ecology of the disease differs by type of schistosome, by local snail ecology, by local economy, and by local customs. Population mobilization and a labor-intensive war on snails decreased and somewhat controlled the disease in China but that could change because of factors such as agricultural modernization, economic liberalization, and growing population mobility. Schistosomiasis is spreading in the different ecologies of the coffee plantations and new settlements of Brazil and the new irrigation works in east, west, and south Africa. The microgeography of the disease can guide local intervention efforts, but aside from the work of Kloos in Ethiopia and the Nile little research has been done.

Tick-Borne Diseases

Ticks vector an array of viral and rickettsial diseases, from Russian spring–summer encephalitis to boutonneuse fever in India and South Africa (see Table 3-1). Each has its own characteristic landscape ecology. The landscape epidemiology of central European encephalitis (CEE), for example, was studied by Wellmer and Jusatz (1981). The encephalitis is caused by a togavirus vectored mainly by the common tick, *Ixodes ricinus*. Wellmer and Jusatz (1981) delimited the temperature, humidity, precipitation cycles, vegetation, animal associations, and other environmental conditions needed for its maintenance. They found that lower mountain elevations with dense and diversified vegetation are required by the disease system, limited by such factors as an annual isotherm of 46 °F (8 °C), homogenous vegetation such as occurs in pine forest biomes, and light soils with humus for sufficient ground moisture. Wellmer and Jusatz determined that the foci are limited to a few square kilometers each, and that a density of only 1 virus-infected tick per 1,000 ticks was required to maintain a natural nidus, which the German geographers called a *standortraum* (multifactor location space). They mapped and analyzed the geoecological conditions for the repeated infection of specific regions by infected ticks and the recurrent infections of people who entered the natural nidus. (See Vignette 3-2, on field mapping.) American studies have not been so specific, although there are two excellent candidate diseases to research: Rocky Mountain spotted fever (RMSF) and Lyme disease.

Tick vectors pose a four-stage ecological puzzle. RMSF is generally vectored by the "dog tick," *Dermacentor variabilis,* and Lyme disease by the "deer tick," *Ixodes scapularis* (now considered to include *I. dammini*). There are important differences between the two disease systems, but they have the basics in common. Three separate blood meals are required for the life cycle. The adult female lays up to 10,000 eggs which hatch into six-legged larvae vernacularly called "seed ticks." These must feed for a week on a small animal, usually a rodent or rabbit. Then the larvae drop off and metamorphize into eight-legged nymphs. Nymphs climb grass and bushes and "quest" vigorously, waving their legs at vibration, heat, or carbon dioxide, for an animal host and another blood meal. After feeding, they drop off and change into adult ticks. According to climate and species, nymphs instead of adults may crawl under leaves or other cover to spend the winter. In spring they emerge hungry for another meal and able to infect new rodents before new tick larvae hatch. Adult ticks need a third blood meal. They may also feed on rodents, rabbits, opossum, or even birds (useful for dissemination), but they tend to be more discriminating in what they latch on to. They prefer deer, raccoon, fox, or other large mammals such as dogs, which can disperse them over a wider territory. Each of these blood meals provides an opportunity for the tick to become infected and in turn infect its next host. Here RMSF and Lyme diverge, however. The agent of Lyme is a spirochete, a bacteria, *Borrelia burgdorferi* (Vignette 2-1, Table 1). Each larva must begin the cycle of infection again and the enzootic disease is maintained by 25–50% infection rates of nymphs. The rickettsial agent of RMSF, *Rickettsia ricketsii,* can pass transovarially in ticks to the new generation. Even less than 10% infection rates among ticks seem adequate to maintain the disease system, because the tick itself is the reservoir. The landscape epidemiology of both rests on the tick's habitat, abundance of small mammals, winter shelter, dehydrating sun, bird predators, and such. RMSF involves the intrusion of people into the natural nidus of the disease (May's silent zone). Lyme seems to result from the expansion of the nidus to include people.

RMSF, sometimes called tick-borne typhus, was first identified in Montana and Idaho (hence its name), but it is most common today in the Piedmont region of the southeastern United States. It has been isolated from the chipmunk, meadow vole, pine vole, white-footed mouse, cotton rat, cottontail rabbit, opossum, and snowshoe hare, and serological (antibody) evidence for infection has been found in many other mammals (Burgdorfer, 1980). Better publicity has enabled RMSF to be diagnosed earlier and treated with antibiotics, sometimes even before diagnosis. Although this complicates statistical reporting, it has brought the case mortality down considerably. The onset of the disease involves fever, chills, aches, nausea, and a rash that spreads from the wrists and ankles. Many of these symptoms are common to other diseases and are easily misdiagnosed without antibody identification. Many cases are so mild they are asymptomatic. Of those who do develop disease symptoms and are not promptly treated, however, 6% to 15% may die.

RMSF has been increasing in the United States, especially in the Southeast. It is hard to determine how much of the increase is due to greater incidence and how much to better reporting. The increase and focus of the disease is attributable to the rapid extension of suburbs into the wooded, open-field habitat of the dog tick. The Piedmont is one of the most rapidly growing regions within the southeastern sun belt. The new suburban houses, parks, jogging paths, and family dog sojourns are in the natural nidus of RMSF. It is normally a zoonosis transmitted among small mammals, but when human residential land use and recreation are extended into the woods, infected ticks can be brought home to houses and yards.

It is not certain whether Lyme disease was relocated from Europe, where the spirochete has been well established, or had an indigenous variant here. It causes initial symptoms of the generic headache/bodyache/fatigue variety. If not treated, serious symptoms of crippling arthritis and heart abnormalities or neurological complications can develop months or years later. The first U.S. cases were identified in 1962 in Lyme, Connecticut. Lyme already has spread to the Pacific and the southeastern coast and Piedmont. It has established three main foci: New England and the surrounding area, the upper Midwest, and the Pacific Northwest (Herrington, 1995). In the east, the reafforestation that has occurred since midcentury has brought the white-tailed deer and other forest animals back to levels not seen in two centuries. Deer, raccoon, and other animals favored by the deer tick (which is somewhat misnamed, as there are ticks that spend their entire life on deer whereas *I. scapularis* needs three separate hosts) are those most quickly domiciliating to suburban residential areas. This is an intense nidus with often more than half the adult deer ticks infected. Diffusion has occurred along deer paths in river corridors and electric pylon corridors into suburban areas. The West Coast nidus is not so dangerous for people. The main tick involved there, *I. neotomae*, is the most infected but feeds on the chief reservoir, woodland rats, not people. A second tick, *I. pacificus*, which feeds on many different hosts including rats and people, is needed to connect the nidus to humans, but because of its diverse diet, as it were, the linking tick's prevalence of infection is low.

The cultural interventions and buffers for the two systems are similar. (No text figure is included: Try to diagram them.) Both diseases can be treated successfully with antibiotics if caught early. Theoretically, reservoir hosts can be destroyed; even if people wanted to exterminate the local deer, however, taking on the white-footed mouse would seem impossible. Because ticks get dehydrated on their questing roosts in the summer sun, by late afternoon they usually have climbed down to the cooler and humid ground. Therefore, walking into the nidus at the end of the day is protective. The different stages of the tick can be killed with insecticide, sprayed in the yard, or put on the dog. Around the house, keeping the lawn mowed short and brushing out of the dog's fenced yard help keep the ticks away. Body buffers while walking into the nidus include long, white pants (for easy viewing) tucked, even taped, into socks and boots, and long sleeves,; repellent perhaps. Because it takes hours of feeding for the tick to pass the infection, the best single body buffer is careful examination of children and dogs a couple times a day. For the pinhead-size nymph of deer tick, this is, of course, easier said than done.

Other Transmissible Diseases

It is not possible in one chapter to discuss many of even the most serious transmissible diseases. Onchocerciasis, or river blindness, is a filarial disease that has for centuries denied some of the most fertile alluvial land to agricultural settlement in West Africa and parts of Central America. The intensive multinational assault of the World Health Organization on its West African nidus is one of the success stories of the past decade. Filariasis (elephantiasis) occurs throughout tropical Asia and Africa and in India and elsewhere is heading to the city with the Culex mosquito. Trypanosomiasis, or African sleeping sickness, affects all efforts of hydroelectric, agricultural, and transportation development in Africa, to which it is confined by its uniquely occurring vector, the tsetse fly. Chagas's disease, or American trypanosomiasis, becomes more serious in South America with every settlement that pushes into the Amazon. It too has spread to the city with migrants, and to the United States; besides expansion of its nidus, it threatens the blood supply for transfusions. Innumerable arboviruses occur whose implications for human health are not even known. The diseases identified by the tables in this chapter are all suitable subjects for analysis using landscape epidemiology.

REGIONALIZATION

In the beginning of this chapter we stated that landscape epidemiology involved four types of regions whose dynamics and locations imparted pattern to the distribution of disease. Let us review some aspects of nidal disease in these terms.

Despite the transportation and mobility transformations of the last few centuries, many nidal diseases are still limited to their realm of evolution. Trypanosomiasis occurs only in Africa because the tsetse fly occurs only there. Schistosomiasis and onchocerciasis must have been introduced to the United States thousands of times, but because the necessary species of snails and blackflies are absent, the diseases cannot establish themselves (although suitable vector substitutes were found in tropical America). Plague, on the other hand, has found enough ecological parallelism in various species of burrowing rodents to have become thoroughly established (by relocation diffusion) in all the grassland biomes.

Biomes, encompassing as they do biotic expression of climate, topography, and soils, broadly categorize the conditions under which a wide variety of nidal diseases flourish, survive, or occur periodically. Mosquito-borne diseases are much more complexly established and intensively transmitted in rain forest and subtropical rice lands than in deciduous forest and cannot be endemic in coniferous regions unless bird migrations or other mediums connect biomes. The disappearance of a disease at a certain elevation in a country's highlands is often the first clue that the disease is transmitted by mosquitoes. Trypanosomiasis disappears as one journeys from the wet savanna to the dry. Mountains and high latitude lands are the favored biome for flea-, louse-, and tick-borne diseases.

The culture realm determines many of the ways the habitat is modified and the population is exposed to or protected from disease. In May's example (1958a), the lowland Vietnamese who built their houses on the ground were part of the Chinese culture realm, not the Southeast Asian realm in which houses are built on stilts. The dispersed settlement form helped prevent malarial transmission in parts of the United States, an advantage the nuclear European villages did not have during many centuries of endemic malaria. Types of clothes and construction materials are cultural characteristics that have profoundly affected the importance of disease transmitted by sand flies, mosquitoes, and lice.

Realm of evolution, biome, and culture realm overlap to delimit broad regions of disease occurrence, but it is at the microscale that one can determine the limiting factors of disease transmission and specify intervention points. A transmissible disease does not occur uniformly across the earth's surface. The dynamics of its occurrence from season to season and year to year are affected foot by foot by the immediate weather, soils, topography, land use, and flora and fauna. People can destroy a nidus of disease by exterminating the reservoir or plowing up the vector's habitat and not know what they are doing. They can also bring in water or clear vegetation and create conditions conducive to intense disease transmission without planning for those consequences. Mapping the exact location and conditions where disease transmission is marginal or most intense is of great significance for breaking transmission paths or protecting the population (Vignette 3-2).

One of the major developments in the study, regionalization, analytical modeling, epidemic surveillance, and prediction of vectored diseases in this century is the ongoing development and application of GIS technology and methodology (Chapter 13). Satellite imagery (remote sensing), field surveys of land and people, and epidemiological data can be combined to detect such habitat changes as extent of flooding (and mosquito outbreaks) or to specify the vegetation, slope, and topographic conditions of a targeted nidus

(Mott, Nuttall, Desjeux, & Cattand, 1995). Efforts are being made to predict outbreaks of Rift Valley fever from water-on-the-land, give early warning of major crop failures and famine, track locust breeding conditions and outbreak paths, and in general monitor and/or model numerous habitat change and vectored disease relationsips. There are serious scale issues that have not yet been worked out, such as how to use vegetation or slope information by the acre when tick density varies by the foot and population data are at a county scale. Nevertheless, remote sensing is becoming vital to landscape analysis and international relief and intervention. Vectored diseases such as dengue and malaria have also been targets of a lot of concern and speculation about the impact of global warming, and research efforts are being made to develop simulations using GIS. The World Health Organization (WHO) is now trying to use its website to encourage such applications and make GIS software and analytical programs accessible to poor countries (Vignette 12-1). The part of its website devoted to control of tropical disease connects to many studies as examples, such as WHO planning and implementation of onchocerciasis eradication in West Africa. The website presents examples of methods of integrating field survey; satellite usage; multiple land use covers of settlement, agriculture, streams, and topography; as well as soils, health service, and more, through use of a GIS. It also encourages the adoption of this methodology elsewhere.

CONCLUSION

North American geographers are not familiar with the approach of landscape epidemiology. They are more used to analyzing the patterns within a city, using socioeconomic, ethnic, and demographic factors to explain the occurrence of phenomena such as homicide, tuberculosis, or heart attacks, and then regionalizing to determine the most efficient locations for treatment given the incidence patterns (see later chapters). Asking many of the same geographic questions but using the methodology of disease ecology, medical geographers can analyze the biogeography of nidal disease systems to specify location and system interaction points that will ease control or eradication. More can be done to minimize transmission of nidal diseases and maximize health education, vaccination, and regulatory protection of targeted groups.

REFERENCES

Ackerknecht, E. H. (1945). *Malaria in the upper Mississippi Valley 1760–1900*. Baltimore: Johns Hopkins University Press.
Benenson, A. S. (Ed.). (1995). *Control of communicable diseases in man* (16th ed.). Washington, DC: American Public Health Association.
Burgdorfer, W. (1980). Spotted fever-group diseases. In J. H. Steele (Ed.), Section A:

Bacterial, Rickettsial, and Mycotic Disease (vol. 2, pp. 279–302). [C.R.C. Handbook Series in Zoonoses]. Boca Raton, FL: CRC Press.

Calhoun, J. B. (1979). *The ecology of the Norway rat*. Bethesda, MD: U.S. Department of Health, Education and Welfare.

Carter, H. R. (1919). The malaria problem of the South. *Public Health Reports, 34,* 1927–1935.

Childs, S. J. R. (1949). *Malaria and colonization in the Carolina low country, 1526–1696* [Johns Hopkins University Studies in Historical and Political Science Series 58, No. 1]. Baltimore: Johns Hopkins University Press.

Daniels, T. J., & Falco, R. C. (1989). The Lyme disease invasion. *Natural History, 7,* 4–10.

Diamond, J. (1997). *Guns, germs, and steel*. New York: Norton.

Drake, D. (1854). *A systematic treatise, historical, etiological and practical, on the principal diseases of the interior valley of North America*. New York: Lenox Hill.

Farid, M. A. (1980). Round table: The malaria programme-from euphoria to anarchy. *World Health Forum, 1,* 8–33.

Gubler, D. J., & Trent, D. W. (1993). Emergence of epidemic dengue/dengue hemorrhagic fever as a public health problem in the Americas. *Infectious Agents and Disease, 2,* 383–393.

Halstead, S. B. (1980). Dengue haemorrhagic fever: A public health problem and a field of research. *Bulletin of the World Health Organization, 58,* 1–21.

Herrington, J. E. (1995). An update on Lyme Disease. *Health and Environmental Digest, 9,* 29–32.

Hunter, J. M. (1980). Strategies for the control of river blindness. In M. S. Meade (Ed.), *Conceptual and methodological issues in medical geography* (pp. 38–76). Chapel Hill: University of North Carolina, Department of Geography.

Jusatz, H. J. (Ed.). (1968–1980). *Medizinische Landerkunde* (vols. 1–6) [Geomedical Monograph Series]. Berlin: Springer-Verlag.

Knight, G. (1971). The ecology of African sleeping sickness. *Annals of the Association of American Geography, 61,* 23–44.

Kucheruk, V. V. (1965). Problems of Palaeo-genesis of natural pest foci with reference to the history of rodent fauna. In A. N. Formasov (Ed.), *Fauna and ecology of the rodents*. Moscow: Moscow Society of Naturalists.

McNeill, W. H. (1976). *Plagues and peoples*. New York: Doubleday.

Markovin, A. P. (1962). Historical sketch of the development of Soviet medical geography. *Soviet Geography: Review and Translation, 3,* 3–19.

May, J. M. (1958a). *The ecology of human disease*. New York: MD Publications.

May, J. M. (1958b). *Studies in disease ecology*. New York: Hafner.

Meade, M. S. (1976a). Land development and human health in West Malaysia. *Annals of the Association of American Geographers, 66,* 428–439.

Meade, M. S. (1976b). A new disease in Southeast Asia: Man's creation of dengue haemorrhagic fever. *Pacific Viewpoint, 17,* 133–146.

Meade, M. S. (1977). Medical geography as human ecology: The dimension of population movement. *Geographical Review, 67,* 379–393.

Meade, M. S. (1980). The rise and demise of malaria: Some reflections on southern landscape. *Southeastern Geographer, 20,* 77–99.

Mott, K. E., Nuttall, I., Desjeux, P., & Cattand, P. (1995). New geographical approaches to control of some parasitic zoonoses. *Bulletin of the World Health Organization, 73,* 247–257.

Pavlovsky, E. N. (1966). *The natural nidality of transmissible disease* (N. D. Levine, Ed.). Urbana: University of Illinois Press.

Pollitzer, R. (1954). *Plague* [Monograph Series 22]. Geneva: World Health Organization.

Prothero, R. M. (1961). Population movements and problems of malaria eradication in Africa. *Bulletin of the World Health Organization, 24,* 405–425.

Rodenwaldt, E., & Jusatz, H. J. (Eds.). (1952–1961). *Welt-Seuchen Atlas.* Hamburg: Falk.

Sandosham, A. A. (1970). Malaria in rural Malaya. *Medical Journal of Malaya, 24,* 221–226.

Shell, E. R. (1997). Resurgence of a deadly disease. *Atlantic Monthly, 280,* 45–60.

Stevens, J. (1977). American mobilization for the conquest of malaria in the United States. *Journal of the National Malaria Society, 3,* 7–10.

U.S. Census Bureau. (1890). *1890 census of population.* Washington, DC: U.S. Government Printing Office.

Weil, C., & Kvale, K. M. (1985). Current research on geographical aspects of schistosomiasis. *Geographical Review, 75,* 186–216).

Wellmer, H., & Jusatz, H. J. (1981). Geoecological analysis of the spread of tick-borne encephalitis in Central Europe. *Social Science and Medicine, 5D,* 159–162.

Wills, C. (1996). *Yellow fever, black goddess: The coevolution of people and plagues.* New York: Addison-Wesley.

World Health Organization. (1999). *The World Health Report 1999.* Geneva: Author.

Wyler, D. J. (1993). Malaria: overview and update. *Clinical Infectious Diseases, 16,* 449–458.

FURTHER READING

Bruce-Chwatt, L. J. (1985). *Essential malariology* (2nd ed.). New York: Wiley.

Crosby, A. (1972). *The Columbian exchange: Biological consequences of 1492.* Westport, CT: Greenwood.

Crosby, A. (1986). *Ecological imperialism: the biological expansion of Europe, 900–1900.* Cambridge, UK: Cambridge University Press.

Fonaroff, L. S. (1968). Man and malaria in Trinidad: Ecological perspectives on a changing health hazard. *Annals of the Association of American Geographers, 58,* 526–556.

Garrett, L. (1994). *The coming plague: Newly emerging diseases in a world out of balance.* New York: Farrar, Straus & Giroux; Penguin Books.

Gottfried, R. S. (1983). *The black death.* New York: Free Press.

Haddock, K. C. (1981). Control of schistosomiasis: The Puerto Rican experience. *Social Science and Medicine, 15D,* 501–514.

Harrison, G. (1978). *Mosquitoes, malaria and man: A history of the hostilities since 1880.* New York: Dutton.

Harwood, R. F., & James, M. T. (1983). *Entomology in human and animal health* (7th ed.). New York: Macmillan.

Houle, J. S. (1991). *Dermacentor variabilis in space.* Master's thesis, University of North Carolina at Chapel Hill.

Hunter, J. M. (1993). Elephantiasis: A disease of development in Northeast Ghana. *Social Science and Medicine, 35,* 627–49.

Hunter, J. M. (1990). Bot-fly maggot infestation in Latin America. *Geographical Review, 80*, 382–398.

Learmonth, A. T. A. (1977). Malaria. In G. M. Howe (Ed.), *A world geography of human diseases* (pp. 61–108). London: Academic Press.

Learmonth, A. (1988). *Disease ecology*. Oxford: Basil Blackwell.

Lederberg, J., Shope, R. E., Stanley C., & Oaks, J. (1992). *Emerging infections*. Washington, DC: National Academy Press.

May, R. M. (1994). Chagas disease in changing environments. In B. Cartledge (Eds), *Health and the environment* Oxford: Oxford University Press.

Maupin, G. O., Fish, D., Zultowskiy, J., Campus, E. & Piesman, J. (1991). Landscape ecology of Lyme disease in a residential area of Westchester, N. Y. *American Journal of Epidemiology, 133*, 1105–1113.

Moulton, F. R. (Ed.). (1941). *A symposium on human malaria*. Washington, DC: American Association for the Advancement of Science.

Palka, E. J., & Crawford, T. W. (1994). North Carolina: Natural nidus for Rocky Mountain spotted fever. *North Carolina Geographer, 3*, 1–16.

Prothero, R. M. (1963). Population mobility and trypanosomiasis in Africa. *Bulletin of the World Health Organization, 28*, 615–626.

Pyle, G. F., & Cook, R. M. (1978). Environmental risk factors of California encephalitis in man. *Geographical Review, 68*, 157–170.

Rahn, D. W., & J. Evans, J. (Eds.). (1998). *Lyme disease*. Philadelphia: American College of Physicians.

Rodriguez, A. D., Rodriguez, M. H., Hernandez, J. E., Dister, S. W., Beck, L. A., Rejmankora, E., & Roberts, D. R. (1996). Landscape surrounding human settlements and *Anopheles albimanus (Diptera: Culicidae)* abundance in southern Chiapas, Mexico. *Journal of Medical Entomology, 33*, 39–48.

Rosicky, B., & Heyberger, K. (Eds.). (1965). *Theoretical questions of natural foci of disease*. Prague: Czechoslovak Academy of Science.

Sauer, C. O. (1925). *The morphology of landscape*. University of California Publications in Geography, *2*, 19–53.

Schulze, T. L., Taylor, R. C., Taylor, G. C., & Bosler, E. M. (1991). Lyme disease: A proposed ecological index to assess areas of risk in the northeastern United States. *American Journal of Public Health, 81*, 714–718.

Singhanetra, R. A. (1993). Malaria and mobility in Thailand. *Social Science and Medicine, 37*, 1147–1154.

Vachon, M. (1993). Onchocerciasis in Chiapis, Mexico. *Geographical Review, 83*, 141–149.

Wellmer, H. (1983). Some reflections on the ecology of dengue haemorrhagic fever in Thailand. In N. D. McGlashan & J. R. Blunden (Eds.), *Geographical aspects of health*. London: Academic Press.

White, G. F., Bradley, D. J., & White, A. (1972). *Drawers of water: Domestic water in East Africa*. Chicago: University of Chicago Press.

VIGNETTE 3-1.   Physical Zonation of Climates and Biomes

The diurnal and annual variations in intensity of solar radiation and the amount and timing of precipitation, temperature, and humidity have been described, classified, and analyzed in dozens of ways. The variations are complicated by the tilt of the earth's axis, the physiography of mountains and depressions, the contrasts of land and sea, and the size of continents. The broad zones of vegetation, or biomes, that result are also zones of agricultural cropping patterns and of arthropod habitat. The schema in Vignette Figure 3-1 of a prototype continent is simplified but provides a general framework for considering the study of health through landscape epidemiology and biometeorology.

Seasons occur as the tilt of the earth's axis alternately exposes the Northern and Southern Hemispheres to more direct rays from the sun. The vertical rays are limited to the latitudes between the Tropic of Cancer and the Tropic of Capricorn, with the highest annual amounts being received at the equator and the least at the poles. Because hot air rises and cold air sinks, the equatorial area is a zone of low pressure as the air rises, and the poles are zones of cold, subsiding, dry air (see Vignette 3-1, Figure 1). Because cold air can contain less water vapor than an equal volume of warm air, water condenses as the air rises at the equator and cools at higher elevations, producing continually high levels of rainfall over the year. Similarly, the subsiding air at the poles is warmed as it approaches the earth's surface, and because its capacity to hold water vapor is increased, there is little precipitation. Due to processes of atmospheric circulation, air also subsides at around 30° north and south latitude, forming a zone of little precipitation. Because of the lack of cloud cover, this zone receives more radiation at the surface than does the equatorial zone. As subsiding air at 30° latitude and subsiding air at the poles move over the earth's surface and converge, air rises along a broad frontal zone in the middle latitudes and creates a wet but cooler zone. There is less precipitation in this midlatitude zone than in the equatorial, but because there is also less evaporation and less transpiration from plants, there is high availability of water.

Different vegetational zones, known as biomes, extend over large areas. The biomes are adapted to differences in temperature and precipitation, as well as to seasonal variation. The complex and luxuriant rain forest needs continually wet conditions and high solar radiation, whereas lichen and other tundra vegetation can grow in cold, dry conditions with a short season of long days of solar radiation. As Vignette 3-1, Figure 1 indicates, moving from the poles to the equator, there is a transition of forest type from needleleaf (coniferous, taiga, boreal) to temperate deciduous forest, which loses its leaves in the cold season, to subtropi-

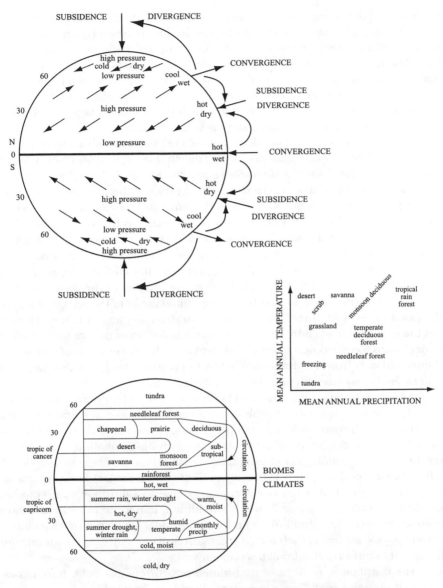

VIGNETTE 3-1, FIGURE 1. Physical zonation of climates and biomes.

cal forests that include evergreen plants such as magnolias and palms, to the tropical rain forest. Desert may be hot or cold, but it is dry; types of desert vegetation such as creosote bush and cactus merge into types of grassland or evergreen scrub as water increases. The savanna biome is grassland, with scattered monsoon deciduous trees, that has adapted to conditions of summer rain and winter drought. At its dry margins the trees are sparse and the grass short, but as it extends toward the equator the trees increase in density until savanna merges into forest. Chaparral is the American name for the biome of evergreen brush that has adapted to the severe conditions of summer drought and winter rain. Grassland, known variously as prairie, steppe, pampas, and veld, extends from short, bunched grass on the arid margins to tall, dense grass on the woodland border.

Broad climatic patterns determine the general pattern of biome location. As can be seen from the prototype continent, the hot, wet equatorial zone coincides with the tropical rain forest biome, and the cold, dry polar zone with tundra. The subsiding zone of air at 30° latitude creates two broad bands of desert, including the Sahara, Gobi (displaced northward by Tibetan mountains), and North American deserts in the Northern Hemisphere and the Kalahari, Australian, and Atacama deserts in the Southern. The rising-air, wet zone is characterized by needleleaf vegetation at its colder latitudes and temperate deciduous at its warmer latitudes. As the climatic zones shift north and south with the sun's rays, they bring wet–dry seasonality to much of the tropics. The area between the equatorial wet and the 30° dry zone supports a savanna or monsoon deciduous vegetation. The area between the 30° subsiding zone and the midlatitude wet zone is characterized by chaparral. Finally, because of the rotation of the earth, air masses revolve and winds blow in ways that bring humid air from the sea into land on the eastern side of continents but bring only overland, dry air to the western side. On the eastern side of continents, there is a transition from tundra to needleleaf to deciduous to subtropical to rain forest, while on the western side of continents the transition is from tundra to needleleaf to chaparral to desert to savanna to rain forest. Grassy biomes cover the transitional areas.

A last complication is introduced by altitude. The atmosphere cools with increasing altitude. Mountains, furthermore, form barriers so that surface air must go up on the windward side, causing precipitation, and come down on the leeward, forming a "rain shadow," or dry area. An altitudinal zonation of vegetation results that is very similar to the latitudinal zonation that was presented earlier. A tall mountain on the equator (as occurs in Kenya and Ecuador) has a vegetation zonation that proceeds from rain forest at its base to subtropoical, deciduous, needleleaf, tundra, and ice on its windward side and rain forest to savanna, thornbush scrub, needleleaf, and tundra on its leeward side. No matter in what climatic zone people are living, therefore, a great variety of vegetation, agricultural, and living conditions exists for human settlements.

The distribution of diseases transmitted by arthropods—ticks, mosquitoes, flies, and so forth—in different parts of the world can be partly understood from biome distribution. Certain nutritional deficiencies are associated with specific staple crops (see Chapter 2), and cultivation of these crops often follows environmental constraints of biome distribution. Conditions of hazard from air pollution (see Chapter 8) or solar radiation (see Chapter 5) also largely coincide with biome distribution patterns. Understanding the location of major earth biomes can provide a useful framework for understanding the spatial patterns of the distribution of many health hazards.

VIGNETTE 3-2.   Field Mapping for Landscape Epidemiology

Broad patterns of the occurrence of transmissible diseases may be generalized from biome distribution, as depicted in Vignette 3-1. Only the largest-scale topographic maps, however, which show the smallest areas, have the necessary detail of slope, vegetation, and water occurrence and flow to be useful in landscape epidemiology. It is one thing to establish that malaria, onchocerciasis, or California encephalitis is endemic in a place. It is another to specify exactly where people are exposed or where factors in the natural nidus are most susceptible to intervention or avoidance.

Field mapping is a valuable technique for such analysis. Often a base map can be constructed from air photos or satellite imagery. Elevation (and therefore slope) can be determined, and detailed contour maps can be constructed for the study area. Sometimes a topographic map of sufficiently large scale is already available. In the past the geographer engaged in fieldwork sometimes had to triangulate between flagged sticks with a compass and construct a base map from scratch. This can now be done much more exactly as well as more easily using geopositioning systems (GPS) off a satellite. Analysis of air photography, composite satellite imagery, and field techniques is taught in many geography curriculums. Products such as topographic maps or land (tax) plats can now often be scanned into a computer system, although detail and complexity can still be problems requiring researcher generalization and categorization. As is commonly the case with GIS and remote sensing, "ground truth" for accuracy and interpretation still needs to be done through fieldwork.

Vignette 3-2, Figure 1 illustrates the importance of such detailed habitat mapping for understanding the transmission of disease. When the water level rose one year, the foundations of houses became islands of higher land. Rats left their preferred sedge nesting areas and moved into close proximity with humans. Thus a change in river level resulted in greatly increased opportunity for the transmission of flea-, mite-, and tick-borne diseases to the human population.

Meade's investigation of health consequences from the resettlement of people in the government's land development program in Malaysia included a study of biotic changes and increase or decrease of transmissible disease risk (Meade, 1976a). A field map for a land settlement scheme and a traditional village was constructed using a Bronson compass and branches stuck in cans of cement, by which to triangulate (Vignette 3-2, Figure 2). In that way, paths, orchards and vegetable gardens, and areas marshy after storms could be mapped as well as houses and particular buildings. Rat traps were set on a spatial sampling frame for fixed periods of time. After the rats were chloroformed, their ears were exam-

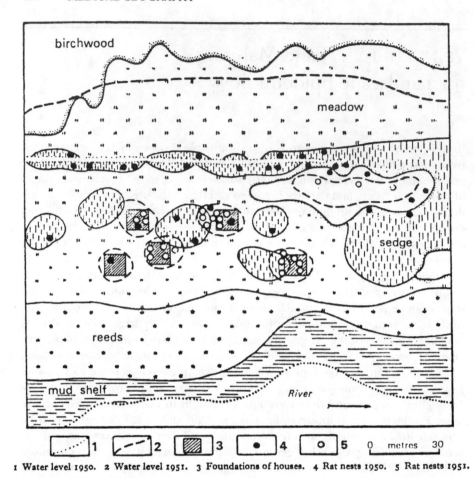

i Water level 1950.   2 Water level 1951.   3 Foundations of houses.   4 Rat nests 1950.   5 Rat nests 1951.

VIGNETTE 3-2, FIGURE 1. Microscale mapping of landscape. From Kucheruk (1965, p. 98). Copyright 1965 by Moscow Society of Naturalists. Reprinted by permission.

ined for the species of mite that transmits scrub typhus. Thus, although laboratory studies could not be done to identify antibodies or to culture the rickettsias, the presence of all other elements necessary for the diseases's transmission and their locational risk could be ascertained. The micromobility of the population could then be studied in relation to dangerous habitat.

The land scheme represented a reversal from the traditional village habitat danger. In the village, most of the *lalang* (*Imperator cylindrica*), a coarse, invasive grass that was preferred rat habitat, occurred in open space associated with the rubber trees where the men tapping latex were occupationally exposed to rat mites. Villagers walked on the road in this linear settlement and had little exposure. The land scheme, however, had created a nuclear settlement containing

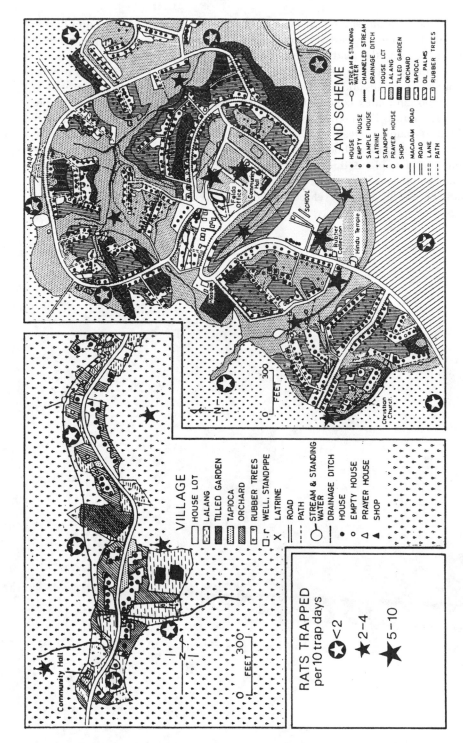

VIGNETTE 3-2, FIGURE 2. Land-use habitat for scrub typhus and the changes resulting from land development.

considerable vacant space that was occupied by *lalang*. The houses had quarter-acre lots that often extended into the ravines, where settlers planted papaya trees and tapioca that the field rats also consumed. Because of the form of the settlement, women and children going to the school, clinic, or store walked on paths through the ravines and fields of grass and were exposed to mites. The area near the school and latex collection station was especially heavily populated by rats and their mites. The men tapping the rubber trees, in contrast, had been disciplined to maintain clean cultivation and control the grass and weeds. Few rats were trapped in the rubber cropland. Much of the vacant land within the settlement had been planned for future development. The *lalang* always invades such vacant, sunny lots. Leaving the undeveloped land under trees, or planting rubber trees there until it was developed, might have reduced the hazard of scrub typhus.

4

Developmental Change and Human Health

The human population of earth, now more than 6 billion, has tripled since World War II. It will increase by more than half again before stabilizing late in the 21st century. After increasing for centuries, population growth peaked at a little over 2% a year in the late 1960s and then began to slow down. Although the present growth rate of 1.4% is likely to continue to decrease, these lower rates are occurring due to a greatly enlarged base, resulting in the absolutely largest population increases in history. The human population will grow by more than 800 million in each of the next three decades. Its age structure will change during this time as a higher proportion become older. The major causes of death will change. The human population of earth will undergo the profound alteration of becoming primarily urban.

The purpose of this chapter is to explain some of the complexity and dynamics of population–habitat–behavior interactions that comprise disease systems and the consequent need for careful evaluation of health consequences in developmental impact analysis. The concepts developed in the chapters on cultural ecology and landscape epidemiology are applied here to show how social and economic change affect disease occurrence. Because population growth and urbanization are among the most powerful forces for change in today's world, models of population transition (mortality, fertility, and mobility) are presented first. Then some ways in which ecological relationships can complicate the transition are discussed. Changes in disease prevalence resulting from development in Africa, Latin America, and Southeast Asia are reviewed. The impact of urbanization and differences from the Western experience are discussed. The final section discusses the implications of global warming, land-use change, urbanization and mobility change, and organizational change with globalization for the emergence of new diseases.

THE CONTEXT OF POPULATION CHANGE

There have been two waves of population growth in recent history. Beginning in the 1700s, European population grew for 200 years, sometimes reaching growth rates of a little over 1% a year. Europeans migrated to the Americas, Australia, and elsewhere so that some of the increased population was redistributed on earth. Today Europeans and their descendants elsewhere have, or are approaching, fertility (birth) below the rate of reproduction which would replace themselves.

The second wave began to build mainly after World War II, when many Third World countries achieved independence. Spreading like a wave around the world, population growth first in Latin America, then Asia, and then Africa crested at more than 3% (in a few countries even 4%) a year before the rate of increase started to decline. There are no "new worlds" to populate, but pressure for redistribution has become evident. Some of the most rapid growth is occurring in places with the most meager environmental and economic resources. A large part of the world's income and wealth has become concentrated in some countries and population growth in others. The World Bank (1993) estimated a few years ago that the "industrial market" high-income countries, with 15% of the world's population, had a per capita gross national product more than 61 times that of the low-income less developed countries, which had 59% of the population but a life expectancy 15 years less. The gap continues to widen.

What we understand of population growth and change is modeled on the European experience, which is not entirely applicable to current circumstances. The following three models of transition—demographic, mortality, and mobility—are interconnected, as shown in Table 4-1.

The Demographic Transition

Mortality and fertility have both been high, fluctuating around each other, for most of human existence. The progression from this state of affairs to the present conditions of low mortality and fertility in the most economically developed countries is known as the *demographic transition*.

The Swedish demographic experience as shown in Figure 4-1 classically illustrates the model. First, mortality declines. For a while fertility continues at its historically high level. During this early stage of the transition, *natural increase,* the difference between births and deaths, accelerates. Then, under conditions usually associated with urbanization and economic demands for a more educated work force, the birthrate begins to fall. In the classic model, the change to a "small-family norm" happens partly because children who add to the wealth of a family in a rural agrarian society drain a family's wealth in an urban manufacturing society. Research in historical demography, however, has demonstrated that in some parts of rural, agrarian France, fertility

TABLE 4-1. Multiple Transitions

Stage	Demographic	Mortality	Mobility
Historic stable	Birthrates and death rates fluctuating at over 35 per 1,000; population increase imperceptible; >45% population aged under 15, <5% over 65	Life expectancy under 35 years; infant mortality >180 per 1,000; death results mainly from infectious diseases	Individual migration almost unknown except for marriage; circulation local for basic agricultural, commercial and religious needs
Early transition	Death rates fall; birthrates remain high; population grows rapidly by natural increase	Infectious diseases are controlled by sanitation, vaccination, suppression of vectors, and medical treatment; young population has low death rate	Migration from rural areas to cities, agricultural frontiers, and foreign countries; circulation increases socially and for labor
Late transition	Birthrates fall as death rates stabilize; population growth slows and population ages	Degenerative diseases become major causes of death; life expectancy exceeds 65 years	Migration to cities and agricultural frontiers slackens; emigration virtually ceases; circulation increases in structural complexity and intensity
Future stable	Birthrates and death rates fluctuating at less than 20 per 1,000; population increase imperceptible or population declining; <20% population aged under 15, >15% over 65	Life expectancy over 70 years; infant mortality <10 per 1,000; death results mainly from degenerative diseases	Multipurpose and vigorous circulation; migration mainly between cities and for retirement; immigration of labor

actually declined sooner than in urban, industrial England. More attention has been paid recently to cultural attitudes about childbearing, to the status and especially the education of women, and to diffusion of the very idea of birth control. Cultural values and societal mores about such critical behaviors as age at marriage, divorce and remarriage, women working for wages, importance of sons, or costs of dowries matter a lot. Social organizational changes from support by extended families to provision of health, family planning, educational, and child-care services transform the social environment. The transition is completed when birthrates fall to meet low death rates, and even below as has happened in several European countries. The total fertility rate, the average number of children a women would have if she went through her life at today's age specific birthrates, has fallen to 1.6 in Sweden, and as low as 1.2 children in Spain and Italy. The Swedish age structure that results from its low birth and death rates now has about the same proportion over 65 as under 15 (18%).

The circumstances of Third World countries today are different in many

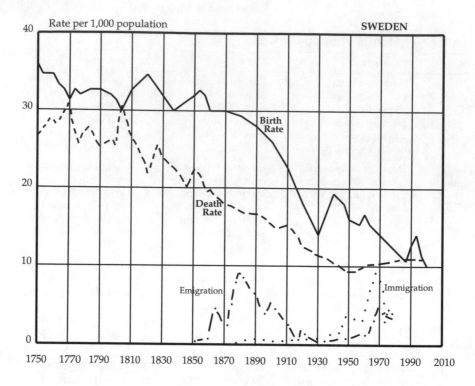

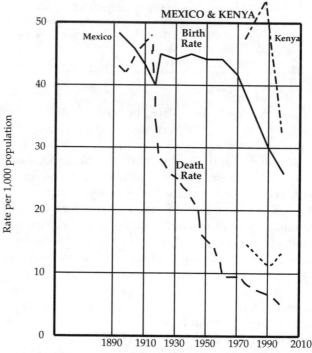

FIGURE 4-1. The demographic transition. Different periods of transition are reflected in the experiences of Sweden, Mexico, and Kenya. Data from Population Reference Bureau.

ways from the context in which Europe went through the transition (Merrick, 1986). The magnitude of population increase is unprecedented. Rates of growth are more than triple those the Europeans experienced because death rates, especially infant mortality, have fallen so rapidly. Such rapid growth places demands on an economy, social institutions, and environment which may threaten to increase death rates again. The decrease in both infant mortality and fertility appeared in the 1980s to have stalled in several countries. Social scientists hypothesized that impact from further advances in technology had diminished and issues of internal distribution, crowding, housing quality, and such become more critical to continued advance. It now seems, however, that there were no prolonged plateaus or upturns in mortality even under conditions of deep economic recession or local war. The progression of the transition now under way everywhere seems relentless, although populations progress at their own rates through their own local problems, causes, and methods. There are *delayed models* in which birthrates remain elevated longer than expected for the levels of urbanization and economic development that have been achieved, as in Mexico (Figure 4-1) until the late 1970s. Mexico today has a total fertility rate of only 3.0 children. There are *accelerated models* in which concerted government programs affecting education, old-age security, women's employment, infant mortality, and contraceptive means and knowledge have resulted in lowered fertility even under agrarian conditions. China, where fertility has been brought down below replacement level even though its society is poor and 70% rural, is the most notorious example because of the means its totalitarian government used in pursuing what was determined to be critical to national survival and development. But Thailand, a poor rural country whose population is less than a third urban, has also brought its fertility down to 2.0 children, without even the suggestion of coercion. With today's technology of contraception and sterilization, given the belief/social will, it is possible for a population to lower its fertility very rapidly. Despite lowered fertility, of course, the size of the population will continue to grow for decades because of "population momentum" that results from current age structure (up to half of the population being children before fertility decline, with their reproductive years ahead). Sub-Saharan Africa, where mortality rates did not fall until after countries became independent, is the region earliest in the demographic transition. Kenya in the 1980s seemed to be paying the price for being well-governed enough to successfully lower its infant mortality below 10%. It had a total fertility rate of more than 8 children and reached an astounding annual population growth of 4.2% with 52% of its population under 15. There was no shortage of voices claiming that Africans were different from other people. Then Kenya's fertility fell, reaching 4.2 children at the end of the century (reduced by half in a dozen years).

The policies by which governments can encourage slower population growth, policies such as educating girl children and lowering infant mortality through vaccination and safe drinking water, have become a global consensus implemented at the United Nations conferences The results of research and policy experience found expression in the 1994 World Population and Development conference in Cairo and the subsequent 1995 Beijing conference on women which focused on how best to implement their empowerment (as in achieving basic literacy everywhere).

The Mortality Transition

One does not expect people in London to be dying by the thousands from malaria or cholera, although they have in the past. Nor would one expect cancer to be a leading cause of death in Nigeria. In any population the major causes of death are related to the levels of economic and institutional development. The changes in health problems that come with economic and social development are often called the mortality, or epidemiological, transition. Again, most of what we know about the mortality transition comes from the experience of Europe and the United States. There are serious questions about its relevance to conditions in the developing world, as well as speculation about the future, next stage, in developed countries that have completed it. Developmental changes have brought many unanticipated consequences.

The Western Experience

In the Western experience, preindustrial populations had high birthrates and death rates. One in five babies commonly died before it was a year old. The death rate for toddlers and small children was almost as high. Life expectancy at birth was about 30 years. Most people, especially in childhood, died from infectious diseases such as smallpox, malaria, pneumonia, typhoid, or whooping cough (pertussis). These diseases were nearly always present in the population. People also died from great epidemics of cholera, yellow fever, and bubonic plague. Some deaths were caused by vectored diseases, but many more deaths resulted from bacteria or viruses that multiplied in filth and were transmitted through water or milk. As the rural poor, displaced by enclosure of the commons and other agricultural changes, flooded the industrializing cities, the combination of crowding in abominable housing conditions, overwork, and malnutrition caused the death rates to soar even higher. For a century the life expectancy of people in urban areas compared unfavorably with the more salubrious countryside. Most cities would have experienced absolute population loss without constant inmigration from the surrounding countryside.

As the negative consequences of industrialization became recognized, perceptual changes led to social movements to improve hygiene and aesthetics. Sewage and garbage were attacked, wells and aqueducts were built, trees were planted, and other improvements were made. The advent and diffusion of germ theory in the late 19th century was followed not only by improved treatment of diseases with new drugs and sterilization but by a public health revolution. Milk was pasteurized, water was chlorinated, and sewage and garbage were removed. New cultural buffers were created to avoid the newly recognized hazard of germs and the need to avoid them: behaviors such as teaching children to avoid eating things which fell on the floor, not to drink in groups from common utensils, and to wash their hands frequently. Children were sent to camp to get clean air and exercise. The newly recognized importance of sunlight and fresh air led to new housing codes and construction of urban parks. Transportation changes allowed the population to spread out and commute to the central city. Death rates declined, population grew, and people who could not be accommodated even by the prosperous, growing industrial economies of Europe poured out to the Americas, Australia, and other parts of the world. After decades, birth rates declined. Not just in a few countries today but in Europe as a whole mortality rates are greater than those of natality. Mortality and natality, it has been supposed in the past, will begin to fluctuate around a new, low level of stabilization, but every indication to date is that population (without inmigration) will continue to decrease. Other countries with advanced economies, such as the United States, Canada, and Japan, have similarly reached the end of demographic transition.

Under conditions of low birthrates and death rates, death results mainly from degenerative and chronic diseases. Only influenza and pneumonia have continued to be mortal infectious diseases of consequence for the population living in the more developed countries, at least until recently when AIDS emerged as a major cause of death for young adults (Chapter 8). Because few children die from infectious diseases, life expectancy at birth is usually over 70 or even 80 years. Heart disease, stroke, and cancer of various kinds become the major causes of death, with kidney disease, diabetes, cirrhosis of the liver, vehicular accidents, and suicide also being very important. The U.S. Centers for Disease Control and Prevention have just now announced marked reduction in death rates from cardiovascular disease; this latest has also been found in Europe (Warnes, 1999).

Other Transitions

Figure 4-2 presents the transition in causes of death from infectious agents to degenerative and other noncommunicable causes. Whether countries are categorized by national income levels or by world regions, the shift to noncommunicable diseases and the importance of cardiovascular diseases and cancer are clear. Lung cancer is increasing as a cause of death in the developing world (as people become affluent enough to smoke cigarettes) and looms tragically in the future of China. Traffic accidents are also becoming a major public health concern in the Americas, Southeast Asia, and the Western Pacific. For developing countries, the dominance of AIDS and malaria in Africa and the continuing importance of diarrhea and tuberculosis throughout the developing world is clear (World Health Organization, 1999).

114

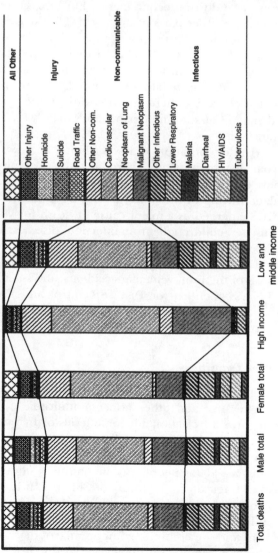

WHO Member States: Percent of Total Deaths

(A)

(B)

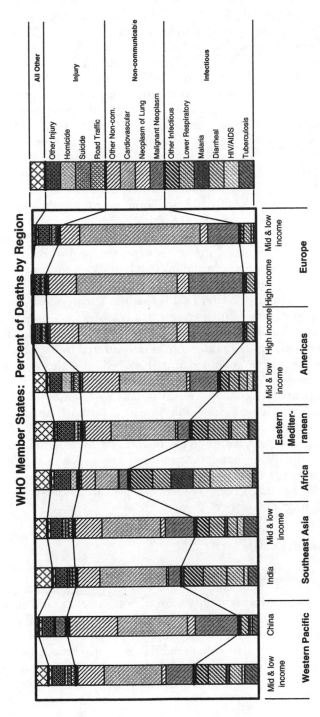

FIGURE 4-2. Causes of death, 1998. Causes of death classified by major infectious, noncommunicable, and violence categories for world countries. Regions are those of the World Health Organization. Data from World Health Organization (1999).

115

After World War II, death rates began to fall rapidly in many newly independent, low-income countries. Infant mortality rates that had been more than 200 per 1,000 fell to perhaps 90, and life expectancy rose to 55 years in many countries. Several factors account for the rather precipitous decline in mortality and consequent growth in population. Antibiotics and other drugs became widely available for the first time. Although biomedical health services are still not available to many rural poor, they are generally accessible in the urban areas. Many countries organized and established programs to vaccinate babies for smallpox, diptheria, and whooping cough. DDT and other insecticides were used to attack malaria, yellow fever, and many vectored diseases, with results that were often dramatic. World Health Organization campaigns to eradicate smallpox and to obliterate yaws (which, having a bacterial agent, responded to a single dose of penicillin) were sensationally successful. Most people concerned with health and development came to assume that the Third World would follow rather closely the Western model and that the demographic problem was controlling births. Death rates, however, have often stopped declining far short of the levels expected on the basis of the Western experience. Development programs that have been successful in increasing incomes have sometimes not reduced mortality but, for some causes, even increased it, as discussed later in this chapter. Furthermore, there is a fragility to the adjusted state of interactions that is seldom perceived. Even well-established declines in death rates can be adversely affected by deterioration of the economy and social organization, as is illustrated by Russia (Table 7-1). When the Soviet system collapsed in the early 1990s, the turmoil in economy and society was quickly reflected in soaring mortality. The increased death from cardiovascular disease is usually ascribed largely to the impact of alcohol. The increase in infectious disease is variously attributed to poor quality control for vaccines and failure of delivery systems, deterioration of nutrition, housing and heat, failure to pay medical personel, and failure to produce and supply medicine or blood products. Epidemics of diphtheria and whooping cough, even in Moscow, affected mostly small children at startlingly high rates. Suicide has become epidemic, especially among those with their pensions and their life's work destroyed.

Water-Related Infectious Disease

Infectious diseases continue to be the leading causes of death and morbidity in the world, especially in infants and children. Tuberculosis killed a million and a half people in 1998, whooping cough almost 300,000, and measles 900,000. Pneumonia is an opportunistic infection which kills (3–4 million annually) weakened elderly and other susceptible people and is one of the two leading causes of child death. The other leading cause, diarrhea, kills (more than 2 million) by dehydration. Although its case mortality has been reduced in the past decade by the diffusion of a simple and affordable new technology, oral rehydration therapy (ORT) (which uses an inexpensive and readily available mixture of salt, sugar, and boiled water to stop dehydration), diarrhea continues to be the leading killer in most of the world. Even in developed countries there is increasing hazard from salmonella and *Escherichia coli* (*E. coli*), ubiquitous intestinal bacterium which are developing antibiotic-resistant strains. Protozoa, such as *Cryptosporidium* from the intestinal tract of cattle and *Giardia*, can survive municipal chlorination unscathed and cause epidemics and mortality even in American cities.

During the World Health Organization's decade of water development in the 1980s, water-related diseases were classified into three development-related categories: water-borne diseases, which were ingested; water-washed (or unwashed) diseases, which were preventable by hand/hair/clothes/floor washing and other hygiene; and water-based diseases, which were vectored diseases requiring water for the vector. As Table 4-2 shows, these include most of the major infectious diseases.

Intervention technology from the developed world has had a major impact on the treatment and prevention of many infectious diseases. Vaccination programs have been especially important. Maternal and child health programs, especially well-baby clinics, have monitored and improved nutrition and promoted child spacing. Much of the decline in infant and child mortality results from the interventions designed for these water-related diseases. Provision of safe and adequate water for drinking and washing, through tube wells and standpipes and municipal water treatment, has been a major and prolonged endeavor (see Table 6-4). Progress in providing safe drinking water in the developing world precipitated increased poliomyelitis as children became exposed to the virus at older ages. Polio is now on a track to eradication through massive mobilization of new vaccines by efforts of the World Health Organization, the Carter Center, and Rotary International. Residual spraying with insecticides, breeding site modification, and new netting and screening. have been undertaken to control the water-based vectors, and perhaps even to eliminate river blindness in the current World Health

TABLE 4-2. Some Major Water-Related Diseases

Water-borne	Water-unwashed	Water-based
Typhoid	Intestinal worms	Malaria (>1 mil./500 mil.)
cholera (6,800/380,000)	Amebic dysentery	Filariasis
Hepatitis A	Colds	Japanese encephalitis (11,000/40,000)
Diphtheria	Typhus (louse vectored)	River blindness
E. coli, salmonella	Plague (flea vectored)	Schistosomiasis (7,000/200 mil.)
Polio (2,000)	Pesticide residue	Dengue/DHF (15,000/560,000)
Cryptosporidium		

Note. Estimates of incidence from Brown (1996, Table 7-1). Mortality data updated from World Health Organization (1999).

Organization campaign. Infant mortality has fallen sharply, largely in response. Changes in social structure, however, such as housing conditions, entitlement to food, and treatment of women, have proven even more difficult to effect. Many of the deliberate changes carried out for economic development, moreover, have had an unanticipated adverse impact on health (Lewis & Kieffer, 1994).

The Mobility Transition

Population movement exists at many scales in space and time and is strongly affected by developmental changes. *Migration* implies the intention of a permanent move, and it is rarely measured unless it crosses an administrative, political border. It may be international in scale, or it may involve moving to another building after marriage. *Circulation* is movement which returns to the original point, but it may involve minutes to go buy some item, a vacation or pilgrimage, or years of absence for long-term study or labor. Mobility affects exposure, introduction, and other aspects of risk and has long been studied by population geographers.

Prothero (1961; 1965) was the first to conceptualize the importance of population mobility in the control of malaria in East Africa; maps of worksheds, animal-herding territories, pilgrimage routes, and other forms of culture-specific population movement were vital to this effort. Gould and Prothero (1975) developed a typology of mobility in which they classified increasing time and scale of movement. By their nature, circulation movements have reverse flows about equal to their forward flows and so have greater potential for disease circulation than does unidirectional migration.

Zelinsky (1971) suggested a mobility transition that adds the dynamic relationship of development to mobility. In a premodern society, with high birthrates and death rates, there is little residential mobility except for that following marriage (see Table 4-1). Circulation is limited to travel for customary religious observances, agricultural needs, local commerce, and warfare. As the demographic transition begins and death rates fall, a massive movement is generated by population growth. People migrate from the countryside to cities, to new agricultural frontiers, and to foreign countries. Social and labor circulation increase. Later in the transition fertility falls, movement to cities and frontiers slackens, and the emigration virtually ceases; however, circulation still increases in intensity and in structural complexity. Later when fertility and mortality have stabilized at low levels, migration is primarily between cities, although there is significant inmigration of unskilled workers. Circulation is vigorous and accelerating and includes pleasure-oriented trips as well as moves for social and economic purposes. Zelinsky suggested that in the future the technolgy of communications and delivery systems may decrease migration and some forms of circulation.

The effects of these changes in mobility, associated with economic development, on patterns of disease diffusion are important subjects for future study, as we will see in the discussion of emerging diseases. Understanding the types of mobility and anticipating their transformations provide a basis for conceptualizing disease diffusion systems at any scale.

MOBILITY AND EXPOSURE

The importance of population movement for the spread of disease has been known since the time of Hippocrates. Recently, the continuing increase in the numbers of international air passengers has been of great concern to health officials. Air travel defies quarantine and other precautions because the trip is accomplished before symptoms appear.

When a *carrier* (a symptomless person passing an infectious agent) moves, he or she can infect people along the way and at the destination. Conversely, if a traveler is susceptible to an infection, he or she will probably become sick if the infection is endemic in the destination area. Figure 4-3 illustrates the most likely transmission patterns. There is always some reverse flow of disillusioned emigrants, return visits, and other purposes. In time the schematized flows may be reversed. Because travelers are usually under some psychological and biometeorological stress (see Chapter 5), they are all the more likely to succumb to infections such as "traveler's diarrhea." An infected person traveling on mass transportation comes into contact with many susceptibles. There used to be a fear, before smallpox was eradicated, that an international visitor would introduce the disease to New York City. By the time symptoms developed and were identified, the traveler could have been in contact with thousands of people in subways, buses, and public places. Important cultural buffers have been created to prevent introduction. Public health quarantine was established centuries ago to prevent the infected traveler from entering the destination area. More recently, vaccination has been used to prevent susceptible travelers from succumbing to infection at their destination. Vaccination, however, is useful for only some diseases, and quarantine has largely become outmoded by the speed of travel. Neither has proved appropriate for rural–urban or other within-country movements.

Perhaps the best way to understand the importance of mobility for disease ecology is to turn to the microscale. Within a district, valley, village, yard, house, or room, areal differences in health hazards can be identified. The child standing in the kitchen next to boiling water is exposed to different hazards than the one across the room tending the cat litter; the man driving his car on a busy street in smog is exposed to different hazards than the farmer driving his tractor through the spore-laden dust. One can visualize surfaces of different kinds of hazards, try to define hazard regions, and then study population mobility in order to understand exposure to them. Vignette 13-2 discusses one method of collecting and analyzing such mobility data.

Roundy (1976, 1978) considered microlevel mobility and exposure to

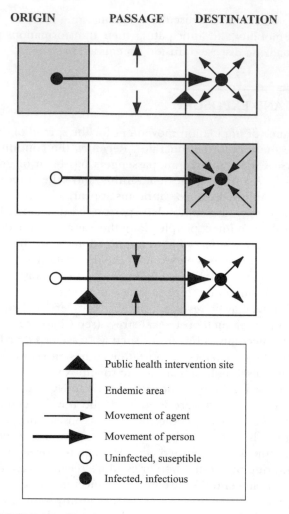

FIGURE 4-3. Mobility and disease agent transmission.

different habitats in Ethiopia. Figure 4-4 shows some of his ways of summarizing exposure. The following are some of the hazards he identified for the areal cells:

- *Individual:* trachoma, scabies, ringworm
- *Household:* tuberculosis, ringworm, tapeworm, ascariasis, salmonellosis, hydatidosis, cutaneous leishmaniasis
- *Compound:* ascariasis, tapeworm. poliomyelitis, hookworm, tetanus
- *Settlement:* tuberculosis, hepatitis, amebiasis, salmonellosis, measles, whooping cough

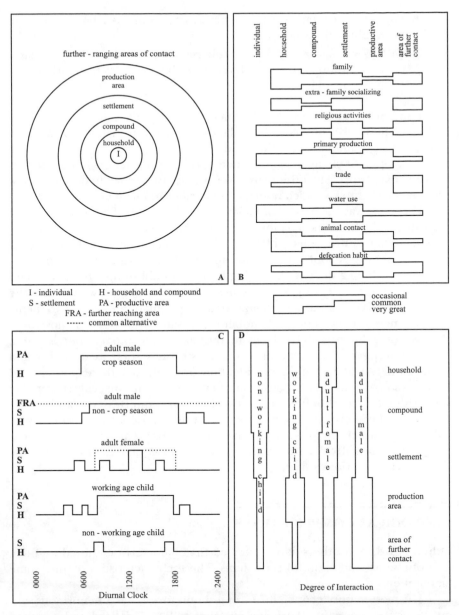

FIGURE 4-4. Cells of exposure in an Ethiopian village. *A* diagrams the areal cells. The width of the bars in *B* signifies the relative exposure of various population groups to different habitats. The line graph in *C* shows time of day of exposure of population subgroups to different habitats. The width of the bars in *D* signifies degree of interaction. From Roundy (1977). Copyright 1977 by Robert W. Roundy. Reprinted by permission.

- *Production area:* tapeworm, amebiasis, schistosomiasis, bovine tuberculosis, rabies, malaria
- *Further-ranging area of contact:* tuberculosis, syphilis, schistosomiasis, malaria, diphtheria, yellow fever, river blindness, yaws, filariasis, visceral leishmaniasis

These and other hazards can be identified with particular habitats. Parts B, C, and D of the figure summarize population exposure to habitats by age/sex role, purpose of mobility, and time of day.

Development changes, Roundy noted, can cause changes in disease hazards and exposures. The Ethiopian government built a road to develop a new regional market town, which it located in a valley to facilitate the road building. The valley was the habitat of malaria, river blindness, filariasis, and other hazards to which the population previously had been only occasionally exposed. In the future, some children might be taken from animal-herding areas and sent to school. Other plans might include planting eucalyptus for firewood, drilling a deep well, digging latrines, establishing a bus route, and increasing the density of grazing animals. All such changes would alter the disease hazards of the various habitats or alter population exposure to them.

An increasingly important mobility exposure results from movement that is not voluntary and subject to our economic models but is *forced.* Whether refugees flee environmental catastrophes such as droughts and floods or flee from war and genocide, they not only face the exposures and transmissions discussed previously but they do so in an especially susceptible state without cultural buffers and stressed by fear, powerlessness, and impoverishment (Prothero, 1994). In some cases, the experience of transit may involve camps which themselves becomes the environments of many years duration (Jacobsen, 1996). The experience and consequences of these disease ecologies await serious study.

ECOLOGICAL COMPLICATIONS

Odum (1978) and others have described the characteristics (listed in Table 4-3) of mature and youthful ecosystems. These characteristics require some elaboration.

The most mature ecosystem, a tropical rain forest, has an enormous variety of species competing. Each species tends to be specialized, to be limited in the number of individuals who can live in its specialized niches, and to grow slowly, reproduce slowly, and disseminate slowly. The different life forms are regulated through feedback stemming from competition, predation, symbiosis, and commensalism. This feedback creates a resilient system that dampens fluctuations while maximizing the use of energy in life support. The system took millions of years to develop its complexities. It is highly vul-

TABLE 4.3. Some Generalized Characteristics of Ecosystems

	Youthful	Mature
Number of species	Few	Many
Number of species individuals	Many	Few
Niche	Generalists	Very specialized
Growth	Rapid	Slow
Reproduction	Frequent, prolific	Infrequent, limited
Dissemination	Wide, fast	Local, slow
Size tendency	Small	Large
Information, feedback	Low	High
Food chains	Linear	Complex
Nutrient conservation	Low	High
Entropy	High	Low
Overall stability	Low	High
Prototype animals	Mice, sparrows	Elephant, chimpanzee
Prototype plants	Dandelion, pine	Mahogany tree

Note. Information derived, for the most part, from Odum (1978).

nerable to human intervention. Once large areas of rain forest are destroyed, as by bulldozers, reestablishment of the intricate relationships by the slow-reproducing, slow-growing, and poorly disseminating life forms will take a humanly incomprehensible length of time. In contrast, a young or simple ecosystem such as a recently colonized landslide has a few generalized species that are able to withstand extremes of weather and soil conditions. They must reproduce and grow quickly and disseminate easily. Although there are few species, each has enormous numbers of individuals. The ecosystems are subject to great fluctuations, as there are few sources of feedback to stabilize them. A flock of birds, a herd or caribou, or a snake passing through can be devastating for plants and rodents in a young ecosystem. Only the sheer numbers, rapid reproduction, and dissemination of species maintain such simple systems.

One of the most profound human influences on the earth has been *ecological simplification*. People create the simplest possible ecosystem for agriculture. When farmers plant a crop, they do not want competition from any bird, insect, or animal; they want it all themselves. They want the crop to grow rapidly, to produce lots of seed, and to be devastated by harvest. Because there are so few of the balances that exist in complex ecosystems, rats, finches, or the wrong kind of rain can also be devastating.

The simple, young ecosystems that people create with their houses, road clearings, farms, meadows, and herds of domesticated animals are ideal for epidemics. When arthropods or disease agents inimical to human health are present in a simple ecosystem, they exists in large, explosively growing numbers with few controls. In a rain forest there may be several species of *Anopheles* mosquitoes capable of transmitting malaria, but they are competing with hundreds of other species of mosquito. Each of the vector species, one of many species that might bite a person passing by, exists in relatively small numbers. Malaria occasionally gets transmitted, but more often it does not, and no focus is developed. When trees are felled, exposing streams to sunlight, conditions similar to a young ecosystem are created. The species of *Anopheles* that breed in those conditions have large numbers of individuals, reproduce rapidly and so take blood meals frequently, have few controls, and create epidemic malaria.

An anthropologist has demonstrated the perils of ecological simplification. Forest-dwelling aborigines in Malaysia have many kinds of intestinal parasites: roundworm, tapeworm, whipworm, fluke, and hookworm. People have only a light infection of any one parasite, however, because they move frequently and foci do not build up. Under these circumstances the parasitic infections seldom result in disease. When people move to the fringes of towns and become sedentary, however, the ecological conditions are simplified, and only a few species of parasitic worms can exist. An intense focus of transmission is formed, which results in high levels of infection involving many individuals of each species. The helminthic infections become diseases (Dunn, 1972).

Humans have created intense transmission of and intimate human exposure to animal diseases by domesticating and herding animals. Animal intestinal worms and fleas, vectored viral diseases, and salmonella infections have become part of the human environment. Besides intentional domestications, humans have also "domiciliated" many animals and arthropods. Audy (1965) uses the term "domiciliated" for creatures that have become closely adapted to living with people and depend on people for their great numbers and success but were not deliberately domesticated and are not kept by people for any purpose. Domiciliated animals include the house mouse and brown and black rats. Domiciliated arthropods include bedbugs and *Aedes aegypti*. The human louse is so domiciliated that it would become extinct without humans. The intimacy with humans is so great, and the house or barn ecosystem so simple, that when a disease than can be vectored or passed by herded animals or domiciliated arthropods is introduced, the intensity of the foci can produce incidence rates like those of the black death.

Audy described the influences that the processes of creating a mosaic vegetation, herding animals, and domiciliating vectors and reservoir animals has had on disease habitat. In Figure 4-5, a virgin forest is cleared by a farmer for cultivation and pasture. What had been a relatively complex ecosystem is replaced by a series of simple ecosystems. The risk of epidemic inherent in a simple ecosystem is multiplied by the number of such systems located in this small area. One additional complication has been introduced. The fringe be-

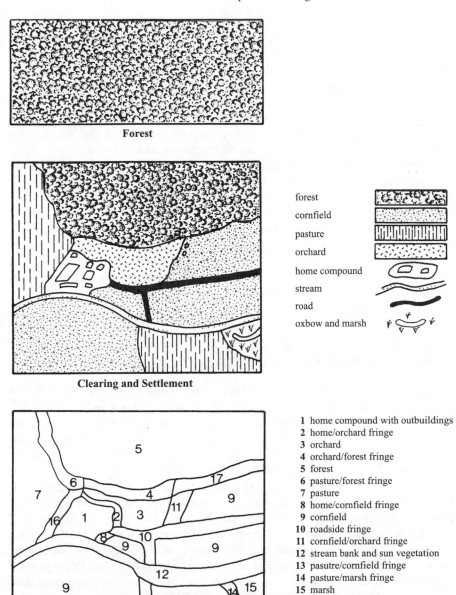

Forest

forest

cornfield

pasture

orchard

home compound

stream

road

oxbow and marsh

Clearing and Settlement

5
6
17
7
4
9
16 1 2 3 11
8 10
9 9
12
9
14 15
13 7

Mosaic Vegetation

1 home compound with outbuildings
2 home/orchard fringe
3 orchard
4 orchard/forest fringe
5 forest
6 pasture/forest fringe
7 pasture
8 home/cornfield fringe
9 cornfield
10 roadside fringe
11 cornfield/orchard fringe
12 stream bank and sun vegetation
13 pasutre/cornfield fringe
14 pasture/marsh fringe
15 marsh
16 home/pasture fringe
17 cornfield/forest fringe

FIGURE 4-5. Ecosystem simplification and multiplication. Epidemic capacity is increased when a complex ecosystem, characterized by diversity of species with few individuals, is replaced by a mosaic of habitats, each characterized by a few species with many individuals.

tween two habitats is itself a habitat conducive to passing infection between ecosystems. For example, birds and rodents might shelter in the edge of the woods and venture out to exploit the cornfield. Birds exposed to forest mosquitoes could pass the encephalitis virus to field mosquitos, which in turn infect field hands. Using the example of African yellow fever (Chapter 3), *Aedes simpsoni* breed in the tendrils of the banana trees that were planted in the forest fringe. Because they bite both forest monkeys and village humans, they are able to pass the virus repeatedly through people to the settlement-dwelling *Ae. aegypti* and so to support an intense domestic focus.

Development obviously changes the ecosystem in ways that affect disease transmission. The potential for disease introduction and human exposure is further altered by changes in human mobility. Although the following section discusses ecological simplification and mobility change and some of their consequences for land development and population resettlement in the Third World, the processes are just as relevant for the most developed lands. Hazards there might include dangerous road curves and toxic chemicals in the ground water instead of insect bites and worm eggs, yet it is microlevel mobility and exposures to precise environments for different durations at different times that result in the pattern or morbidity.

LAND DEVELOPMENT AND HEALTH CONSEQUENCES

Throughout the Third World the increase in population has led to attempts to increase food production by expanding agricultural land and to industrialize by harnessing hydroelectric power from local rivers. The efforts to exploit the resources of Siberia and the coal fields of the western United States have previously led to both planned and spontaneous resettlement on undeveloped lands. Landscape epidemiology was developed in the first place in the former Soviet Union largely as a response to the problems of settling Siberia. Let us review some of the cultural and ecological changes that affect the exposure of the population to disease hazards.

As the transition in birthrates and death rates proceeds, there is an increase in migration to agricultural frontiers and cities and a continual increase in circulation. The diffusion of different strains of old and new disease agents takes on new dynamics as susceptibles, infectives, and immunes mix on a new scale. The density of human-host foci increases as villages and cities grow. Often there is a change in house type and/or settlement form. Not only does shelter in the city slums tend to use material different from that in farming villages, but available material for frontier housing is often limited. On the other hand, as affluence increases, screens and window glass become more common, letting light into previously dark interiors. Throughout the developing world corrugated iron ("zinc") roofs have been replacing thatch because they last longer. A secondary consequence is that the nesting sites of many disease-bearing arthropods and rats, as well as the snakes that control them, are being destroyed. Villages that traditionally were nuclear may become elongated, linear villages along roads. People who lived in nuclear villages may move to a dispersed pattern on the frontier. Such changes alter the exposure to arthropod-borne disease and to fecal contamination of water. The provision of water itself is often profoundly altered. Deep tubewells may make safe, abundant water available for bathing, laundry, and drinking to people who previously had access only to scummed, hand-dug wells during the dry season. In cities people will have flush toilets, sewerage systems, and chlorinated water. Even if a government expands such systems as fast as the budget will allow, however, a large portion of the city's population will likely consist of inmigrants living in squatter areas without any amenities for hygiene. The circulation of population in a city and the roles of peddler and pedicab driver, frequently assumed by migrants, ensure that the disease focus of such squatter slums is a problem for the whole city. Improved and extended transportation systems contribute to growing population circulation. They ensure that motor vehicle accidents will increase, that disease agents will spread more widely more quickly, and that tsetse flies, schistosomes, and other components of disease systems will travel long distances for relocation. Transportation systems also ensure that food from outside sources will be available to alleviate local crop failures or other disasters and that existing health service facilities will become more accessible.

Agricultural development affects the cultural–ecological process of animal herding. There is increased penning, control of breeding, and higher-quality feed. The nature of barns and enclosures often changes. Animals do less scavenging. They are harvested, or culled, more regularly so that the age structure of the herd becomes younger, and the proportion of immune animals to susceptible ones changes. The socioeconomic role of contact with animals may change. It may come to involve more men than boys and become an occupational specialty rather than a source of general population exposure. When men are away for wage labor it may become women's work. Replacement of draft animals by machines may deprive mosquitoes of their source of blood meals and displace them to less favored meals of people, causing new or intensified disease transmission. As developmental changes affect the quality and resistance of animal and human hosts, increase the intensity of animal herding, displace animals, change occupational connections, modify water and food pathways, and alter habitat for arthropod vectors, the significance and distribution of various diseases transmitted from animals to humans will also be affected. What these effects will be, what can be planned, what needs to be studied, and what kinds of intervention can be made remain unanswered.

Irrigation and Water Impoundment

Nothing except the use of fire can compare with the ecological consequences of the human ability to control water. The health hazards resulting from impoundment of water and irrigation of crops have long been recognized, although not often evaluated by engineers and economists. Much of the present appreciation of their importance stems from the construction of the Aswan High Dam in Egypt and the spread of schistosomiasis.

Basin irrigation is ancient practice in upper Eqypt. The basins constructed to store the floodwater of the Nile were eventually drained to supply irrigated fields, subsequently planted to crops, and eventually dried up completely before again being flooded. At the height of Ethiopia's rainy season, the flooding Nile brought vital silt and water to the lower river valley. It also washed out the snails and their eggs that had survived the dry season, and physically damaged the snails' gills, thus serving to control the snail population. With the coming of the Aswan High Dam and perennial irrigation, the snail population expanded greatly. Because the nutrient-rich irrigation water flowed only slowly through the agricultural fields, was cleared of silt by reservoir sedimentation, and often supported aquatic vegetation, it was an excellent snail habitat. As predicted by health professionals, schistosomiasis, which had been endemic at low levels in the region from the time of the pharaohs, exploded to become a universal scourge. The same situation has been repeated monotonously, from the Gezira irrigation scheme in the Sudan to Lake Volta in Ghana. Africa is a dry continent. Irrigation is absolutely crucial to countries' hopes of feeding their growing populations, but the price is high. In Kenya, in a district on the shores of Lake Victoria, the rate of schistosomiasis infection for children entering elementary school went from virtually nothing to 100% in less than 10 years.

Kloos (1985) has shown how complex and dynamic the ecology of schistosomiasis can be and also the important part human behavior plays (see Figure 3-7). In Ethiopia's Awash Valley, water resources development is increasing *Schistosoma mansoni* in irrigation schemes in the upper valley by improving the habitat for its *Bulinus* snail intermediate host; these snails, however, remain territorially limited by temperature, silt, and other habitat conditions. The same development, by decreasing flooding, is decreasing *Biomphalaria* snails that host *S. haematobium* in the river lowlands. Endangering behavior, such as using the canals for laundry, bathing, and swimming, remains unchanged even by the provision of safe well water. At the same time, alterations in mobility are increasing the prevalence of *S. mansoni* among pastoralists, who come to the irrigated farmland partly to get health care, and of *S. haematobium* among migrant laborers.

In Brazil, too, expanding irrigation means expanding the territory of schistosomiasis. In Southeast Asia there are only a few foci, including a small but critical one in the Mekong River. As some of the plans for damming and controlling that great river materialize now that there is peace and many dams on tributataries are completed, one of the feared consequences is the spread of schistosomiasis throughout the Mekong River basin.

Water impoundment also has important implications for several water-based, vectored diseases. As discussed in Chapter 3, malaria was an important consideration in building the Tennessee Valley Authority dams in the southeastern United States. Government rice irrigation projects as well as small village dams have led to establishment of hyperendemic foci of lymphatic filariasis in northeastern Ghana (Hunter, 1993). The significance of irrigation for encephalitis is less often recognized. One of its best-known consequences was the relocation–diffusion and intensification of encephalitis in southern California as the Culex mosquitoes, vectors of the virus, bred in the organically polluted irrigation water (Reeves & Hammond, 1962). Similarly, the expansion of rice irrigated lands in Southeast Asia have been important in the increase of Japanese encephalitis. In Thailand, perennial irrigation of rice fields and intensified husbandry of pigs has led to intensified Japanese B encephalitis, because the pigs are hosts that carry high levels of viremia and amplify the transmission. In Southeast Asia, impoundments also served to concentrate such parasitic diseases as clonorchiasis (see Table 3-5).

There are also disease systems that are adversely affected by impoundments and irrigation. Around many of the reservoir impoundments in West Africa, the blackfly *Simulium damnosum* has decreased as its breeding sites in rapids and fast-flowing streams have been eliminated by flooding reservoirs and altering river gradients. Consequently, river blindness has often decreased, and the World Health Organization has been able to build on this in its drive to eradicate onchocerciasis in West Africa. Furthermore, irrigation water can be important for hygiene, supplying abundant water for bathing and laundry in areas in which water previously was too precious for such uses during the dry season. Their universal role as sewage collector, however, can make irrigation ditches major sources of infection.

Tubewells, or boreholes, have usually been considered great assets for health, whatever they did to water tables and salination in agriculture. Holes are drilled, or bored, sometimes a 100 or more feet deep and a small copper tube is inserted. A hand pump for domestic water or a diesel engine for irrigation then brings to the surface water uninfected by schistosomes, fecal bacteria, or other surface contamination. In parts of India and Bangladesh there have been disastrous results for health, however, as arsenic has been pumped to the surface over large areas. Now arsenic contaminates the only drinking water available as well as agricultural fields.

Population Resettlement

Countries in Southeast Asia and South America are vigorously promoting population resettlement in wilderness areas as a way of developing their national resources and relieving population pressure on declining land resources (Zelinsky's migration to the agricultural frontier). The Federal Land Development Authority (FELDA) in Malaysia has resettled hundreds of thousands of farmers who needed land on development "schemes," or projects, carved out of rain forest to grow rubber trees and oil palms. Although not without political and economic problems, the land development schemes have become models for other countries. They have played an important role in making Malaysia internationally dominant in palm oil production, and for a generation they have created decent livings for poor farmers who otherwise might have gone to the urban squatter slums. They have been much studied by political scientists and economists for their costs and benefits and for their organizational successes and failures in increasing human capital. Interested in the alterations being wrought worldwide by land development programs, Meade (1976, 1977, 1978) studied the FELDA schemes' impact on health.

People who had applied for land were admitted from all over Peninsular Malaysia. They spoke different dialects, and in those schemes to which Chinese and Indian Malaysians were admitted along with Malays, they had different religions, diets, and other cultural practices. Most were far from their home villages for the first time. For the first few years, while the tree crops matured, they faced raw land that had to be cultivated, fertilized, drained, and planted. Some settlers could not speak to their neighbors and in any case were not used to mixing with strangers. It took 2 to 3 years for communities to form. Occasionally, before that time some lonely settlers, unable to get to town or visit home villages, left the schemes. Women, accustomed to giving birth to their first child in their mother's house, were especially stressed. Malay women did not traditionally hoe plantation fields or work on roads, but they did these and other jobs on the land schemes. Sometimes older children had to stay home from school to take care of small children while the mother worked, leaving the children to eat plain cold rice for lunch. The men were required to report to work early in the morning even in poor weather, a kind of regimentation previously unknown to many of them.

Settlers' houses at first were too small for large families, but later houses were enlarged and smaller families selected. The corrugated iron roofs were long-lasting and vermin-free, but because the whole area had been clear-felled and was exposed to tropical sun, the houses frequently heated to over 110 °F (43 °Celsius) during the afternoon. Each house had land around it for gardening. It takes years for fruit trees to mature, however, and it was difficult for government agents to get the Malay settlers to grow vegetables (which are usually provided by Chinese farmers in the highlands). Almost all the adults used the latrines, although most of them were not previously used to it, but because toddlers are not diapered, some house compounds were fecally contaminated. A few children's play groups maintained helminthic infections until school age, and the school became a focus for infecting the children who had grown up in more sanitary homes. Every few houses shared a standpipe that brought chlorinated water. Although the system often broke down because of leakage and siltation problems, the enteric infections and fevers in one scheme, studied in detail, were clearly reduced compared to those in the nearby traditional village.

There were five kinds of increased hazards. The worst was malaria. Many of the schemes constructed in rain forest areas repeated the experience of early rubber plantations. The ecosystem was simplified: Trees were cut down and the vegetation was burned, exposing the streams to sunshine and creating breeding habitat for *Anopheles maculatus*. Houses were sprayed with insecticide twice a year as part of Malaysia's rather successful campaign against malaria, but the success of chloroquine and insecticides led to neglect of traditional concern for drainage, shading, oiling, and other techniques that had orginally been developed in Malaysia. The mosquitoes were becoming resistant to the insecticides and the malaria plasmodia resistant to chloroquine. The clinics serving the areas of low-density population where remote schemes were established were not enlarged before the settlers came: Their capacity was adequate for the presettler population. Settlers sick with malaria were therefore driven in landrovers for hours over rutted and flooded land to clinics with no capacity to treat them, were given chloroquine pills, and sent home. The resulting underdosage, combined with new strains, led to increased prevalence of chloroquine-resistant malaria and its unusual expressions. In at least one scheme, rare cerebral malaria led to the perception of spirit possession and consequent abandonment of the land. As the schemes matured and crop trees grew to shade the water, the epidemic receded.

In the center of a land scheme, vacant land was often left for future post offices, bus stations, and shops. This land was quickly invaded by a coarse grass. Located amidst growing trees, tapioca plants, and human waste material, the grass made an excellent habitat for rats. As discussed in Vignette 3-2, a reversal of traditional population exposure to the risk of scrub typhus occurred in the land scheme. Women and children were exposed instead of men, who had been occupationally exposed in the rubber forest.

The settlers who stayed until their trees were mature and producing generally achieved a higher income than did their relatives in the villages. Because of their more remote location, however, everything cost more, and nutritional circumstances had changed. The FELDA store stocked dried and canned food only. The settlers did little fishing or hunting, and fresh fruit and vegetables were limited. In the study scheme, settlers had almost given up trying to raise chickens because, having been raised to scavenge and range freely, the chickens were constantly stricken by epizootics and repeatedly wiped out. The settlers had come from small villages of a few hundred people to a scheme of thousands, but the consequences of urbanization (herding of humans and animals) for contagion were best reflected in the chicken population.

Remote location and higher income also meant proliferation of motorcycles. Roads were winding, hilly, and frequently wet; overloaded lumber trucks were frequently uncontrollable; and many cycle drivers were unlicensed and helmetless. Motorcycle accidents and mortality became a definite factor in the health of the scheme population.

Finally, changes in mobility lay behind not only vehicular accidents but also diffusion of infectious disease. In the traditional village, almost everyone walked or rode bicycles to visit and go marketing on a daily basis. On the scheme, usually the male head of the household rode a motorcycle into town on Saturday to do shopping and go to the mosque, sometimes taking small children with him. Most other people stayed on the scheme for years at a time. When people did leave, it was not for local mobility but to take an inter-state bus back to their home villages. At the time of the study there was a cholera epidemic on the coast. Despite the poor wells of the village and the safe water supply of the scheme, it was probably the scheme that was most at danger of having cholera introduced, because its settlers were more likely to take trips into infected areas, and bring back such gifts as seafood.

One of the advantages of studying land development in Malaysia is that subtle changes can be identified. Elsewhere, such major vectored diseases as hyperendemic trypanosomiasis, malaria, and schistosomiasis can overwhelm everything else.

Development of the Amazon

The agricultural frontiers in South America attract settlers mainly to the Amazon basin from the Andes Mountains and the Brazilian coast. This basin land was long protected from settlement by the presence of yellow fever and malaria. Gade (1979) suggests that diseases such as leishmaniasis prevented the Incas from extending their hegemony into the tropical lowlands. Leish-maniasis certainly is one of the curses of settlers today, although malaria and yellow fever have been controlled sufficiently to make settlement attractive for the first time since the Colombian Exchange.

Again, mobility patterns are critically important. Much of the movement into the Amazon basin is really circulation. People move seasonally to take advantage of different altitudinal zones in the Andes or to work on planta-tions or road construction. There is special concern that onchocerciasis may be spread from endemic areas along the northern border into the basin, where three species of *Simulium* exist. Schistosomiasis is also spreading with the new agricultural developments.

There are special health problems for population mobility in this re-gion. People migrating from the Andes are adapted to living at high eleva-tions. Respiratory and circulatory problems can develop in these settlers in the wet lowlands. Water impoundment, deforestation, and other ecological simplifications have increased some disease hazards. In a pattern reminiscent of Malaysia, forest clearance is creating conditions for a new malarial vector, *Anopheles darlingi*, and faciparum malaria is now becoming epidemic in the Peruvian Amazon. Helminthic infection levels have increased, and fecal con-tamination of water has spread enteritis. Game has been depleted, and diets are often poor in protein.

As Weil (1981) points out, however, many of the health problems of the settlers are simply those of protracted poverty. Many settlers are faced within a few years with nutrient depletion of the soil, laterization, weed invasion, and other losses. They sell out to cattle ranchers and move to a new frontier. Little health care is available. Those involved in capital-intensive agribusiness have money to buy food from afar, to get vaccinations and prophylactic drugs, and to have protective housing, deepei wells, less dangerous work, and access to health care when they do get sick. Their actions can induce different adverse disease ecologies, however. In Central America, increased cultivation of cotton for export to Japan has led to a greatly increased use of insecticides. The contaminated environment is now producing vectors of malaria and arboviruses highly resistant to control by multiple insecticides.

African Development and Unintended Changes

The medical geography of developmental changes in Africa has been the most investigated of any region. Multiple infections with different types of helminths and protozoa are common. Much of the rural African population has close contact with vectored disease. The three diseases that can render land totally uninhabitable—malaria, river blindness, and sleeping sickness— seem to have evolved in the African realm. They still deny expanses of good agricultural land to the growing and sometimes malnourished population. Much of the pastoral mobility and labor movement to plantations and mines is international in scope, to a degree reached on no other continent. While African peoples go through the demographic transition, the circulation that characterizes the mobility transition continues to grow and to have a profound impact on the diffusion of disease agents (including HIV) and relocation of nidal systems. It is here that the spread of schistosomiasis first made politicians and development specialists concerned about adverse ecological and health consequences of development. It is here that the emergence of HIV became a modern plague, and where ebola repeatedly threatens to do so.

The comprehensive review by Hughes and Hunter (1970) of the literature on development and health in Africa sensitized a generation of scholars and experts. Hughes and Hunter described, for example, how the evacuation of tribes from their agricultural and grazing land was carried out by colonial governments because of outbreaks of rinderpest or smallpox or in order to stop tribal warfare. Such evacuations allowed brush and tsetse to claim the abandoned territory, so that returning herdsmen or farmers years later found the land denied them by trypanosomiasis. They described how roads had become linear transmission sites for disease. Tsetse, blackflies, mosquitoes, and disease agents of many kinds become concentrated where roads cross streams or rivers and people stop to eat, wash, and urinate. New reservoirs and roads mean new trading paths and new exposures and transmissions. They described some of the nutritional and social–psychological consequences of development.

Hughes and Hunter explained the difficulty of intervening in the complex disease systems and multiple levels of infection. They emphasized most of all, however, the need for a comprehensive, ecologically informed approach to the developmental projects designed to break the synergism be-

tween poverty and disease. Since then, examples of the inadvertent consequences of developmental changes in Africa and everywhere else have multiplied.

It should be evident that the old assumption of positive association between economic development and improved health is not necessarily true. By
far the most common inadvertent consequences result from changes in nutrition.

Nutritional Changes

Many people assume that most of the malnutrition in the world is a consequence of poverty, and that economic development that increases people's
income will improve their nutritional status. Certainly for those suffering
from absolute deficiency of calories and protein, the economic ability to "demand" food can mean the difference between life and death. For malnutrition, however, the evidence is that increased prosperity can have an adverse
effect, at least initially.

Food preference plays a crucial role in nutrition. The excess calories and
fat of the American diet and the consequent obesity and serum cholesterol
are sometimes considered a new kind of malnutrition. Except for those people who are vegetarians for religious reasons, however, the evidence is that
those whose diets are based on vegetable protein and grain are happy to increase their meat consumption at the first economic opportunity. Japan is
the most obvious example, but the preference for meat when accessible has
become obvious from China to India. Other changes in preference are more
problematic. Often the first purchase made with increased income is Coca-
Cola or alcohol. Sugar consumption increases, from soft drinks especially,
and consequently dental cavities increase in places where dental care belongs
only to the rich. Diabetes may increase. Colonialism and the continuing power of the Western world have led many people to give bread a status higher
than the locally produced staple. New members of the technocratic class and
residents of cities will buy bread when they can, even when the indigenous
millets and other grains are more nutritious. Highly polished white rice is
prized. Chapter 2 describes the association of beriberi and the spread of rice-
milling technology.

The changes in diet consequent upon developmental alterations take
many forms. When the Tonga people were moved in order to construct the
Kariba Dam in Africa, they were resettled in land where their traditional
crops did not grow. They resisted the strange new seeds the government gave
them, and they no longer caught fish and rodents along the river to balance
their diet: Consequently, they endured severe malnutrition. Similarly, people
in Southeast Asia who used to gather a few leaves to garnish their staple rice
have to learn in frontier areas to grow vegetables.

There are many ways that technology and development affect nutrition.
Roads, bridges, electricity, and refrigeration can have tremendous beneficial

results. Food can be delivered to areas where crops fail. Varieties of food can be supplied year-round rather than seasonally. Intestinal diseases can be curbed. Modern processing and storing can deny the rodents and vermin their free meals and save more food for people. Alternatively, as discussed in Chapter 2, such food processing can spread beriberi. Information on weather, farming practices, or new strains of food crops can be disseminated quickly. Just a few years of education, basic literacy, can increase nutritional knowledge and improve child care. New foods and fish cultivation can be introduced, and poultry and livestock diseases can be controlled.

Adverse effects of development are deeply intertwined with societal changes. Women, drawn into economic activities outside the house, have fewer children. Usually they also stop breast feeding and start bottle feeding. Other women do so simply because bottle feeding becomes associated with higher status. For monetary reasons powdered milk is often overdiluted with unsafe water in bottles that cannot be boiled because of fuelwood shortage. The consequences of these practices can be epidemics of enteritis and high infant mortality.

By far the most profound, baffling, and frustrating deterioration in nutrition often follows the successful development of the cash economy and improvement in local incomes. If a cash crop is introduced and processing, transportation, and marketing for it are arranged through great effort, some of the best and most powerful changes of the developmental process are begun. Incomes may increase, accessibility to health care and education may improve, and loyalty to the central government can be cemented. It is still assumed by most planners that if the economic basis of the standard of living is improved for the peasantry, their nutritional status and disease status will improve too.

Repeatedly it has been found that cash cropping and monoculture displaces local cultivation of food. People may devote to the cash crop all their land or all their labor, if they are involved as laborers in agribusiness. Local millets or vegetables are not grown. Chickens are neglected. No one goes hunting. Money is available to buy food from the store, and because of roads and development, food can now be available year-round. But people who are not used to working in a money economy tend to spend all their money soon after they earn it. They often spend it on alcohol, consumer goods such as radios and cloth, and treats such as ice cream and soft drinks. The result commonly is that households are soon out of money and reduced to the cheapest, poorest of foods long before the next harvest of their cash crop. Food preference is important: People choose status foods and sweets and no longer have access to the nutritious but coarse homegrown fare. People in villages that have planted remunerative cash crops, such as cocoa in Ghana or coffee in Central America or Kenya, often are wealthier than neighboring villagers but also more apathetic, sick, and malnourished. Plantations and agribusiness are sometimes criticized for demanding that all of their laborers' attention be devoted to the cash crop and for providing no land for vegetables, fruit, or staple foods. As one travels in developing areas, however, one sees many private farmers who devote all their land to a remunerative cash crop and who suffer the same consequences.

URBANIZATION

Our present-day city is inhuman. . . . It is becoming more so with every day that passes. If it is inhuman it cannot be better for the health of mankind; it creates grave problems for man.

—C. A. Doxiadis (1967, quoted in Weinstein, 1980, p. 72)

One of the most profound demographic changes, comparable only to population growth, is the current urbanization of the world's population. In the mid-19th century, England was the only majority urban country in the world. By 2020, the human population of earth will become urban. Most Latin American countries are already more than 70% urban. Sub-Saharan Africa and monsoon Asia are now about a third urban. Where populations are growing 3% a year, capital cities are often growing at 8% a year. The process of urbanization in the developing world intensifies most of the types of change discussed in this chapter. Boyden (1970), McKeown (1988), and Dubos (1965) have described historically how urbanization can change the state of everything. The dimension of the present global urbanization is comparable to only two other changes: the domestication of plants and animals and the cities that subsequently developed and the onset of the industrial revolution. The agricultural revolution created systems of cities in which disease agents could cross species, like protomeasles (from canine distemper and bovine rinderpest), and find enough interacting susceptibles to become established. The creation of many contagious diseases evolved from the herding of domestic animals. That revolution also created extensive hierarchies of power, new organization, and changes in empowerment of people and in gender role.

The sheer growth of the urban population today has major consequences for patterns of disease and health. Table 4-4 presents some of the dimension of change looming ahead. The author estimated and included absolute numbers of people involved because the usual percentages are at once too familiar and too removed from impact.

It needs to be said upfront that the net impact of urbanization on health in the developing world is good. It can be measured in the decline of child mortality. Despite the difficulties and adverse effects discussed later, most of the health changes that accompany urbanization, related to the demographic transition, are positive. Health services become more accessible, infectious diseases more controllable, sewage and water more treatable, the population

TABLE 4-4. Dimensions of Urban Change

	Population 1995 (mil.)	% urban	Number urban	Population 2020 (mil.)	% urban	Number urban	Absolute increase 1995–2020
World	5,607	45	2,523	8,378	62	5,194	2,671,000,000
More developed	1,164	74	861	1,259	81	1,020	159,000,000
Less developed	4,443	35	1,555	7,119	59	4,174	2,619,000,000
Asia							
Japan	3,267	30	980	4,891	56	2,739	1,759,000,000
China	1,192	28	334	1,504	56	842	508,000,000
Mother India[a]	1,155	25	288	1,863	55[a]	1,025	737,000,000[a]
Africa	700	34	238	1,538	54	831	593,000,000
Latin America	470	71	334	679	83	563	230,000,000

Note. Population estimates from Population Reference Bureau; urban projections from United Nations (1989).
[a]Our estimate from combined figures for Bangladesh, India, and Pakistan.

easier to reach with vaccination. As more children live and the population grows older, the diseases of developed economies gradually come to the fore. Despite how bad conditions in urban slums can be, the migrants there have chosen them over the worse conditions for their lives in rural origins.

The consequences of the inadequate, crowded, and often windowless housing for the rural migrants pouring into the cities are congruent with the Western experience. Tuberculosis has become a scourge in the cities of Asia and especially in Africa. Measles is a fatal disease in many populations. These and other infectious diseases have become raging epidemics as people's immune systems have become compromised by HIV infection, so that instead of dying later of AIDS people die from tuberculosis quickly. Bubonic plague periodically flares up in cities. In 1994 temperatures of over 120 °F in India had left many animals prostrate and people crowded into slums where grain was stored. Excess fleas, stored food, crowded people and the plague bacilli demonstrated again that such conditions can create the panic of pneumonic plague transmission. Contagious diseases thrive with urbanization.

Given the rapid growth and the impossibility of new sewerage and potable water supplies keeping pace with new dwellers and settlements, water-borne diseases are again a major health hazard. El Tor cholera was introduced from Asia into South America in the 1980s to become a serious public health problem. In 1992 a new vibrio cholera, 0139 Bengal, emerged in India and threatens now an eighth pandemic of cholera as it displaces El Tor. Animals, too, have been urbanized and the herding process is introducing a variety of antibiotic-resistant bacteria and zoonotic protozoa into human water supplies, especially in developed countries.

Malnutrition is a problem in the new cities. More urban women bottle-feed their babies. More urban people turn to corn or cassava flours and other food sources that can be quickly prepared, and turn their backs on the millets, sesame seeds, groundnuts, and other wholesome foods of the countryside. Mineral and vitamin deficiencies proliferate.

Everywhere, mobility changes are at the heart of health changes. Vehicular accidents increase and have become a major cause of death. Migration into cities and circulation between village and city disseminate tuberculosis, cholera, and sexually transmitted disease. Agricultural families suffer at planting and harvest time from the loss of good workers, with nutritional consequences to both rural and urban populations. Female-headed households are increasingly impoverished. With men gone to cities and mines for wage labor for years at a time, all the agricultural chores of cultivation and harvest and marketing fall to women already spending longer time gathering fuelwood and caring for children who have lived.

The mental and social stress of such rapid and extreme change, of culture conflict between ethnic groups and generations, of despair, isolation, loneliness, and crushed hopes, lead to mental and social diseases. Alcoholism increases. Sexually transmitted diseases increase. Infertility consequent to gonorrhea can result, adding to the social stress, or AIDS can increase, leaving villages of orphans (Chapter 10). Suicide in many places is epidemic. Mental illness has become a serious problem in many rapidly growing cities and has added substantially to the recognition of the important role that the indigenous health practitioners of various cultures have to play in coping with ill health.

Urbanization of Vectored Diseases

The health hazards discussed previously as part of the urbanization process today are not very different in kind from the Euro-American experience of the past century. One important difference developing, however, is the urbanization of vectored diseases. The European model of urbanization assumes that the city population is removed from vectored diseases except, initially, for those vectored by rat fleas and human lice. This is not necessarily true today (Schriefer, 1994; Azad, Radulovic, Higgins, Noden, & Troyer, 1997). Surtees (1971) was prescient in his concern for urbanized vectors.

What Audy called the "domiciliated" animals and arthropods (such as mice and cockroaches and Ae. aegypti) have been urbanized too, along with dogs and cats and other pets. Their infections are thus subject to the process of "herding" as well as those of people (see Chapter 2). Open drainage and septic ditches, construction sites, garbage mountains, and water storage have created simple ecosystems with abundance of vectors. In India, Anopheles stephensi likes to bite people, has become highly insecticide resistant, and breeds prolifically in the gravel-mining, construction, garbage pooling of the periurban area. Assisted by population mobility and some other Anopheles, it has created epidemic urban malaria. Culex fatigans especially likes the polluted drainage and septic systems. As Surtees had foreseen, it made Brugian filariasis such an endemic urban vectored disease that Indian scientists (Dhanda, Das, Lal, Srinvasan, & Ramaiah, 1996) recently remarked that filariasis, considered to be an urban disease, was rapidly emerging as a major problem in rural areas. As discussed in Chapter 3, dengue fever transmitted by the domiciliated *Aedes aegypti* seems to have been transformed into a hemorrhagic form through the intense transmission found in urban areas. It is now spreading in the Caribbean and Central America. Yellow fever remains an urban threat in Africa, but it is appearing again in tropical America with the spread of reintroduced *Ae. aegypti*. Chagas disease has gone with people to the cities where the reduviid bugs thrive in poor urban housing and domiciliated animals. Controlling its spread through the blood supply has become a problem reaching, through population mobility, even into the United States.

New Urban Forms

Urban areas are not only growing, they are changing form and structure. The U.S. population, for example, has become more suburban than "city." The urban areas have become "green," intermingling domesticated, domicilitated, wild, and human animals in new ways. One result has been the emergence of rabies as danger to human health again in the eastern United States. In the southeastern region, raccoons, supplemented by the occasional bat, bring the disease into backyards, domestic animals, and people. In the North, foxes are more involved, and in the Midwest skunks, but the result is a new contact between a deadly disease of wild animals and humans. Lyme disease and Rocky Mountain spotted fever (Chapter 3) continue to spread and intensify as population decentralization pushes housing into wooded areas and agricultural fields are converted to support resurgent deer, and rodent, populations. It seems that urban park rats may be better for feeding and infecting ticks, being larger with higher viremia and longer life, than the rural white-footed mice (Steere, 1994). In some western states, murine typhus has been brought into human contact by cat fleas. Perhaps the biggest and least appreciated development is the spread of *Aedes albopictus*, the Asian tiger mosquito, which was brought by a shipload of tires for recylcing to Texas. In less than 10 years it has spread to the Carolinas and Pennsylvania. Although in Asia *Ae. aegypti*, which is so domiciliated and people-loving, displaced *Ae. albopictus* to become the most dangerous vector of dengue and other viruses, in the United States the development of new urban forms seems to be reversing the relationship. *Ae. albopictus* is thriving in the vegetation and wildlife of suburban sprawl. The species is capable of surviving winter conditions, with a range in Asia north to Japan and Korea, and so it may extend and intensify the range of dengue in the United States. Perhaps more important, however, the facility with which it feeds on opossum, raccoon, birds, dogs, and rodents as well as people raises a much greater risk of cross-species transmission of viruses and consequent new disease hazards.

In Asia, a new urban form that McGee, Ginsburg, and Koppel (1991) refer to as *desakota* (Malay for villagecity) seems to be developing. In regions of
wet rice cultivation the rural density of population can be 300 per square mile.
As cities grow and commerce and transportation spread along roads going
from them, the cities come to enfold large rural areas and activities. High-rise
apartment buildings, elementary schools, and shophouses surround wet rice
fields, intense pig and chicken production, and large mosquito populations;
intensively cultivated vegetable plots are fertilized with human nightsoil; industrial chemicals and sewerage drain into irrigation ditches: Such new combinations of habitats and activities under dense and mobile human populations promise the emergence of whole new disease ecologies.

EMERGING DISEASES

The demographic transition, described in the section of the same name early
in this chapter, may well be ending by ushering in a stage of renewed parasitic and infectious disease. Infectious agents are newly discovered to be involved in everything from ulcers to hardening of the arteries. Instead of disappearing at the end of the demographic transition, we find diseases once
almost eradicated now opening new hospital wards. The most notorious of
these is the multiple-drug-resistant new tuberculosis; but strains of staphylo-
coccus in hospitals threaten to again make them places to get sick. Children
again die from intestinal fauna acquired in the meat and water of the most
developed places. There are several dimensions to this emergence and resurgence of infectious disease, most of which develop from the cultural ecology
that has been discussed in the Chapters 2, 3, and 4.

The first dimension is not geographical: the technological changes of
medical and iatrogenic practice. The widespread use of, and demand for, antibiotic treatments even when useless, as against viruses, and the general over-
prescription of drugs have helped create drug resistance. Inadequate medical follow-up and patient compliance has helped create drug resistance. New
technologies of transferring human organs and tissues have created new
means for agents to pass, xenographs; future use of pig and other animal
parts will create xeno-zoonoses. Use of immunosuppressant drugs to prevent
tissue rejection or fight the rapidly growing cells of cancer has allowed a new
set of infectious agents to be unsuppressed. Most of the dimensions of
change are, however, very geographical (Haggett, 1994; May, 1994; Meslin,
1997).

Land Use Change

The changes in habitat, species, feedback regulation, and human exposure
that attend deforestation, agricultural conversion, irrigation, dam building,
agricultural intensification, road building, and urbanization have been cov-

ered in this chapter and 2 and 3. It might be useful, therefore, to focus on the species our ecological simplification seems to have benefited most, the thriving and growing worldwide population of rodents.

Rodents are the supreme opportunists and creatures of simple ecosystems. They have short lives, multiply rapidly, grow quickly, and disseminate widely, and so adapt quickly immunologically to disease agents and to poisons. Furthermore, they eat anything people eat—and are reported to consume up to 20% of the human harvest and food supply—and they thrive on contamination. They are, aside from ourselves, probably the greatest beneficiaries of recent human modification of the earth.

Rodent zoonoses that have been increasingly infecting people include leptospirosis, murine typhus, bubonic plague, Rocky Mountain spotted fever, Lyme disease, and a variety of Central European and Asian hemorrhagic fevers. More dramatically, dust contamination from their urine and other excretions has recently caused outbreaks of Hanta virus pulmonary syndrome in the United States, Lassa fever in Africa, and Bolivian hemorrhagic fever (Machupo) in South America. In Bolivia, Malaysia, and elsewhere serious crop destruction and epidemic disease have resulted from the loss of rodent predators because of intensified agriculture's use of pesticides. When new arboviruses, such as ebola, emerge from disturbed areas, the role of rodent as host is at the top of the hypothesis list.

A new set of ecological connections seems to be emerging in marine ecosystems. The excess of minerals and nutrients resulting from agricultural runoff and urban sewerage, perhaps abetted by coastal warming, is causing algae blooms and proliferation of species of dinoflagellates and cyanobacteria and, probably pfisteria, which make the deadly toxins that have decimated seals and sea lions and endangered people.

Technological impacts abound in this context. The destruction of some of the ozone layer by gases of human manufacture has caused the mutation of microbes through increased ultraviolet radiation and probably has prevented the "germicidal layer" from eliminating some of them. Pollution, whether of chemicals from the Green Revolution and other agricultural intensification or from the industrial growth and international shipment and dumping of toxic chemicals, has contaminated water supplies in parts of the world least able to regulate or remove the poisons. Currently, the most famous technological impact of all is global warming.

Global Warming

There are public health concerns that global warming will expand the area in which tropical vectored diseases can occur (Epstein, 1997). It is true that a lessening of winter's severity might allow a species of mosquito, for example, to expand its range into new territory, or to higher altitude. Under warmer conditions, arthropods reproduce faster and hence take more frequent blood meals, and this could result in transmission to more people. In most cases, however, the arthropod is already present in that territory (in which the disease of concern does not occur) and the disease can currently be transmitted there. The mosquito *Anopheles quadrimaculatus*, for example, is still widespread in the United States and quite capable of transmitting malaria, as it did intensely in the 19th century from Minnesota to Arizona (Chapter 3). The changes in behavior and habitat which eliminated malaria from most of the United States are still protective buffers. One effect of the concern for global warming, unfortunately, is to remove attention from the cultural, socioeconomic side of things. The greatest danger of reestablishment of malaria in the United States, for example, probably comes from the new population of homeless people who sleep outdoors, especially in parks where the mosquitoes can find them.

The pattern of precipitation and availability of water affected by climate change is much more wide-reaching an issue than warmer temperatures themselves. Any global changes in climate are likely to cause some areas on earth to become wetter and others dryer than they now are. Drying of the land will affect not only agriculture but sanitation and hygiene: the water-borne and water-unwashed diseases. Wetting of the land will affect breeding areas for many arthropods and snails, some of which vector human diseases. A sharp illustration of what could happen occurred in Arizona/New Mexico in 1993, when the Pacific oceanic changes of El Niño caused an exceptionally wet winter and spring, a greening of the desert, a profusion of piñon nuts, and an explosion of mice, whose urine people were exposed in their spring mobility and cleaning: An epidemic of Hanta virus emerged. Future changes in impoundment and irrigation technologies, social organization, or the built environment are likely to be more important to expansion of malaria than a few degrees of warming per se. More impoundment of water behind dams to provide for perennial irrigation would create open, stagnant, sunny bodies of water suitable for several species of *Anopheles*. If sea levels rise, hundreds of millions of people would be displaced from tropical deltas and river valleys. The mass migration of environmental refugees could introduce any infection any of them have to new populations of people and mosquitoes. Enough social disruptions might enable malaria to spread to middle latitudes again as the cultural buffers (mosquito-proof housing, indoor water supply, etc.) break down. It is more likely than these grand scenarios, however, that warming a couple of degrees over a few decades would cause subtle relationships to be altered. For example, the reproductive and other biological clocks of various arthropods would be differentially affected by warming, which would likely cause disruption in predator–prey life-cycle feedback and possible vector explosions.

Organizational Change and Globalization

A new wrinkle in this cloth of cultural interactions with the environment is being created by the globalization of urban society, trade, industry, technology, and socioeconomic organization. Globalization has many profound effects, whether on wage structures and employment, information flow, belief systems, or scale of the pollution syndrome (Chapter 6). One of the most profound for the ecology of disease has been the qualitative escalation of international migration and circulation (Martin & Widgren, 1996). Any given year, more than 200 million people are moving internationally for wage labor: Africa to Europe, tropical Asia to the Persian Gulf, Pacific Islands to New Zealand, South America to the United States of course, but also from Indonesia to Malaysia, the Philippines to Japan, Paraguay to Argentina, Zambia to South Africa. There are countries in which more than a fifth of the labor force consists of foreign workers (Switzerland, Côte d'Ivoire) and even more than half (Saudi Arabia and other Gulf states). The United Nations recognizes more than 5 million refugees who often live in the most desperate conditions, susceptible to disease. Population circulation from developed midlatitude countries to the tropical world for purposes of tourism and business also exceeds 200 million annually. The emerging social, political, and economic organization of the world combined with the technologies of fast transportation have created a world in which the agricultural disturbances in the most remote regions of the world may have pandemic consequences almost instantly.

Consider, as one example of new development changes, what has to be called the industrialization of food animal production. Like the urbanization of the human population, the herding of animals into enormous, densely packed populations reprises the ecological consequences of the first domestications. Cattle in feedlots at the giant slaughterhouses and meat-processing plants can be penned hundreds of thousands at a single facility. Chicken raising has been specialized into brooders, egg production, chicken (broiler) raising, and assembly-line slaughter, cleaning, parts production, packaging, and marketing. Fowl being raised for food are penned so densely that their beaks commonly must be cut. Following the business success with chickens and turkeys, in recent years swine production (according to "the North Carolina model") has followed suit. Piglets are now nursed through bars on trapped sows, raised densely packed tens of thousands to a facility, fed by conveyor belts, wastes flushed into septic "lagoons" and eventually sprayed on the land. Food contamination from such industrialized production and marketing poses new challenges for inspection and for risks of pandemic. Food thus produced is shipped not only across the United States but internationally, as from Thailand to Japan.

Putting aside for text purposes ethical issues about the treatment of animals or the exploitation of labor, serious public health consequences need consideration. The waste discharge and spills thus produced have attracted a lot of attention through putrefaction of streams, river and offshore fish kills, and recently pfiesteria (a dinoflagellate protozoa) attacks on fish and production of neurological toxins. Animals cannot be herded so densely without massive use of antibiotics, which are passing newly resistant strains of microbes on to people. The salmonella and other intestinal fauna are increasingly contaminating carcasses and parts in the mass, speeded-up assembly-line processing. The combination of birds and pigs close together at such densities raises several red flags. The influenza virus is thought to "shift" when avian flu and other strains get combined in pigs, producing the pandemics. Emergence of a few cases of what seemed a new flu strain from chickens in Hong Kong in 1998 caused a panic and the slaughter of all the chickens. Avian encephalitis viruses, such as Japanese encephalitis (and probably Eastern equine encephalitis), can be amplified by the high viremia in pigs into major epidemics. The animals are not raised on grain grown on that farm anymore but by agribusiness production that spans continents. When cattle in Britain began to get Bovine spongiform encephalopathy (BSE; mad cow disease), it was traced epidemiologically to feed that included sheep brains and body parts (although cows are famous as vegetarians). This British feed had already affected cows in Italy and other European countries in trade. Although the string of protein molecules that seems to be involved (prions) defies any definition of life, it seems to reproduce the same brain destruction in chains of animals that consume it. Epidemiologists make an analogy with Kuru previously among cannibals in Papua New Guinea. The Western public's alarm, however, is with the rare human brain disease, Creutzfeldt-Jacob, which may be part of the same food chain as BSE. More common, if little understood, health challenges from animal feed and raising include synthetic estrogens, growth hormones, and similar elements of high-tech mass production. In such ways, new technologies of agricultural production, processing, and marketing internationally are creating a new disease ecology.

FRAMEWORKS AND ARGUMENTS

Although most of the changes discussed in this chapter have been concerned with the developing world, readers should not think that the process of change is not as consequential for health in the industrialized world. New industries and economic bases, such as the food production described previously, bring with them new occupational exposures, waste products, and hazards. Settlement changes resulting from migration to nonmetropolitan areas lead more people into contact with natural foci of vectored disease. Water systems and sewerage sysems interlock in new ways and water is reused many more times. Toxic chemicals enter groundwater, offshore fish are poisoned with heavy metals or toxins from fertilized algae blooms, and agricultural runoff carries potent chemicals into municipal drinking water. Social diseases such as alcoholism and homicide, sexually transmitted diseases, and mental diseases continue to evolve. Many of these influences are considered in Chapters 6 and 7, on the pollution syndrome and diseases in developed places.

Some geographers have criticized the efficacy of looking at the impacts, usually unintended, of developmental changes on disease ecology, as this chapter has done. Stock (1986), for example, argued that Hunter's concern for development impacts on disease in Africa had little effect. There has been, he points out, a fundamental shift away from modernization theories of socioeconomic change to dependency and Marxist theories which recognize that many health problems are integral to the expansion of capitalism rather than just unanticipated side effects of development initiatives. Stock notes how little work has been done by geographers relating patterns of ill health to capitalist underdevelopment. Political economists decry the lack of focus on political considerations. The growing approach of political ecology does indeed offer an important theoretical framework for gaining understanding for human environment interactions, considering as it does the "hidden agendas" of individuals and groups in political context as well as the large-scale social, economic, and political structures that shape events (Mayer, 1996). There certainly are vaulting structures of international economics and social and political organization, as well as such transcendent and powerful ideas as religious values, nationalism, or simply male power and status struggles (àla sociobiology theory).

These arguments are discussed elsewhere. This chapter is not about ultimate political/economic causations but about the local interactions of cultural ecology that create and maintain disease systems. There would be such kinds of interactions and disease would exist whatever the higher political and economic structures, whether feudal or tribal, pure communist, or unrestrained capitalist. There is, for example, movement of people in space, although the origins and destinations and purposes and characteristics of movers change in time and place. Scientists concerned with health also need basic facts, greater knowledge and understanding of how the processes of interaction between people and their habitat affect health and disease. What role does settlement form or building material play in exposure, what effects do different kinds and durations of population mobility have, how does human simplification of the ecosystem affect species relations, and how do all these effect the dynamics of epidemic? This chapter has been about microscale facts and effects, about individual acts of exposure, and about cultural learning for protection.

Medical geographers need to become involved in developing prospective medical geographies of health and disease. Much is known of the etiology of specific diseases. Many consequences of specific types of changes are collectively understood among the biological, medical, and social sciences. These include the consequences of changing age structure through fertility behavior and immigration, changing house type, changing contact with natural foci of vectored diseases, changing transportation systems and population circulation, changing occupational hazards, changing exercise and food habits, changing recreational habits, and changing demands on the environment for cleansing human sewage and industrial wastes and providing safer water for consumption and hygiene. The projection of present trends is not enough. Their integration, from a geographic perspective, is crucial everywhere to sound planning and health promotion. The emergence of new infectious diseases, for example, may ultimately result from the globalization of the world economy and urbanization of world population, but it requires development of global surveillance systems together with technology transfer and institution building for vaccine development and delivery to the remotest places. Developing such prospective medical geographies will require frameworks founded in political ecology informed by the cultural ecology of disease.

REFERENCES

Audy, J. R. (1965). Types of human influence on natural foci of disease. In B. Rosickt & K. Heyberger (Eds.), *Theoretical questions of natural foci of disease: Proceedings of a symposium* (pp. 245–253). Prague: Czechoslovak Academy of Science.

Azad, A. F., Radulovic, S., Higgins, J. A., Noden, B. H., & Troyer, J. M. (1997). Flea-borne rickettsioses: Ecologic considerations. *Emerging Infectious Diseases, 3,* 319–327.

Boyden, S. V. (Ed.). (1970). *The impact of civilisation on the biology of man.* Toronto: University of Toronto Press.

Brown, L. R. (Ed.) (1996). Populations affected by various infectious diseases 1993. In *State of the World, 1996.* New York: Norton.

Dhanda, V., Das, P. K., Lal, R., Srinvasan, R., & Ramaiah, K. D. (1996). Spread of lymphatic filariasis, re-emergence of leishmaniasis and threat of babesiosis in India. *Indian Journal of Medical Research, 103,* 46–54.

Director-General. 1995. *The world health report 1995: Bridging the gaps.* Geneva: World Health Organization.

Dubos, R. (1965). *Man adapting.* New Haven, CT: Yale University Press.

Dunn, F. L. (1972). Intestinal parasitism in Malayan aborigines (Orang Asli). *Bulletin of the World Health Organization, 46,* 99–113.

Epstein, P. R. (1997). Climate, ecology, and human health. *Consequences, 3,* 3–19.

Gade, D. W. (1979). Inca and colonial settlement, coca cultivation and endemic disease in the tropical forest. *Journal of Historical Geography, 5,* 263–279.

Gould, W. T. S., & Prothero, R. M. (1975). Space and time in African population mobility. In L. A. Kosinski & R. M. Prothers (Eds.), *People on the move.* London: Methuen.

Haggett, P. (1994). Geographical aspects of the emergence of infectious diseases. *Geografiska Annaler, 76B,* 91–104.

Hughes, C. C., & Hunter, J. M. (1970). Disease and development in Africa. *Social Science and Medicine, 3,* 443–493.

Hunter, J. M. (1993). Elephantiasis: A disease of development in Northeast Ghana. *Social Science and Medicine, 35,* 627–649.

Hunter, J. M., Rey, L., Chu, K. Y., Adekolu-John, E. O., & Mott, K. E. (1993). *Parasitic diseases in water resources development: The need for intersectoral negotiation.* Geneva: World Health Organization.

Jacobsen, K. (1997). Refugees' environmental impact: The effect of patterns of settlement. *Journal of Refugee Studies, 10,* 19–36.

Kloos, H. (1985). Water resources development and schistosomiasis ecology in the Awash Valley, Ethiopia. *Social Science and Medicine, 20,* 609–625.

Lewis, N. D., & Kieffer, E. (1994). The health of women: Beyond maternal and child health. In D. R. Phillips & Y. Verhasselt (Eds.), *Health and development* (pp. 122–137). New York: Routledge.

Martin, P., & J. Widgren (1996). International migration: A global challenge. *Population Bulletin, 51.*

May, R. M. (1994). Changing diseases in changing environments. In B. Cartledge (Ed.), *Health and the environment* Oxford: Oxford University Press, 150–171.

Mayer, J. (1996). The political ecology of disease as a new focus for medical geography. *Progress in Human Geography, 20,* 441–456.

McGee, T., Ginsburg, N., & Koppel, B. (Eds.). (1991). *The extended metropolis: Settlement transition in Asia*

McKeown, T. (1988). *The origins of human disease.* Oxford: Basil Blackwell.

Meade, M. S. (1976). Land development and human health in West Malaysia. *Annals of the Association of American Geographers, 66,* 428–439.

Meade, M. S. (1977). Medical geography as human ecology: The dimension of population movement. *Geographic Review, 67,* 379–393.

Meade, M. S. (1978). Community health and changing hazards in a voluntary agricultural resettlement. *Social Science and Medicine, 12,* 95–102.

Merrick, T. W. (1986). World population in transition. *Population Bulletin, 41.*

Meslin, F. X. (1997). Global aspects of emerging and potential zoonoses: a WHO perspective. *Emerging Infectious Diseases, 3,* 223–228.

Mott, K. E., Desjeux, P., Moncayo, A., Ranque, P., & de Raadt, P. (1990). Parasitic diseases and urban development. *Bulletin of the World Health Organization, 68,* 691–698.

Odum, E. P. (1978). *Ecology: The link between the natural and the social sciences* (2nd ed.). New York: Holt, Rinehart & Winston.

Omran, A. R. (1977). Epidemiologic transition in the U.S.: The health factor in population change. *Population Bulletin, 32.*

PAHO. (1996). New emerging and re-emerging infectious diseases. *Bulletin of the Pan American Health Organization, 30,* 176–181.

Palloni, A. (1981). Mortality in Latin America: Emerging patterns. *Population and Development Review, 7,* 623–649.

Phillips, D. R., & Verhasselt, Y. (1994). *Health and development.* London: Routledge.

Prothero, R. M. (1961). Population movements and problems of malaria eradication in Africa. *World Health Organization Bulletin, 24,* 405–425.

Prothero, R. M. (1965). *Migrants and malaria.* London: Longmans.

Prothero, R. M. (1994). Forced movements of population and health hazards in tropical Africa. *International Journal of Epidemiology, 23,* 657–664.

Reeves, W. C., & Hammon, W. MD. (1962). *Epidemiology of the arthropod-borne viral encephalitides in Kern County, California, 1943–1952* (Publications in Public Health 4). Berkeley: University of California Press.

Roundy, R. W. (1976). Altitudinal mobility and disease hazards for Ethiopian populations. *Economic Geography, 52,* 103–115.

Roundy, R. W. (1977). *Hazards of communicable disease transmission resulting from cultural behavior in Ethiopian rural highland-dwelling populations: A cultural–medical study*

(Doctoral dissertation, University of California, Los Angeles). Ann Arbor, MI: University Microfilms.

Roundy, R. W. (1978). A model for combining human behavior and disease ecology to assess disease hazards in a country: Rural Ethiopia as a model. *Social Science and Medicine, 12,* 121–130.

Schriefer, M. E. (1994). Murine typhus: Updated roles of multiple urban components and a second typhuslike rickettsia. *Journal of Medical Entomology, 31,* 681–685.

Service, M. W. (Ed.). (1989). *Demography and vector-borne diseases.* Boca Raton: CRC Press.

Sharma, S. N., Subbarao, S. K., Choudhury, D. S., & Pandey, K. C. (1993). Role of Anopheles culicifacies and Anopheles stephensi in malaria transmission in urban Delhi. *Indian Journal of Malariology, 30,* 155–168.

Steere, A. C. (1994). Lyme disease: A growing threat to urban populations. *Proceedings of the National Academy of Science, 91,* 2378–2383.

Stock, R. (1986). "Disease and development" or "the underdevelopment of health": A critical review of geographical perspectives on African health problems. *Social Science and Medicine, 23,* 689–700.

Surtees, G. (1970). Effects of irrigation on mosquito populations and mosquito-borne disease in man, with particular reference to rice field extension. *International Journal of Environmental Studies, 1,* 35–42.

Surtees, G. (1971). Urbanization and the epidemiology of mosquito-borne disease. *Abstracts on Hygiene, 46,* 121–134.

Tabibzadeh, I., Rossi-Espagnet, A., & Maxwell, R. (1989). *Spotlight on the cities: Improving urban health in developing countries.* Geneva: World Health Organization.

United Nations, Department of International Economic and Social Affairs. (1989). *Prospects for world urbanization, 1988.* New York: Author.

Warnes, A. M. (1999). UK and western European late-age mortality: Trends in cause-specific death rates, 1960–1990. *Health and Place, 5,* 111–118.

Weil, C. (1981). Health problems associated with agricultural colonization in Latin America. *Social Science and Medicine, 15D,* 449–461.

Weinstein, M. S. (1980). *Health in the city: Environmental and behavioral influences.* New York: Pergamon Press.

Wolfe, B. L., & Behrman, J. R. (1983). Is income overrated in determining adequate nutrition? *Economic Development and Cultural Change, 31,* 525–549.

World Bank. (1993). *World development report 1993: Investing in health.* New York: Oxford University Press.

World Health Organization. (1992). *Our planet, our health: Report of the WHO commission on health and environment.* Geneva: World Health Organization.

World Health Organization. (1999). *World Health Report 1999.* Geneva: Author.

Zelinsky, W. (1971). The hypothesis of the mobility transition. *Geographic Review, 61,* 219–249.

FURTHER READING

Akhtar, R. (Ed.). (1987). *Health and disease in tropical Africa.* London: Harwood Academic.

Desowitz, R. S. (1981). *New Guinea tapeworms and Jewish grandmothers.* New York: Norton.

Doxiadis, C. A. 1974. *Anthropopolis: City for human development.* Proceedings of a symposium with Rene Dubos. New York: Norton.

Dunn, F. L. (1968). Epidemiological factors: Health and disease in hunter–gatherers. In M. H. Logan & E. E. Hunt, Jr. (Eds.), *Health and the human condition: Perspectives on medical anthropology* (pp. 107–118). North Scituate, MA: Duxbury Press.

Farvar, M. T., & Milton, J. (Eds.). (1972). *The careless technology: Ecology and international development.* New York: Tom Stacey.

Garrett, L. (1994). *The coming plague: Newly emerging diseases in a world out of balance.* New York: Farrar, Straus & Giroux; Penguin Books.

Gelbard, A., Haub, C., & Kent, M. M. (1999). World population beyond six billion. *Population Bulletin, 54.*

Groupe de recherche et d'echanges technologiques. (1994). *Water and health in underprivileged urban areas.* Paris: Water Solidarity Network.

Fidler, D. P. (1996). Globalization, international law, and emerging infectious diseases. *Emerging Infectious Disease, 2,* 77–84.

Harpham, T. (1994). Urbanization and mental health in developing countries: A research role for social scientists, public health professionals, and social psychiatrists. *Social Science and Medicine, 39,* 233–245.

Howe, G. M. (1972). *Man, environment and disease in Britain.* New York: Barnes & Noble.

Howe, G. M. (Ed.). (1977). *A world geography of human diseases.* London: Academic Press.

Hubbert, W. T., McCulloch, W. F., & Schnurrenberger, P. R. (Eds.). (1975). *Diseases transmitted from animals to man* (6th ed.). Springfield, IL: Charles C. Thomas.

Hunter, J. M. (1990). Bot-fly maggot infestation in Latin America. *Geographical Review, 80,* 382–398.

Jamison, D. T., Mosley, W. H., Measham, A. R., & Bobadilla, J. L. (Ed.). (1993). *Disease priorities in developing countries.* Oxford University Press.

Kalla, A. C. (1995). Health transition in Mauritius: Characteristics and trends. *Health and Place 1,* 227–234.

Karlen, A. (1995). *Man and microbes: Diseases and plagues in history and modern times.* New York: Putnam's Sons.

Lee, Y. S. (1994). Urban planning and vector control in Southeast Asian cities. *Kaohsiung Journal of Medical Sciences, 10,* S39–S51.

Matuschka, F. R. (1996). Risk of urban Lyme disease enhanced by the presence of rats. *Journal of Infectious Diseases, 175,* 1108–1111.

Moeller, D. W. (1997). *Environmental health* (rev. ed.). Cambridge, MA: Harvard University Press.

Murray, C. J. L., & Lopez, A. D. (Eds.). (1996). *1990 global burden of disease: A comprehensive assessment of mortality and disability from diseases, injuries, and risk factors in 1990 and projected to 2020* (Global burden of disease and injury series, vol. 1). Harvard School of Public Health, World Health Organization, and World Bank. Cambridge, MA: Harvard University Press.

Mutatkar, R. K. (1995). Public health problems of urbanization. *Social Science and Medicine, 41,* 977–981.

Phillips, D. R. (1994). Epidemiological Transition: Implications for health and health care provision. *Geografiska Annaler, 76B,* 71–89.

Platt, A. E. (1996). *Infecting ourselves: How environmental and social disruptions trigger disease* (Worldwatch Paper 129). Washington, DC: Worldwatch Institute.

Rodriguez, A. D., Rodriguez, M. H., Hernandez, J. E., Dister, S. W., Beck, L. A., Rejmankora, E., & Roberts, D. R. (1996). Landscape surrounding human settlements and *Anopheles albimanus* (Diptera: Culicidae) abundance in southern Chiapas, Mexico. *Journal of Medical Entomology, 33*, 39–48.

Sharma, V. P. (1996). Re-emergence of malaria in India. *Indian Journal of Medical Research, 103*, 26–45.

Schofield, C. J., Briceno-Leon, R., Kolstrup, N., Webb, D. J. T., & White, G. B. (1990). The role of house design in limiting vector-borne disease. In S. Cairncross, J. E. Hardoy, & D. Satterthwaite (Eds.), *The poor die young* (pp. 189–212). London: Earthscan.

Singhanetra, R. A. (1993). Malaria and mobility in Thailand. *Social Science and Medicine, 37*, 1147–1154.

Stanley, N. F., & Alpers, M. P. (Eds.). (1975). *Man-made lakes and human health*. New York: Academic Press.

Stone, R. (1995, February 17). If the mercury soars, so may health hazards. *Science, 267*, 957–958.

Takemoto, T., Suzuki, T., Kashiwazaki, H., Mori, S., Hirata, F., Taja, O., & Vexina, E. (1981). The human impact of colonization and parasite infestation in subtropical lowlands of Bolivia. *Social Science and Medicine, 15D*, 133–139.

Thompson, K. (1969). Insalubrious California: Perception and reality. *Annals of the Association of American Geographers, 59*, 50–64.

Thompson, K. (1969). Irrigation as a menace to health in California: A nineteenth century view. *Geographical Review, 59*, 195–214.

Vachon, M. (1993). Onchocerciasis in Chiapis, Mexico. *Geographical Review, 83*, 141–149.

Williams, B. (1990). Assessing the health impact of urbanization. *World Health Statistics Quarterly, 43*, 145–152.

Wills, C. (1996). *Yellow fever, black goddess: The coevolution of people and plagues*. New York: Addison-Wesley.

World Health Organization. (1976). *Water resources development and health: A selected bibliography* (Document MPD/76. 6). Geneva: Author.

World Health Organization. (1993). *The urban health crisis: strategies for health for all in the face of rapid urbanization: Report of the technical discussions*. Geneva: Author.

5

The Biometeorology
of Health Status

Biometeorology considers how variation and change in the physical and chemical characteristics of the atmosphere affect variation and change in the physicochemical systems of living organisms. The human mammal is sensitive to a far wider range of atmospheric characteristics (insults, or stimuli) than is commonly realized. These include not only temperature, humidity, air movement, atmospheric pressure, solar radiation, sound, and gaseous pollution but also infrasound, magnetism, and electrical charge. In addition, a host of indirect influences derive from the biometeorology of each location on earth. A knowledge of climate is necessary to understand what crops are grown with what reliability or to find pattern in the occurrence of arthropod habitats and vectored diseases, topics considered in earlier chapters (Vignette 3-1 explains some patterns).

Biometeorological conditions affect the health status of the population. In terms of the triangle of population–habitat–behavior interactions, this chapter is especially concerned with influences of the natural environment. Elements of the built environment, such as microwaves or buildings' central heating, can also be important influences on the physiological status of the population, that is, on the body's chemical–electrical system. Physiological status is influenced by the time of year and the time of day; it responds to the light, temperature, and altitude of a place. The susceptibility of a person to disease, toxins, and pharmaceutical drugs can be altered by biometeorological changes. Although there is a tendency in medicine to treat all people as a homogeneous population, in fact human physiological characteristics differ from place to place as well as individual to individual. Some of the most talked about influences of the weather, such as a long, hot summer, can be as much constructs of social rhythms in employment and school vacation, sports, and what might be called the political economy of air conditioning as consequences of the weather itself.

This chapter surveys the effects of weather and of electromagnetic radiation on human health. Biological rhythms and acclimatization to temperature and altitude are examined. The physiological basis of climatic influence is described in some detail: sound geographical hypotheses and choice of relevant variables depend on an understanding of the disease process. The influence of elements of weather and their change and passage is described. This chapter also considers the effect of biometeorological influences on the seasonal occurrence of death and birth.

DIRECT BIOMETEOROLOGICAL INFLUENCES

The Radiation Spectrum

Figure 5-1 illustrates he spectrum of electromagnetic radiation. Electromagnetic radiation is propagated through space in the form of packets of energy called photons, which travel at the speed of light. Each photon has a frequency, wavelength, and proportional energy. Short wavelengths of radiation are known as *ionizing* radiation because they can detach electrons and damage atomic structure. These photons of the higher-energy ranges, cosmic, gamma, and X rays, can penetrate into genes and disrupt DNA sequences, which are the body's blueprints. X rays are principally a human-made health hazard; the atmosphere shields us from their natural sources.

Ultraviolet light is best known for causing sunburn. Because the damage it does depends on the intensity and duration of exposure, it creates some important occupational hazards. Welding, for example, produces such intense ultraviolet radiation that an instant's unshielded exposure can cause severe inflammation of the eye's membrane. Only a small band within the range of ultraviolet radiation can penetrate the atmosphere to any extent. Ultraviolet radiation interacts with oxygen to produce ozone and form what is called the "germicidal band" within the stratosphere. In this zone, air-borne bacteria and fungus spores are killed, and the atmosphere is cleansed. This ozone layer, which is threatened by chemofluorcarbons and other technological creations, also partially blocks ultraviolet radiation and so shields life on earth from its more harmful effects.

Ultraviolet radiation also activates a human enzyme to produce vitamin D. The dependence of the human body on ultraviolet radiation to catalyze the body's synthesis of vitamin D posed something of a dilemma for human evolution as people spread over the globe. Too much ultraviolet radiation can cause skin cancer and genetic mutation; not enough can cause a lack of vitamin D, which is necessary to the proper metabolism of calcium. The calcium deficiency disease, rickets, is characterized not only by bowed legs and misshapen backs but also by deformed pelvic bones, which can cause women

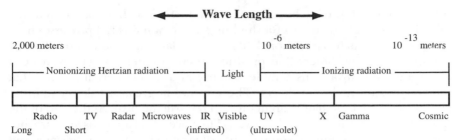

FIGURE 5-1. The spectrum of electromagnetic transmission. Radiation, from cosmic to radio, is a continuum of wavelength.

to die in childbirth. Some radiation must penetrate the skin; too much must be kept out. Yet people live from the equator to the Arctic Circle, with great variation in both annual and seasonal levels of radiation. The evolutionary solution is the deposition of melanin, a dark pigment, in the skin surface of people who live in regions of high radiation and its absence in the skin of people in high-latitude areas of low overall radiation. This adaptation to radiation shields people of equatorial lands and exposes people of the high latitudes. Tanning is the solution for people who live in changeable environments with great fluctuations in radiation levels. The ultraviolet radiation mobilizes pigment that is deposited during times of excessive radiation and removed during seasons of low radiation. Behavioral interference with this rather elegant solution, however, is culturally widespread. In parts of England during the industrial revolution buildings were shrouded in palls of black coal smoke, with the result that children were exposed to little sunlight. In some Moslem lands, women in purdah are so cloistered indoors and shrouded outdoors that rickets can be a problem even though there is intensive solar radiation. The greatest interference with this evolutionary design is continual human migration. Slavery moved tropical Africans to high latitudes, and northern Europeans colonized Australia, the southern United States, and other sunny places. Some negative health consequences followed.

Visible light is biologically very powerful. It stimulates photoreceptive tissue, such as the retina in human eyes. It also changes the electrical charge of protoplasm (the physical base of all living activities) and the viscosity, permeability, and colloidal behavior of proteins. It thereby causes living things to turn toward light and energizes photosynthesis. Light seems to be the most important factor influencing biological rhythms. Only photons in the intermediate range of electromagnetic radiation can be detected by human senses.

Infrared and longer-wave radiations are important for heating the earth's atmosphere and surface and cold-blooded plants and animals, either directly or through reradiation by the earth. The health hazards of these long-wave radiations result from their function as penetrating heat sources.

Infrared radiation used to be a cause of blindness in such occupations as the manufacture of glass, but careful shielding and new industrial processes have removed most such occupational hazards. Today, microwaves are of some concern as the machinery that produces them proliferates. The waves can penetrate the body at considerable distance and cause internal heating that the body's sensors do not detect. The eyes are at greatest risk because the lens of the eye has no blood circulation to remove the heat. At the end of the spectrum are the longer radio waves. They are all around us but are not known to have ever done anyone harm, not even to people intensely exposed because of their occupation.

All of these types of electromagnetic radiation vary over the surface of the earth. The earth's magnetism affects the path and concentration of much radiation. The tilt of the earth results in the seasonal and latitudinal differences described in Vignette 3-1. High elevations that project through thousands of feet of atmosphere experience different amounts and constitution of radiation. Human-made sources of several kinds of radiation are becoming important, and they have a very irregular distribution. Consequences of radiation have been much studied in terms of cell chemistry, microbiology, and physiology, but the spatial distribution of hazards and effects has received little attention, except for skin cancer.

Biological Rhythms

The presence or absence of light is one of the oldest and most universal selective pressures to which all living things have to adapt. An important part of that adaptation has been the development of daily and seasonal rhythms of many body processes. It is clearly beneficial to an organism to be able to anticipate when cold, night, rain, high tide, or spring flowers and grass are going to come so that the slow physiological processes of growing hair, losing leaves, storing food, or coming into rut can be initiated in good time. The precise synchronicity of breeding swarms of many sea creatures and insects, the beaching and egg-laying of turtles and crabs that travel great distances to appear simultaneously at a specific place, and the migration of birds and bats are phenomena that have long fascinated scientists and testified to the existence of biological clocks. The equivalent body rhythms of human beings have been recognized much more recently.

The existence of endogenous "clocks" is now well established for a wide variety of animals, including humans. Even in constant temperature and total darkness some biological processes continue to oscillate rhythmically. The rhythms with a span of about 24 hours are known as *circadian*. In humans they include sleep and wakefulness; body temperature; cognitive performance; serum hormone levels; urinary cycles and excretion of ketosteroids, chloride, sodium, and urea; and ionization of blood calcium and phosphate, which affects regulating hormones. It is clear that the physiological state of individuals is constantly changing. Tenfold differences in the susceptibility of mice to bacterial toxins at different times of night have been demonstrated, and it is likely that human circadian rhythms also influence susceptibility to infection and toxins.

The study of circadian and other rhythms can help us understand the ways in which environment directly affects and alters the status of a population. Reception and interpretation of environmental stimuli influence virtually all the body's major organs and endocrine systems (Figure 5-2). There have been major advances in understanding the nature of the body's clock (Barinaga, 1999; Somers, Devlin, & Kay, 1998; Thresher et al., 1998). A recently discovered cluster of nerve cells in the brain, *the suprachiasmatic nucleus* (SCN), is now believed to be the organ responsible for synchronizing body rhythms with environmental light. Pigments called cryptochromes have been found in the eye, skin, and part of the brain, and they are believed to drive the body's clock. The two forms of cryptocrines located in a part of the retina absorb blue light and transfer the light signal to the SCN, a process for which the individual does not have to be awake or conscious. In individual neurons there, two proteins alternately build up and turn on and off each other's

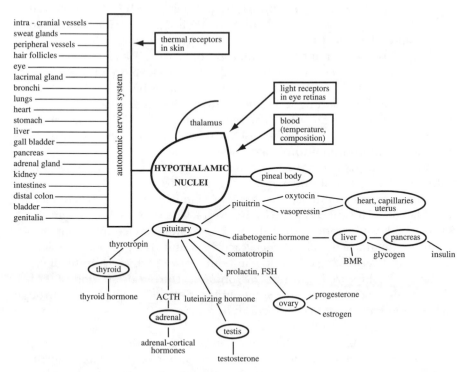

FIGURE 5-2. Hypothalamic environmental mediation. Sensing the environment, the hypothalamus acclimatizes the body through its direct neural connections to many organs and through the hormones it induces the pituitary to send.

gene for production, forming an accurate internal clock in each of tens of thousands of cells in the SCN. This oscillation also turns on and off a gene for production of vasopressin and maybe other endocrines. The photoreception of the cryptochromes sets the body's elegant master clock of oscillating proteins. Individual light sensitivity can result in seasonal affective disorder (SAD; winter depression) and sleeping problems of the elderly, as well as difficulties adjusting to changes in longitude.

The main body mediator, the hypothalamus, controls the pineal gland in mammals, which acts as an endocrine transducer (that which converts one form of energy to another). It synthesizes and secretes the hormones melatonin and serotonin, two of the most powerful chemical transmitters in the brain which can penetrate everywhere in the body. During the day, the pineal gland synthesizes serotonin. As darkness falls, the pineal gland produces a surge of melatonin. The cycle in the pineal gland is implicated as the clock that controls the development of puberty (Fellman, 1985). A sharp decline in melatonin production at puberty seems a trigger. Middle-age adults secrete only half as much melatonin as children. Besides causing sleepiness, melatonin dampens release of estrogen (and is being worked on as a contraceptive) and so may be related to timing of conception.

The hypothalamus also controls the pituitary, the body's master gland, and so it can adjust most of the body's metabolism, endocrine system, blood vessels, and other organs as appropriate for environmental conditions. As we shall see, this is important for acclimatization. In the 1980s SAD was recognized: the winter blues, with depression, excessive sleep, weight gain, loss of interest in daily activities. The major therapy that has been developed is phototherapy, simply bright lighting for a short period in the morning, to communicate with the pineal gland. The recent research on the cellular clocks of the SCN and the photoreception of the cryptochromes will result in new therapeutic interventions within a decade.

Most people become aware of circadian rhythms when they travel longitudinally. The physical and mental effects of desynchronizing the body's rhythms from those of the environment are familiar as jet lag. It is not a matter of fatigue: The effects are the same even if one slept well on the airplane. Rather, body temperature and kidney and hormone cycles are no longer appropriate for the schedule of social activities and daylight. Each biological clock is reset, advancing or slowing an hour or two each cycle, until all cycles are again synchronized with the environment. During the period of jet lag, however, the body may be more susceptible to infectious agents and, through impaired judgment and coordination, to accidents. There is growing use of melatonin to help reset the clock.

The large volume of international travel has made circadian rhythms and their adjustment a matter of concern to business, sports, and tourist industries as well as to diplomats and the military. One topic of interest is the importance of circadian rhythms for work shifts. When people continuously work at night, first the sleep cycle, then the body-temperature cycle, and eventually, it is thought, all the other cycles will be appropriately set to the social activity pattern. In some professions, however, shifts are regularly changed around or even rotated. This means that nurses, policemen, and other 24-hour-service personnel may frequently be involved in critical situations while effectively in a state of jet lag.

Most research on circadian rhythms has been medical. There has been no study of their spatial variation, their effects on population mobility, or the impact on them from cultural transformation of the environment. Are people who live in the long winter nights of high latitudes, for example, more susceptible to infectious agents than those in equatorial lands? Light is used today to induce chickens to lay more eggs and to bring cattle and sheep back into estrus after a miscarriage or failed fertilization. Does nighttime electric lighting affect human fecundity at all? Reading under bright light until late at night, as academics do, delays sleep onset by changing the circadian rhythms. Geographically designed studies of circadian rhythms would include contrasts between places and cultures (and occupations, activities by gender and class) and could be very illuminating.

Acclimatization

Acclimatization is the genetically given capacity of humans to adapt their physiological systems over long periods to heat, cold, and altitude. People are adapted to living in an extraordinary range of temperatures and other environmental conditions. They live and reproduce in hot deserts and Arctic tundra, as well as in the high Andes and Himalayas.

Behavioral and genetic adaptations are of great importance to acclimatization. Cultural geographers have studied adaptive differences in house-type design and construction, the materials and design of clothing, and the cultural rhythms of daily activity patterns. Genetic adaptations often involve the morphology of the body. In many animal populations, for example, long limbs and slimness serve to dissipate heat efficiently, while squat bodies with a low surface-to-volume ratio serve to conserve heat. Physical anthropologists have identified some such tendencies among human populations, but extensive migration has created as much exception to the rules (tall Norwegians in the Arctic and compact Chinese in tropical Asia) as conformity (compact Eskimos in the Arctic and tall, slender Tutsi in tropical Africa). As important as genetic and behavioral adaptations are, this chapter looks at the physical processes of acclimatization and the implications for health that result from variations in physiologic status of the population.

The physiological processes of thermoregulation are known in some detail. The human body must maintain a temperature of around 98.6 °F (37 °C) regardless of the environmental temperature. Over short periods, people react by shivering to generate heat from muscle movement and sweating to cool the body by evaporation. People everywhere sweat and shiver at the same skin temperature. Acclimatized people, however, use other physiological means to control body temperature. Their skin temperatures may not reach the threshold values for sweating or shivering.

The hypothalmus learns about environmental temperature from nerve channels to thermoreceptors in the skin, and about body temperature from nerves and the hypothalamic blood vessels. The hypothalamus causes the peripheral blood vessels to dilate (vasodilation) under heat stress, so that more blood can be brought to the surface for cooling, and to constrict (vasoconstriction) in protection against heat loss, so that more blood is held in the core of the body. Over time, the density of the capillary network near the skin will change. Most animals sweat from a few sites (armpits, for example) controlled by the sympathetic nervous system. Humans have evolved an unusual capacity for eccrine (excretory) sweating by glands located all over the body. This involves excreting dilute solutions of water, salts, urea, sugar, and lactic acid for purposes of cooling the surface of the body through evaporation. Under conditions of prolonged heat, the efficiency of this sweating may be greatly increased. The acclimatized person sweats from the body's entire surface; the flux of water can reach several liters in an hour. The consequent drain of blood electrolytes (such as magnesium and sodium) is enormous, even though urinary output is considerably diminished.

By far the most complex adaptations to temperature involve the endocrine system (see Figure 5-2). Through the thyroid gland, the basal metabolic rate is altered to generate more or less heat from food. Because different kinds of food, such as fats or carbohydrates, have different capacities for heat generation, dietary needs change. Levels of thyroxin, which regulates carbohydrate metabolism, change, as do levels of iodine required to make thyroxin. Thus, someone living at a cold, high elevation would need more iodine to maintain a high basal metabolic rate and would be more at risk of goiter than someone in a warm place, even if iodine were equally available in the environment. In fact, iodine is less available in glaciated mountains, which have soils deficient in iodine and are usually remote from the transportation systems that would facilitate trade and the import of seafood, so goiter is often a serious problem of such areas.

Another endocrine system, the adrenocortical system, stimulates the pancrease to produce more or less insulin and controls the metabolism of the liver. It also affects capillary resistance and the removal and excretion of waste products from the blood. Even the relative amounts of the types of cells that comprise blood change from winter to summer. Blood volume also increases under heat stress and decreases under cold stress. An important adaptation to cold is deposition of a layer of fat under the skin.

The work of the heart, deposition in the blood vessels, blood-clotting time, blood sugar levels, and innumerable other physiological characteristics differ in people acclimatized to different degrees of heat or cold and even in an individual in different seasons.

Acclimatization to high altitude affects far fewer people but in some ways is more dramatic than adaptations to heat or cold. The greatest adaptive stress is from low oxygen tension in the rarified atmosphere: More red blood cells must be produced, and hemoglobin (and iron nutrition) must be increased. The body must change its endocrine balance to prevent acidosis resulting from changed levels of carbon dioxide in the blood. Permeability of cell and capillary walls and the facility with which red blood cells give up oxygen to body tissue must be increased. Lung size, surfaces, and permeability are altered. When fully adjusted to elevations of over 10,000 feet (3,000 meters), the physiology of people alters sufficiently to create much more susceptible, and often hazardous, reactions to therapeutic doses of drugs. Fecundity seems to be lower at high altitudes. When people acclimatized to high altitudes descend to sea level to seek work, they may be susceptible to respiratory infections.

THE INFLUENCES OF THE WEATHER

Weather, as distinct from climate, consists of atmospheric conditions experienced by people on an immediate basis. It changes hour by hour and mile by mile. The frequency and amount that it changes—the variability of weather—are its most important characteristics. The extremes of conditions reached are also significant for health.

Air masses, huge chunks of relatively homogeneous air flowing over the earth's surface with a depth of up to a few kilometers, are as familiar to television weather report watchers as the fronts that separate air masses. Although tremendous energy exchanges occur at the fronts, the air masses do not generally mix. They retain their own characteristic temperature, humidity, atmospheric (barometric) pressure, and other properties. The fronts that separate them are accompanied by winds and, especially if associated with squalls and thunderstorms, the generation of ionization, extremely low frequency (ELF) waves, and infrasound (too low in frequency for humans to hear). Let us review these individual elements and their health implications before considering what happens when fronts pass or extreme conditions develop.

Temperature, Humidity, and Air Movement

Temperature, humidity, and movement of air together determine how readily the human body loses its heat. Such heat is generated by metabolic activity, even when the body is at rest. We have considered the major physiological processes by which the body controls the generation, conservation, and dissipation of heat during acclimatization. The ability of the body to radiate heat depends on the surrounding temperature. The effectiveness of evaporative cooling depends on the surrounding humidity and air movement. Temperature–humidity, "comfort," and wind-chill measures portray environmental stress much more accurately than a simple measurement of temperature, which is commonly used by medical scientists.

The most obvious health impact of the weather attends extremes of heat and cold. Death from exposure to cold involves no mysterious mechanisms: When the body's core temperature falls below a certain point, its chemical reactions cease. Heat causes increased peripheral circulation, which can be stressful in its own right, and copious sweating can drain the body of electrolytes. In heatstroke, the sweating mechanism shuts down, allowing body temperatures to rise rapidly. Certain proteins in the brain can permanently change, even if the body is cooled before death results.

Heat waves have long been associated with increased mortality. Persistently high temperatures seem more closely related to mortality than do the peak temperatures reached. The most consistent predictors seem to be the average temperature and the number of successive hot days. Increased mortality usually occurs in the first 2 or 3 days following the heat wave's peak. Greenberg, Bromberg, Reed, Gustafson, and Beauchamp (1983) studied the 1980 Texas heat wave and compared it with the heat wave of 1950 and the period from 1970–1979. Temperatures of over 100 °F (37.7 °C) existed for 61 of 71 days, and 107 deaths were attributed to heat. The risk of death was highest among males, blacks, those engaged in heavy labor, and the elderly. Death rates were higher during heat waves of former years. Greenberg et al. presume that is because of the increased prevalence of air conditioning today. In terms of our triangle, the lack of access to the technological intervention of cooling in the built habitat is a killer. Yet climatologists, who are geographers, can so focus on the natural habitat that they fail to consider cultural buffers or even the built environment. Kalkstein and Davis (1989), for example, conclude that "regional acclimatization" appears to be especially important in summer, since the strongest associations of heat with mortality occur where hot weather is uncommon (Northwest Pacific and Continental North) and the weakest associations occur where heat is most common (the Southeast and Continental South). This they took to be evidence that people respond to weather in a relative rather than absolute fashion, because where hot weather occurs rarely the population responds more dramatically. They also found in their models of nonwhites, however, strong mortality responses to heat in southern cities (Atlanta, Birmingham, Memphis) despite lack of association in white models. This they took to indicate that nonwhites may be more sensitive to heat. Several social risk factors may be involved. Today these include the increased numbers of elderly (whose physiology is less efficient at cooling) living alone, the risk of living alone compounded when people decline to open their windows for improved circulation because of fear of crime, and, of course, lack of money to buy cooling technologies. Chicago, St. Louis, and many other cities have responded to these risks by organizing the provision of fans and warning family and neighbors to check on the elderly.

There are several population predisposing factors for suffering heatstroke. These include the presence of such degenerative diseases as cardiovascular disease, renal (kidney) disease, and hypertension; preexisting acute diarrheal or febrile disease; salt deficiency and dehydration; and the use of drugs that affect the thermoregulatory system—alcohol, amphetamines, and such therapeutic drugs as diuretics and anticholinergics. People who undertake sustained activity in the heat are at risk, as are people whose lack of fitness or acclimatization makes their cardiovascular systems less able to cope with the necessary heat dissipation.

Heat waves have also been associated with increased crime, especially homicide, but the pattern is not systematic or consistent. A plausible biological pathway is that heat interferes with sleep and therefore with dream cycles. This topic cries out for some behavioral-vertex research.

An increase in the number of deaths following heat waves has been repeatedly observed. It is not clear, however, how much of the increase in mortality occurs to those about to die from degenerative disease anyway. Several studies have reported less than normal mortality shortly after the peak associated with the heat wave, but the decrease does not always offset the previous increase. There is some concern that people surrounded by air conditioning may be losing their acclimatization to heat so that they are less able to cope with extreme heat stress. Mortality, however, is certainly higher among those socioeconomic groups least likely to enjoy air-conditioned homes.

Air-Borne Life

The air is charged with living things. The transport and survival of bacteria, viruses, fungi, and allergens such as pollen depend on certain conditions of atmospheric temperature, humidity, condensation, and movement. Agents of human disease are injected into the air by coughing and sneezing, by the shedding of hair and dead skin, and by the spray of cooling towers, air conditioners, and irrigation systems. Soil bacteria, fungi, and pollen are picked up by the wind. Dispersal depends on atmospheric turbulence. To all such life forms, ultraviolet radiation ultimately is lethal.

Temperature and humidity are the limiting factors for survival in air; they act together with different effects on different organisms. Bacteria often can withstand extremes of temperature but may be seriously affected by humidity. The ubiquitous intestinal bacteria *Escherichia coli* survives for less than 3 hours at 68 °F (20 °C) and 50% relative humidity, but mycoplasma of human pulmonary origin survived up to 5 hours at 82 °F (28 °C) and 50% humidity. Viruses can multiply only in living organisms, but they can survive in the air anywhere from a few seconds to a few hours. Polio viruses have been shown to be progressively desiccated in the air but to have sufficient longevity for dissemination over several miles. Tolerance and preference for environmental conditions are highly specific to the type of organism. In one study, for example, polio virus survived best at 80% relative humidity, but vaccinia virus survived best at 20% (Hyslopo, 1978).

Air-borne bacteria and viruses have caused epidemics miles from their sources. An outbreak of Q fever in San Francisco, for example, was traced to the fumes from the fat-rendering plant of a slaughterhouse. The combined effects of temperature and humidity are thought to result in different survival times for air-borne microorganisms in summer and winter and thus to be a critical factor in the seasonal incidence of disease (described later in this chapter).

Both fungi and pollen are suspended in the air. A few fungal infections of the lungs are serious diseases, especially histoplasmosis and coccidioidomycosis. Their distribution is clearly related to temperature, humidity, rainfall, and local winds, which pick up the fungi from disturbed soil. The distribution of human disease may be limited by prevailing winds as well as soil temperature and moisture. Ragweed, the most common pollen source for the hayfever that afflicts more than 6% of the U.S. population, grows best on cultivated land. Again, rain, wind, and humidity affect dispersal.

Atmospheric Pressure

The weight of the atmosphere presses on the surface of the earth. Subsiding air exerts more pressure than rising air. One atmosphere of pressure, usually defined as 1,013 millibars (mb), is felt as 14.7 pounds per square inch (1,034 grams per square centimeter) at sea level. Atmospheric (barometric) pressure changes are slight in equatorial zones. Over North America normal pressure changes between air masses are on the order of 25 mb. At high latitudes pressure changes may reach 120 mb. The most extreme low and high pressures ever recorded on earth amount to a difference of about 3 pounds per square inch (211 grams per square centimeter). (Altitudinal changes, such as those encountered in balloons or depressurized aircraft, can cause much greater pressure difference).

The major mechanism postulated for why normal changes in atmospheric pressure affect the body's biochemistry is that body volume expands slightly, leading to retention of water and therefore to alteration of electrolyte balance. Eventually, levels of disequilibrium are reached that trigger intervention by higher homeostatic control systems to restore proper fluid levels. These changes would result in water storage in certain parts of the body—in joints, eyes, and so forth—and could cause joint pain, glaucoma pain, increased blood pressure, blood clotting, and general irritability.

Winds

Winds blow between the different atmospheric pressures that characterize air masses and between zones of subsiding and rising air (Vignette 3-1) as part of the heat balancing of atmospheric circulation. The strength, frequency, and duration of winds vary greatly from place to place.

Air movement is important for cooling the body and for dispersing disease agents. A "red" snow that fell in Sweden in 1969 was caused by high concentrations of bacteria later traced through winds between a low-pressure air mass over Scandinavia and a high-pressure air mass over the Soviet Union, to sandstorms north of the Black Sea. Not only microorganisms ride the winds. Hunter (1980) has shown that the blackflies that are the vectors of onchocerciasis can be disseminated over hundreds of miles by the wind systems associated with the arrival of the wet season in the savanna lands of West Africa. This monsoon effect is a major obstacle to the World Health Organization's attempts to control onchocerciasis over a large area of the Ivory Coast, Mali, Ghana, and Burkina Faso (formerly Upper Volta).

Winds have another effect. The movement of air, especially air with low humidity, promotes the ionization of atmospheric gases. Electrons are stripped from their atoms, producing positive and negative charges. In the extreme form associated with convective buildup of cumulus clouds, segregation of electric charges may result in lightning. The degree of atmospheric electrical charge is one characteristic of an air mass.

Dry winds, such as the Chinook, Santa Ana, foehn, sirocco, and harmattan, are associated across cultures with irritation, bad temper, accidents, and violence. Despite an extraordinary richness of folklore, however, there has been little in the way of controlled studies. The heat itself used to be implicated, but suspicion is now directed at ionization.

Atmospheric Ionization

Ionization in the atmosphere has several sources. It results from radiation impact as well as the friction of movement. The charged molecules are electrical and chemical stimuli with undetermined consequences for human health. Persinger (1980) has reviewed and explained many of the phenomena involved with the "electromagnetic stimuli of the weather matrix." Much of the following discussion draws on his book.

Atmospheric ions could react with chemical processes in the body by giving or taking electrons if they had access to biochemical pathways; therefore, their potential to be culprits in the etiology of suicide, homicide, aggression, infection, migraines, conjunctivitis, and respiratory congestion needs to be considered seriously. Their physical influence as environmental electrical stimuli is generally dismissed on the grounds that any current the ions might induce in the human body by their presence in the atmosphere would be too small to have an effect, even around the brain neurons' electric field. Chemically, however, there is a pathway for possible interaction: by absorption into the blood stream through the lungs, the ions might alter the pH by acting as oxidizing or reducing agents. This could influence a host of chemical pathways and homeostatic sensors and controls.

The serotonin irritation syndrome of migraines, nausea, irritability, edema, conjunctivitis, and respiratory congestion has been correlated with the accumulation of positive ions that occurs as much as a day before the weather changes. The serotonin hypothesis, in brief, is that in the brain a major chemical transmitter whose activities are associated with aggression, sexual activity, pain sensitivity, and other functions is affected by bursts of atmospheric ions. The mechanism is not explained yet, but if it exists, it would be relevant to depression, irritability, suicides, report of pain, and other cross-cultural correlates of the weather.

Unpleasant effects have usually been correlated with positive ions, whereas negative ions are generally associated with feeling good. Positive ion charges occur naturally before thunderstorms, and they accompany hot, dry winds. Humans generate positive ions by such means as heating systems, in which cold, dry air is heated, making it drier, and blown through metal pipes. Dry throats, mouths, and membranes, which become more permeable to virus, may result from sleeping and living in heated environments. Therapeutic claims made for machines that generate negative ions for bedrooms have not been proven.

Extremely Low Frequency Waves and Infrasound

A few scientifically sound studies have been done on the effects of geomagnetic storms upon moods or brain function. Most of these have focused on reaction times, which are quantifiable measures. It is possible that the intensity and quantity of ELF waves (3 Hz to 3 kHz or so) generated by such storms could influence the brain because they include the frequencies of the brain's own transmissions. Most ELF energy (generated, for example, by lightning and human-made sources) remains between the earth and the ionosphere and travels long distances without appreciable attenuation. The major variations in the number and intensity of ELF waves and their sources result from diurnal and seasonal changes.

Infrasound shares some of these ELF characteristics in that it can travel long distances with little loss of energy. At frequencies too low for humans to hear, the waves have the potential to generate whole-body vibration by resonance. They are generated by severe weather disturbances and, traveling at the speed of sound, could be detectable weather precursors. In laboratory studies of infrasound, 10 Hz at 115 decibels can cause lethargy, euphoria, and loss of time judgment; these are frequencies generated inside closed automobiles traveling at 100 kilometers an hour. At other frequencies, infrasound is associated with nausea and dizziness. The research literature, however, is sparse. There are few weather stations that measure infrasound and fewer correlation studies under controlled conditions.

Passage of Fronts

The passage of a front marks a change of air mass. Especially when the passage is accompanied by squalls, it entails winds, electric charge, and the generation of ELF waves and infrasound. As the air masses change, so do many of the environmental conditions that have been affecting people: temperature, humidity, brightness or cloud cover, suspended living organisms, and atmospheric pressure. The body must cope with all these stimuli and their changes. Accumulated stresses can lower the level of health so that individuals fail to rally (Chapter 2). It is thus not surprising that the passage of fronts has often been related to increased mortality.

There have been numerous studies on the influence of frontal passage and weather changes on morbidity and mortality rates. Weather types have been classified in many ways, and various weather elements have been examined singly or together. The best correlations have been attained when weather is treated as a complex of elements. Those variables most often found to be important include mean temperature, diurnal change, mean dew point, mean visibility, mean barometric pressure, day-to-day change in barometric pressure, mean wind speed, and various comfort indices used to adjust temperature for humidity and wind speed. The most consistent relationships of the rates have been to intensity of change in the weather. The most consistent mortality and morbidity associations with weather conditions have been overall mortality, cardiovascular disease, and asthma; diabetes, respiratory illness, and psychiatric conditions also have some associations with weather.

SEASONALITY OF DEATH AND BIRTH

Death Seasonality

It has been known for at least 2,500 years that some causes of death occur more often in one season than in another. A hundred years ago it was common knowledge in the United States that in summer people died of malaria, yellow fever, cholera, typhoid, gastroenteritis, and tuberculosis. In winter people died of influenza, stroke, and cold-related causes.

The literature on seasonality of mortality has been dominated by one person, Masako Sakamoto-Momiyama of the Meteorological Research Institute in Tokyo. Her work over 25 years discovered, explained, and popularized the importance of seasonal patterns and how they are changing.

After analyzing the seasonal pattern of occurrence of scores of diseases at various latitudes, in various climates, and among different age, socioeconomic, race, and ethnic groups, Sakamoto-Momiyama developed general models of variation (Figure 5-3). Mortality patterns in most countries have been bimodal; that is, they have had both winter and summer peaks. With economic and social development, the summer peak has disappeared, and mortality now has its highest incidence in winter. Sakamoto-Momiyama differentiates several types of shift in seasonality. In the *transitory type* (cancer in Figure 5-3), the summer peak of incidence gradually shifts into autumn as it decreases, perhaps moving toward a winter peak. The *reversing type* reverses from a summer to a winter peak. It has two subcategories: diseases for which the former summer peak becomes a trough and a new winter peak is created

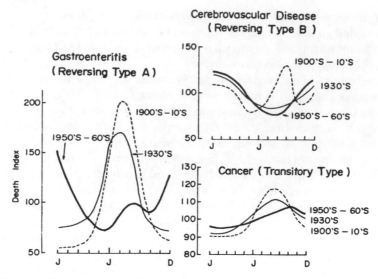

FIGURE 5-3. Models of seasonal shifts in mortality. When the death index by month is plotted for several time periods, the peak of mortality for some diseases reverses from summer to winter; for others the summer peak gradually disappears, leaving a previous winter peak as the only seasonality; for still others the summer peak decreases and shifts toward fall. From Sakamoto-Momiyama (1977, p. 33). Copyright 1977 by University of Tokyo Press. Reprinted by permission.

(reversing type A) and diseases that formerly had both a winter and a summer peak but lost the summer one (reversing type B). Gastroenteritis, tuberculosis, and beriberi are type A; many of the degenerative diseases associated with aging are type B.

As Sakamoto-Momiyama (1977, p. xiv) relates, while doing research in 1965–1966 in New York she was surprised to find the winter peak disappearing for many causes of death in the United States. Her detailed studies of infant mortality in particular led her to revise her previous idea that technological progress would lead to concentration of mortality in winter, as she had concluded from her experiences in Japan. Instead, she hypothesized that a "deseasonalization" of mortality would occur. Her latest works note that Japan and western Europe are following the United States and Scandinavia into this deseasonalized pattern of mortality (Sakamoto-Momiyama, 1977).

There can be many reasons why mortality incidence loses seasonality under conditions of economic and technological development. Heavy labor and exposure to the elements decrease. Diet changes and a variety of nutritious foods become available all year. Medical technology advances, and health care becomes more accessible. For some causes of death one can point to specific sociotechnological developments: Refrigeration and the chlorination of water supplies control summer gastroenteristis, for example;

the conquest of polio means that swimming pools no longer start summer epidemics; changes in house type, screening, occupation, and other factors have led to the eradication of diseases such as malaria and yellow fever in some countries. Sakamoto-Momiyama (1977) has advanced the hypothesis that much of the deseasonalization of mortality is due to central heating and air conditioning. She points to the relationships between temperature and cerebrovascular disease (Figure 5-4). Sweden and New York City, which have widespread central heating, show consistent linear relationships without changes of slope at high temperatures, while Western Europe and Honshu in Japan, where many houses are not heated, have seasonal changes of slope. Hokkaido, which is cold in winter, uses heating systems that are turned off when the temperature reaches 54 °F (12–13 °C); the winter slope is small until that point and afterwards resembles Honshu's (represented by Tokyo in Figure 5-4).

Much research has been stimulated by these studies: Vignette 5-1 discusses some of the statistical procedures essential to seasonality research. Although many diseases have been analyzed in detail by epidemiologists, few studies have been done on geographical patterns, and few national studies have been completed by geographers. Kevan and Chapman (1980), for example, confirm the deseasonalization of many diseases in Canada but find great seasonality continuing for bronchitis, pneumonia, influenza, and circulatory diseases (winter) and violence, accidents, and poisoning (summer).

Influenza continues to be a winter disease. The association of cooling winter temperatures with increased influenza mortality, after a certain lag, is

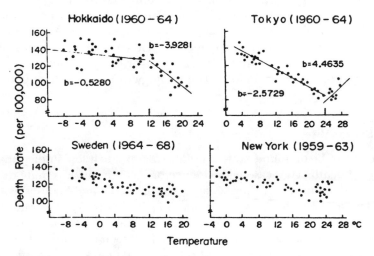

FIGURE 5-4. Association between cardiovascular mortality and temperature. In Hokkaido (northern Japan), Sweden, and New York, deseasonalization of mortality seems to be associated with use of central heating. From Sakamoto-Momiyama (1977, p. 165). Copyright 1977 by University of Tokyo Press. Reprinted by permission.

indubitable. The association persists over widespread locations and different climates. The reason is unknown. Speculation blames several factors:

1. Biometeorological conditions cause the nasopharynx and trachea to be dry, and membranes become more susceptible to virus penetration.
2. The virus can survive in the air, between hosts, more easily when the air is relatively dry and cold than when it is hot and humid.
3. The lower solar radiation, and hence ultraviolet radiation, promote virus survival.
4. The body's metabolic changes make it more susceptible.
5. People gather indoors in closer proximity for longer periods in winter, schools are in session, and even recreation tends to be indoors— a point emphasized by the importance of room density as a correlate in many influenza epidemic studies.

Any explanation of influenza's seasonality must account for its winter incidence in Florida and Hawaii, on the Great Plains and in New England, and in perpetually crowded institutions such as prisons.

Mortality from heart disease is negatively correlated with temperature in several midlatitude countries. Between 30 and 70 °F (−1 and 21 °C) correlation coefficients of −.95 have been found. A 2.5% increase in mortality has been estimated for each degree Celsius decrease in mean monthly temperature, although the exact relationship differs by climate area. Sometimes mortality from ischemic heart disease but not cerebrovascular disease, and sometimes the reverse have been correlated with temperature change.

In general, respiratory disease shows the strongest association with winter, and cancer shows the least seasonality—which is hardly surprising given its long incubation period. The meteorological conditions and physiological stresses of acclimatization are undoubtedly involved in seasonality, but so are culture rhythms and technology. The etiology of most seasonal patterns of mortality remains puzzling.

Birth Seasonality

Seasonality of birth, found everywhere, has been much less studied than seasonality of death. The seasonal incidence of birth in Japan is quite different from that in countries of Europe, and that of the United States is again distinct. The index of birth (see Vignette 5-1) in Figure 5-5 illustrates the bimodal pattern that has persisted in the United States for decades but showed signs of changing lately. There have been a few good descriptions of the seasonal patterns by region, race, and other population characteristics in the United States and Europe, including at least one study in which no seasonality was found in a population (Arcury, Williams, & Kryscio, 1990). In some studies, the amplitude (height above and below the index line) has been

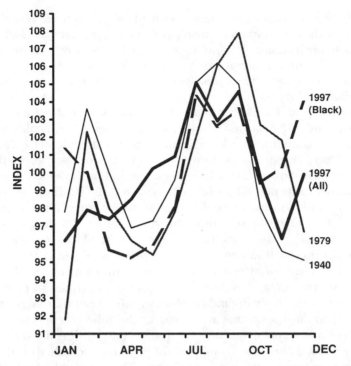

FIGURE 5-5. Seasonality of birth in the United States. The bimodal pattern has remained remarkably constant for decades. In recent years, the April trough (summer conceptions) and February minipeak have been lost overall, but African Americans still retain the southern pattern.

found to be greater for illegitimate births and births to the poor, to the less educated, and to blacks, although there are a few indications that these relationships may be changing. Despite minor differences in the amplitude of seasonality among population subgroups in the United States, however, the pattern of seasonality has been remarkably similar. The relative peaks vary in magnitude and timing across the country; they have changed over time, but the manner of this change has not yet been studied.

One possible reason for birth seasonality is that high temperatures may have an effect on spermatogenesis (the creation of sperm). High temperatures may also injure sperm. As with other biometeorological effects, threshold and range are presently unknown. How high a temperature over how long is necessary to affect fertility? Is a single episode, such as playing tennis in tight athletic clothing on a hot day, enough exposure? Is birth, like mortality, also becoming deseasonalized?

The seasonal patterns of birth may have nothing to do with temperature. They may be a result of agricultural patterns, school calendars, the timing of holidays and vacations, Christmas–New Year celebrations, and leisure time in the United States, and of equivalent events in other cultures. When people migrate, does their seasonality of birth pattern change relatively suddenly under the new environmental conditions or gradually, over a generation or more, through cultural adaptation? Vignette 5-2 discusses the various hypotheses about the cause of seasonality of birth and its relevance to the triangle of human ecology.

There are innumerable consequences for health and disease from birth seasonality. The most obvious is the variable need for health services. Obstetrical wards built for peak periods will have many idle beds during the trough. Birthing classes and maternity leaves from work are affected. More significant effects, however, may lie with congenital birth defects, premature births, and neonatal mortality (Keller & Nugent, 1983). There is considerable seasonal variation in neonatal mortality, but its correlates are not clear. The point often made by scientists who study congenital disease is that if there is seasonality, the condition is not the result of genetics alone. Something in the environment after conception, whether in the womb, at birth, or after birth, must actually cause the expression of the disease. As bones, nerves, palates, and endocrine systems form at different times in the development of the fetus, biometeorological influences that might be relevant to congenital disease may not occur at the time of conception at all. This is especially true for one mental disease that universally shows a seasonality of birth. There is a strong peak of birth for individuals with schizophrenia during late winter and early spring. These individuals would have been fetuses in their third month, when the central nervous system is forming, during the late summer heat that is associated (in the United States) with the minimum of conception. This, of course, is also, especially at high latitudes, the time of maximum sunlight and effect on serotonin production and other hormone cycles.

The problem of separating environmental and cultural factors is complex. Mothers are likely to be eating different foods, exercising in different ways, and following different work and sleeping habits during summer than they are in winter. It is suspected that for some congenital diseases, seasonality may result from the activity of a viral agent. This is an analogy to the congenital effects of rubella (German measles) infections. Most physicians studying a seasonal pattern in a congenital disease will look to changes in food, drink, sickness, and medicines before they will consider the weather.

Other Biometeorological Effects

There are many other, more indirect, biometeorological effects on mortality and natality. Chief among these is the effect of climate on agricultural cycles and cropping patterns, and hence on many nutritional problems. The "hunger season" recognized in wet–dry climatic zones of Africa, for example, creates nutritional susceptibility to infectious diseases and other stresses. In many places the weather cycle creates periods of high and low employment, of transportation difficulties and poor access to health services, and of stagnant air or atmospheric inversions and intense pollution episodes. Chapter 6 considers some pollution effects.

CONCLUSION

There is a vast store of folklore on weather sensitivity. Old war wounds, creaking joints, and restlessness are notorious for being able to predict changes in the weather. Mood swings, migraine headaches, asthma, rheumatism, and heart problems are popularly associated with various weather conditions. As we have seen, it is certainly possible that popular wisdom is not pure myth. Changes in barometric pressure, temperature, ionization, sunlight, and other weather elements may plausibly affect the biochemistry of the body.

There is remarkably little proof, however, of the effects of weather on health, aside from temperature extremes. The connections between weather conditions and human biochemistry and behavior are complex matters. Among the difficulties facing the researcher are the classification of morbidity and mortality data, the range and location of weather conditions, and the limitations on doing controlled studies with human beings as subjects. Conditions and data vary with age, season, socioeconomic status, and cultural buffering through the use, for example, of air heating and cooling. Most of the research done so far has been accomplished in Europe with its generally moderate marine climate. The climates of the United States and the seasonality of its latitudes vary in more substantial ways and offer many opportunities for research.

The present status of research is such that little is known of the relevant periodicities. The body's clocks vary from seconds and hours to days, months, and possibly years. Variations in temperature, pressure, or other weather elements and their rates of change occur over seconds, minutes, hours, days, months, and years. Finding the pathways for influences is difficult because of the problem of specifying the relevant periodicity (should one correlate heart attacks with temperature change in a day or over a number of days, with passage of a front or with the number of fronts that passed within a limited time) and our ignorance of threshold or relevant range (is a temperature change from 80 to 60 °F the same in effect as one from 40 to 20°; can winter in countries whose mean daily temperatures never get below freezing be compared with that in countries whose temperatures stay below freezing for weeks). The general scientific law of initial value, applied to biometeorological studies, would state that any weather influence is going to differ with both the level from which it started and the level of the physiology it is affecting. For example, if a certain influence raises blood pressure, the health result depends to a large degree on the initial level of the blood pressure. At what point, then, can we detect effects? The tremendous range of individual variation in physiology further complicates study.

In sum, health effects from biometeorological changes are believed to occur, and plausible pathways for many influences exist. There is a clear need for broad-based, multifactorial, methodologically sound research.

REFERENCES

Arcury, T. A., Williams, B. J., & Kryscio, R. J. (1990). Birth seasonality in a rural U.S. county, 1911–1979. *American Journal of Human Biology, 2,* 675–689.

Barinaga, M. (1999, April 16). The clock plot thickens. *Science, 284,* 421–422.

Bovallius, A., Roffey, R., & Henningson, E. (1978). Long range air transmission of bacteria. *Applied and Environmental Microbiology, 35,* 1231–1232.

Calot, G., & Blayo, C. (1982). Recent course of fertility in western Europe. *Population Studies, 36,* 349–372.

Campbell, D. E., & Beets, J. L. (1979). The relationship of climatological variables to selected vital statistics. *International Journal of Biometeorology, 23,* 107–114.

Cech, I., Youngs, K., Smolensky, M. H., & Sargent, F. (1972). Day-to-day and seasonal fluctuations of urban mortality in Houston, Texas. *Biometeorology, 23,* 77–87.

Cowgill, U. M. (1966). Season of birth in man: Contemporary situation with special reference to Europe and the Southern Hemisphere. *Ecology, 47,* 614–623.

Dalen, P. (1975). *Season of birth: A study of schizophrenia and other mental disorders.* Amsterdam: North Holland.

Driscoll, D. M. (1971). The relationship between weather and mortality in ten major metropolitan areas in the United States, 1962–1965. *International Journal of Biometeorology, 15,* 23–39.

Driscoll, D. M. (1983). Human biometeorology in the 1970's. *International Journal of Environmental Studies, 20,* 137–147.

Fellman, B. (1985). A clockwork gland. *Science, 85,* 76–81.

Folk, G. E., Jr. (1974). *Textbook of environmental physiology.* Philadelphia: Lea & Febiger.

Greenberg, J. H., Bromberg, J., Reed, C. M., Gustafson, T. L., & Beauchamp, R. A. (1983). The epidemiology of heat-related deaths in Texas—1950, 1970–79, and 1980. *American Journal of Public Health, 73,* 805–807.

Hansen, J. B. (1970). The relation between barometric pressure and the incidence of peripheral arterial embolism. *International Journal of Biometeorology, 14,* 391–397.

Hollander, J. L. (1963). Environment and musculoskeletal diseases. *Archives of Environment and Health, 6,* 527–36.

Hunter, J. (1980). Strategies for the control of river blindness. In M. S. Meade (Ed.), *Conceptual and methodological issues in medical geography* (pp. 38–76) Chapel Hill: University of North Carlina, Department of Geography.

Huntington, E. (1938). *Season of birth.* New York: Wiley.

Hyslopo, N. S. G. (1978). Observations on the survival of pathogens in water and air at ambient temperatures and relative humidity. In M. W. Loutit & J. A. R. Miles (Eds.), *Microbial ecology* (pp. 197–205) Berlin: Springer-Verlag.

Kalkstein, L. S., & Davis, R. E. (1989). Weather and human mortality: an evaluation of demographic and interregional responses in the United States. *Annals of the Association of American Geographers, 79,* 44–64.

Keller, D. A., & Nugent, R. P. (1983). Seasonal patterns in perinatal mortality and preterm delivery. *American Journal of Epidemiology, 118,* 689–698.

Kevan, S. M., & Chapman, R. H. (1980). Variations in monthly death rates in Canada: A preliminary investigation. In F. A. Barrett (Ed.), *Canadian studies in medical geography* (pp. 67–77). Downsview, Ontario, Canada: York University, Department of Geography.

Krueger, A. P., & Reed, E. J. (1976). Biological impact of small air ions. *Science, 193,* 209–213.

Moeller, D. W. (1997). *Environmental health* (rev. ed.). Cambridge: Harvard University Press.

National Center for Health Statistics. (1998). *Births. Final data for 1997.* Bethesda, MD: NCHS.

Persinger, M. A. (1980). *The weather matrix and human behavior.* New York: Praeger.

Rodgers, J. L., & J. R. Udry (1988). The season-of-birth paradox. *Social Biology, 35,* 171–185.

Rosenberg, H. M. (1966). Seasonal variation of births in the United States. 1933–63. In *Vital and Health Statistics* (Series 21, No. 9, pp. 1–42). Washington, DC: U.S. Department of Health, Education and Welfare.

Sakamoto-Momiyama, M. (1977). *Seasonality in human mortality.* Tokyo: University of Tokyo Press.

Sakamoto-Momiyama, M., & Katayama, K. (1967). A medical–climatological study in the seasonal variations of mortality in the United States of America. *Papers in Meteorology and Geophysics, 18,* 209–232.

Sakamoto-Momiyama, M., & Katayama, K. (1971). Statistical analysis of seasonal variation in mortality. *Journal of the Meteorological Society of Japan, 49,* 494–509.

Somers, D. E., Devlin, P. F., & Kay, S. A. (1998, November 20). Phytochromes and cryptochromes in the entrainment of the Arabidopsis circadian clock. *Science, 282,* 1488–1490.

States, S. J. (1976). Weather and death in Birmingham, Alabama. *Environmental Research, 12,* 340–354.

States, S. J. (1977). Weather and deaths in Pittsburgh, Pennsylvania: A comparison with Birmingham, Alabama. *International Journal of Biometeorology, 21,* 7–15.

Takahashi, J. S., & Zatz, M. (1978). Regulation of circadian rhythmicity. *Science, 217,* 1104–1110.

Thresher, R. J., Vitaterna, M. H., Miyamoto, Y., Kazantsev, A., Hsu, D. S., Petit, C., Selby, C. P., Dawnt, L., Smithies, O., Takahashi, J. S., & Sancar, A. (1998, November 20). Role of mouse cryptochrome blue-light photoreceptor in circadian photoresponses. *Science, 282,* 1490–94.

West, R. R., & Lowe, C. R. (1976). Mortality for ischaemic heart disease: Inter-town variation and its association with climate in England and Wales. *Internationl Journal of Epidemiology, 5,* 195–201.

FURTHER READING

Barry, R. G., & Chorley, R. J. (1982). *Atmosphere, weather, and climate* (4th ed.). New York: Holt, Rinehart & Winston.

Critchfield, H. J. (1983). *General climatology.* Englewood Cliffs, NJ: Prentice-Hall.

Jusatz, H. J. (1966). The importance of biometeorological and geomedical aspects in human ecology. *International Journal of Biometeorology, 10,* 323–334.

Kavaler, L. (1981). *A matter of degree: Heat, life, and death.* New York: Harper & Row.

Rapoport, A. (1969). *House form and culture.* Englewood Cliffs, NJ: Prentice-Hall.

Terjung, W. H. (1966). Physiologic climates of the conterminous United States: A bioclimatic classification based on man. *Annals of the Association of American Geographers, 56,* 141–179.

Tromp, S. W. (1980). *Biometeorology.* London: Wiley/Heyden.

VIGNETTE 5-1.   Monthly Indexes

The study of seasonality of events is complex because the pattern of the whole year has to be compared, whether as months or as weeks. Various, often complex, statistical analyses (such as correlation–regression, Box–Jenkins ARIMA modeling, and spectral analysis) have been used to study seasonality. Beware. It is easy to summarize and compare patterns in a careless and invalid manner. Whatever methods of analysis are used, three methods have proved essential to preparing the pattern for analysis or comparison. These are smoothing, adjustment, and indexing.

Smoothing serves to tone down random fluctuation and other "noise," which can be especially important when total numbers are small. A pattern that was clouded and confused in the raw numbers often shines through smoothed data. There are several methods of smoothing. The simplest and most common is to create a running average. For example, 1980, 1981, and 1982 yield a mean value used for 1981; 1981, 1982, and 1983 yield a mean value for 1982; and so on. Smoothing in this manner is more appropriate for yearly running totals, however, than for months, because of the variation in the number of days in a month. When smoothing monthly data in this manner, one ends up with periods of 92 days for one average and 89 days for another. The irregular pattern of month length increases such period differences rather than smooths them. Another method of smoothing, illustrated in Vignette 5-2, Figure 2, involves trigonometric functions such as sine waves (in harmonic analysis) to identify the periodicity and strength of variation.

The most important step is to *adjust* for the number of days in a month. Comparing deaths in February and August will not do. There are different types of adjustment formulas, but they all do essentially the following:

$$A_i = \frac{M_i}{D_i} \times \frac{365}{12}$$

where i is the month, A is the monthly adjusted number of cases or deaths, M is the number of cases or deaths, D is the number of days.

The adjusted monthly deaths (or morbidity cases) may be used to create monthly adjusted death rates by dividing by the total population. The procedure also works for age categories, and can be used to create age-adjusted monthly rates.

Indexing portrays each month's incidence as the percentage above or below what would be, under conditions of even distribution throughout the year, the monthly average after adjustment for the number of days (Figure 5-5). When the

VIGNETTE 5-1, TABLE 1. Monthly Adjustment and Indexing

1994 month	Number of days	Cases of aseptic meningitis	M_i	Adjusted D_i	Number index
January	31	351	11.3	344.4	46.3
February[a]	28	322	11.5	349.8	46.9
March	31	423	13.6	413.0	55.4
April	30	516	17.2	523.2	70.1
May	31	497	16.0	487.4	65.4
June	30	690	23.0	699.6	93.7
July	31	1,043	33.6	1,022.0	136.9
August	31	1067	34.4	1,046.3	140.2
September	30	1,030	34.3	1,043.3	139.8
October	31	1,086	35.0	1,064.6	142.7
November	30	718	23.9	727.9	97.5
December	31	1,189	38.4	1,166.6	156.3
Total	365	8,932			

[a]Beware of leap years.

above equation is multiplied by $(1,200/TM)$, where TM is the total mortality, the result is an index, I, based on 100.

$$I_i = \frac{M_i}{D_i} \times \frac{365}{12} \times \frac{1,200}{TM}$$

Vignette 5-1, Table 1 illustrates the results of using these three methods.

VIGNETTE 5-2.   Seasonality of Birth

The presence of seasonal patterns in the occurrence of human birth is ubiquitous on earth. The patterns of northern Europe are quite different from those of tropical Africa. In the United States the pattern has been consistent throughout the twentieth century: a minor peak of births in February–March (spring conception); a great concentration of births August–September (early winter conception), and a deep trough of births in April–May (hot summer conception) (see Figure 5-5) There has been spatial variation in the exact timing and sharpness of this pattern between north and south, or between depression and growth decades, but the overall pattern has held for at least half a century. This, despite the fact that the population has become overwhelmingly contraceptive, has seen massive migration from South to North, has become three-quarters metropolitan instead of rural, and has seen origin of immigration shift from eastern and southern Europe to Asia and Middle America. Only in the last 20 years has the pattern of seasonality begun to alter (Figure 5-5).

The fact that there is seasonality to human birth which has a spatial pattern; varies in associations by scale of analysis; and reflects the complex interactions of biology, environment, socioeconomic and demographic structure, and behavior poses a challenge to interpretation and explanation in human ecology and medical geography. Those researching and publishing in biometeorology, anthropology, biological reproduction and fecundity, demographic sociology or epidemiology do not read each other; they lack geographical integration. This vignette summarizes Meade's research on the subject.

METHODS

Since the efforts of geographer Ellsworth Huntington (1938), there has been remarkably little research on the etiology of seasonality of birth. Although his statistical methodology would not pass in an undergraduate term paper today (he did not even adjust for the number of days in a month (Vignette 5-1), he asked some profound questions about the seasonal patterns he documented with data collected from all over the world. He ran latitudinal transects (straight lines along which data is collected) through the United States and Japan to examine climatic change in different cultures. In the former Soviet Union he compared the same ethnic groups in different locales and different ethnic groups in the same locale. He was interested in the effect of climate on people and was the most famous and accomplished proponent of a school of thought known today as environmental determinism. Probably because of the subsequent discreditation of environmental determinism, geographers have ever since ignored the questions he raised.

The main method used to draw out the patterns was harmonic analysis, which has been used by climatologists to analyze such things as weekly or monthly precipitation. The most common way that medical researchers, especially in Britain, address seasonality of death, birth, or congenital malformation is to divide the year into four groupings of 3-month seasons for testing with chi square. In a country as large as the United States, however, these groupings are too arbitrary. March in Minnesota is not the same as March in California or Florida, for example. Given the bimodal pattern, furthermore, even regression by month would miss the pattern of the whole cycle. Imagine the monthly births as a snaking rope. If you push down the monthly births in February, those births are not uniformly redistributed. They may decrease the April trough or raise the September peak, or not. The purpose of harmonic analysis is to express any curve, however complex or irregular, as the algebraic sum of a series of simple sine curves. The first harmonic is one sine curve fit to the monthly data so that the sum of the squares of the difference between them is minimized. This adjusts the height of the curve (amplitude) and shifts the curve (horizontally, or through the calendar) until the height of the curve best fits the maxima in the data distribution, and the point (degree of a circle, day of the year) at which this occurs gives the phase angle of best fit. The second harmonic then fits two sine waves, which best catch a bimodal pattern. Altogether, six harmonics are considered to exhaust variation. When this was done to 1980 births in a transect from Connecticut to Florida, the amplitude of annual seasonality consistently decreased and the phase angle shifted earlier in the year. This matched closely what Huntington had found.

MODELS OF COMPLEXITY

The first dimension of complexity is that influences affecting what is a long process are usually measured with only a single outcome, birth, for which data are collected. The first influences are on genesis and storage of the egg and on genesis of the sperm and maturation in the epididymis. Then, in sequence, influences act upon conception, egg division, zygote growth and movement through the fallopian tube, implantation in the uterus, maturation (fetal loss in first two trimesters; miscarriage in third) as part of the mother's body, sharing most of her nutritional and immunological health and more, birth (stillbirth or live) and then variation in birth weight, gender (sex ratio), congenital disease, neonatal death, and survival. Various influences of infection, diet, emotional stress, altitude change, activity and much more act on this whole process. More than a third of the fertilized eggs will not survive to be a 12-week fetus (many of them because of errors in genetic replication; a few, because of an incompatability with the mother's body that cannot be walled off). Yet, from the single measure of day of live birth, seasonal factors are implicated and analyzed through disciplinary perspective. The triangle of human ecology can help integrate them and focus the points of difference (Vignette 5-2, Figure 1).

Environmentally mediated sociocultural effects have received the most attention. Geographers and anthropologists working especially in developing countries with wet–dry climatic seasonality have noted the importance of separation for wage labor during the dry, nonfarming season. Alternatively, the religious and family celebrations that are usually held after harvest during the dry season provide leisure and raised libido to encourage conception then, an effect perhaps enhanced by the lower coitus during the intense labor periods of plowing, transplanting, or harvesting with their supposed exhaustion. In the United States, the seasonal cycle of school year and vacation would fit this model.

An argument can be made for direct cultural effects over environment. It is clear from births that Ramadan, the Moslem month of fasting during daylight and self-denial of pleasures in general, is a period of low conception. In Malaysia, Moslem Malays, Buddhist Chinese, and Christian Indians all share the same uniformly hot equatorial environment but have different birth periodicity that re-

ENVIRONMENTALLY MEDIATED SOCIOCULTURAL EFFECTS

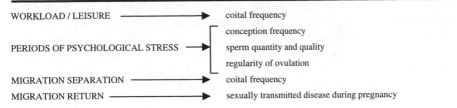

WORKLOAD / LEISURE ──────▶ coital frequency

PERIODS OF PSYCHOLOGICAL STRESS ──▶ conception frequency
sperm quantity and quality
regularity of ovulation

MIGRATION SEPARATION ──────▶ coital frequency

MIGRATION RETURN ──────▶ sexually transmitted disease during pregnancy

DIRECT CULTURAL EFFECTS

RELIGIOUS HOLY DAYS ──────▶ more or less coitus, conception

MARRIAGE TIME PREFERENCE ──────▶ first parity timing

SOCIOCULTURALLY MEDIATED CLIMATIC EFFECTS

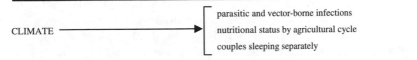

CLIMATE ──────▶ parasitic and vector-borne infections
nutritional status by agricultural cycle
couples sleeping separately

HEAT

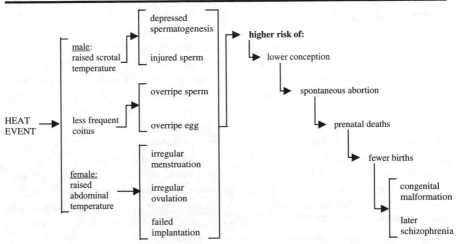

VIGNETTE 5-2, FIGURE 1. Models of seasonality of birth.

flects Ramadan and Chinese New Year (as well as low births during astrological bad-luck years). The most common reaction upon hearing of the September peak of births in the United States is a giggle of "Christmas!"

Seasonal climatic patterns directly affect when mosquitoes and other vectors are active and when crops are grown and harvested and food abundant or in short supply and low nutrition. During the hot season in many places it is common for men to sleep in the courtyard or on the roof, in the open air (or in old New York, on the fire escapes). People may be more exposed to disease vectors. Couples often are separated.

There is some literature on these patterns, but as the reader can see the influences are often both highly localized and often contradictory. There is a universal phenomenon involved. At high latitudes, it would be surprising if light periodicity did not affect human fecundity (see earlier in Chapter 5). Animal breeding suggests, however, that the strongest influence is heat, an hypothesis not entertained by behaviorists in social science.

The scrotum is not enclosed in the safety of the abdominal cavity because it must be a little cooler. Experiments on monkeys, soldiers, and other subjects has clearly demonstrated the capacity of heat to lower sperm count and even totally destroy spermatogenesis. Indeed, sperm counts done in vasectomy clinics are lower in southern cities in the summer. Heat could affect every step in the process of birth, from menstrual cycle to implantation, and activity pattern with its exposure to hazards and access to medical care.

TESTING HEAT

The trough of births in April–May in the U.S. pattern corresponds with conceptions in July and August. This is a national pattern. If heat is involved in lowering conception, variation across the nation and within states should show spatial variation associated with climatic variation. It is not known, however, whether absolute temperature experienced (as by jogging) or length of hot weather to which people are exposed matters. What lags between temperature and birth, or what periods of temperature, should be compared; what extremes or averages?

In Vignette 5-2, Figure 2 birth indices for the mountain, Piedmont, and coastal plain regions of North Carolina have been converted into the first harmonic curves. These are certainly the patterns one would expect if the higher temperatures of the coastal plain, intermediate temperatures of the Piedmont, and lower temperatures of the mountains made any difference to conception. Temperature data averaged over weeks and regions was inversely correlated with births 38 weeks later. Shifting the scale of analysis to state, the first harmonic curve was fitted to 12 months of births for each of the 48 states in 1980. The day of the year when the curve reached its peak amplitude, simply converted from the phase angle, was mapped using SURFER software (Vignette 5-2, Figure 3). The resulting isoline map of human conception in the United States, 1980, shifts from early September in the North to December in the Deep South with al-

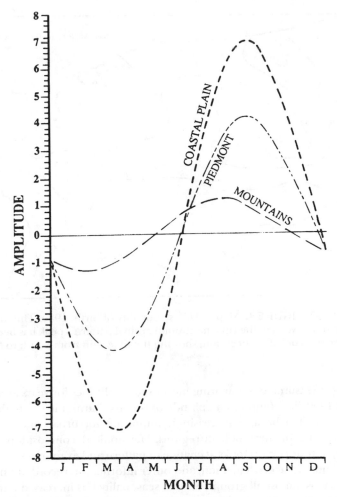

VIGNETTE 5-2, FIGURE 2. Births by region in North Carolina, 1969–1971. The sine waves of the first harmonics show a greater amplitude of seasonality, but similar timing, that might be associated with heat as an etiological factor.

lowance for the mountains. It shows such climatic association that it resembles the Department of Agriculture's map of planting zones.

ASSOCIATIONS AND DEVIATIONS

The patterns of seasonality just discussed could probably not be mapped today. "Noise" and deviation began to become pronounced at the county level in the late 1980s. Within North Carolina, sociocultural factors were addressed at county level

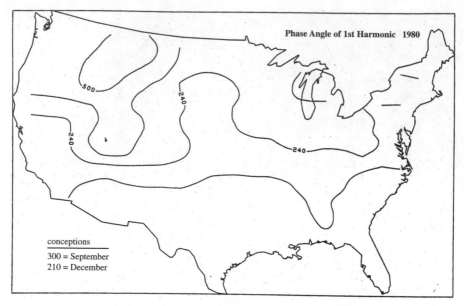

VIGNETTE 5-2, FIGURE 3. Map of U.S. seasonality of birth, 1980. The phase angle, changed to day of year, of the (first harmonic) annual pattern's peak has been mapped as an isoline map of U.S. conception, showing the time shift from South to North.

and change measured by comparing harmonic amplitudes for years around 1970, 1980, and 1990. The (annual) amplitude of the first harmonic was highest always for rural areas but became increasingly important for urban and dramatically more important for metropolitan regions. Harmonic decomposition (i.e. using two, three, or four curves) looks at change in pattern and examines such factors as parity, legitimacy, race, occupation, and other information recorded on birth certificates. Across almost all groups, annual seasonality has increased and bimodal seasonality decreased: Annual seasonality has increased for married women, for example, but births out of wedlock remained bimodal. Some relations were surprising: The more educated a woman, the higher the annual amplitude, for example. As can be seen in Figure 5-5, the bimodal pattern has partly disappeared.

Both a bimodal seasonality of birth and a regular spatial pattern has persisted for decades across this land, but both seem to be declining in recent years. The diffusion of air conditioning may be responsible for ending the April–May trough of births associated with low summer conception, even as central heating changed the pattern of mortality. This has been suggested by some regional-level studies. Almost universal contraception offers a likely hypothesis for the disappearance of the minor February peak, associated with May conceptions and perhaps the sap of spring. What remains most remarkable is the strong, and stronger, pattern of annual seasonality of birth (perhaps now July–September), which becomes stronger the more urban and metropolitan, the more educated, and even the more contracepting the population.

6

The Pollution Syndrome

Since the beginning of the industrial revolution, exponentially increasing kinds and amounts of metals, gases, and chemicals have been added to the air, water, and soil in earth's industrial regions. Many of the chemicals have never existed on earth before. Because biological processes to break them down have not yet evolved, some chemicals persist for long periods. A major source of pressure on the environment today is the desire by newly industrializing countries (NICs) for a lifestyle approximating that of developed nations. New transportation and economic activities are quickly consuming what remains of earth's fossil fuels. The purpose of this chapter is to survey environmental processes and their spatial context as a background for research on diseases and health policies in developed countries and NICs.

Dubos (1965) points out that humankind is now adapting, genetically and culturally, to the environments that humans have built. We spend most of our time in our homes and workplaces. In industrialized countries most people live in cities, but even in rural areas cultivated land and settlements create the environmental stimuli that surround people. Coping with these new stimuli is largely under the control of culture, because genetically we as a species change very slowly. Dubos notes, for example, that there is no reason to think that our eardrums are any more able to withstand vibration than those of cavemen 200 generations ago. Yet, noise levels have increased dramatically.

Normally audible sound consists of vibrations from 30 to 20,000 cycles per second. Loudness is measured in decibels (dB), a logarithmic scale based on sound pressure levels in which a doubling of the intensity of the sound is represented by an increase of 3 dB. Because the ear is more sensitive to sounds in the 4,000-to-6,000 cycle range, it takes less intensity to injure it in these ranges than at higher or lower frequencies. The "A scale" (dBA) was constructed to assess total noise by measuring four frequencies and adjusting for their different effects. Exposure to levels above 90 dBA can produce deafness. Legally, therefore, the maximum occupational noise exposure for 8 hours in a day has been set at 90 dBA. Hearing loss, however, is thought to occur in susceptible individuals exposed to 75 dBA over an 8-hour daily exposure for a working lifetime and in a considerable portion of those similarly exposed at 85 dBA. According to the World Resources Institute (1996), an estimated 100 million people in industrial nations are exposed to traffic noise in excess of 65 dbA.

Although this chapter focuses on chemicals and radiation, other serious health consequences, such as the effects of noise, are also associated with the environmental changes that accompany economic development. Few nations face more environmental degradation due to industrial development than China (World Resources Institute, 1994, p. 74). Most of that nation's rivers, especially in urban areas, are seriously polluted. Dust and chemicals foul the air of many cities and cause widespread health problems. Chronic obstructive pulmonary disease, linked to exposure to particulate matter, sulfur dioxide (SO_2) and cigarette smoke among other factors, accounted for 26% of all deaths in China in 1988. Indoor exposure to emissions from poor-quality coal used for cooking and heating is also a major health risk, increasing the incidence of both pulmonary disease and stroke. In some areas of the country, the uncontrolled irrigation of market crops with raw sewage may cause intestinal worm disease among children. There have been some reports of arsenic poisoning caused by drinking city water in Beijing. If the chemical and physical insults described in the discussion of Audy's definition of health (Chapter 2) were mapped, the surfaces of the industrialized countries would appear as jagged mountain ranges and stratospheric plateaus.

TOXIC HAZARDS OF NATURAL AND ECONOMIC ORIGINS

Toxic hazards to health and life are nothing new. In fact, they occur naturally in the environment. Poisonous and carcinogenic gases are emitted by swamps and volcanoes. Toxic chemicals are produced by fungi parasitic on rye, wheat, peanuts, and other crops, especially in wet years. One such fungal toxin that causes ergotism, for example, has been blamed by scientists for everything from the medieval Saint Vitus's dance to the Salem witch trials. Food plants, such as soy beans, cabbage, and wheat, produce an array of chemicals, designed to protect themselves from fungi and arthropods, that can damage the liver, destroy red blood cells, block the absorption of protein or iodine, cause allergies, and generally poison livestock and humans. Nature produces many chlorine-containing chemicals (Abelson, 1994). The smoke of burning wood contains more than 100 organochlorine compounds, including the extremely toxic dioxin. Forest fires, domestic wood burning, and slash-and-burn agriculture all create large amounts of these polychlorinated chemicals. Adding to these and other naturally occurring pollutants, however, humans are exponentially increasing pollutants of their own creation.

Table 6-1 lists a few of the pollutants and health effects of current con-

TABLE 6–1. Some Environmental Pollutants and Health Effects

Pollutant	Affected organs	Health effects	Source
Mercury	Brain, bowels, transplacental transmission	Minamata disease; liver and kidney disease; diarrhea; lack of coordination; numbness; convulsions; death	Chloralkali plants; pulp and paper processing; electrical industries; fungicides in water and food supply
Cadmium	Blood vessels; kidney	Hypertension; bone softening and fractures; kidney disease; cadmium emphysema	Mining many metals; electroplating; stabilizer for polyvinyl chloride; batteries, cigarettes, pigment
Chlorinated hydrocarbons	Fat tissue; liver	Hydrocarbon toxicity	Processing, storage and transfer of petroleum products; organic solvents; rubber, plastics, paints, lacquer; dry cleaning
Organophosphates	Nerve–muscle synapses	Dizziness; headache; muscular weakness; incoordination; liver and cardiovascular diseases; convulsions; bone-marrow disease; blocks breakdown of acetycholine, which transmits nerve impulses; accumulation leading to convulsions, blurred vision; diarrhea; stillbirth	Insecticide (DDT, lindane, dieldrin, aldrin, chlordane, toxaphene); hexachlorophene (shampoos, deodorants, insecticides, herbicides)
Polychlorinated biphenyls (PCBs)	Fat tissue; liver	Inhibit growth of cells and interfere with enzymes; enhance action of organophosphates; yusho disease; growth disturbance; fatigue; nausea; jaundice; diarrhea; cough; asthma; acne; loss of hair; numbness; nervous system disturbance; joint deformity at birth	Used as heat-transfer media in transformers and capacitors; solvents in adhesives, sealants and anticorrosives; paints and rubber; ink; brake linings
Dusts of quartz, silica, carbon, asbestos, cobalt, and iron oxides	Respiratory interstitial tissue	Pneumonconiosis (scarring of lungs); silicosis; black lung	Mining; sandblasting; quarrying; pottery and ceramics; stone masonry
Hydrogen sulfide	Respiratory center in brain	Paralysis of respiration; consequent edema, hemorrhage, deathdecay in sewers and mines	Oil wells and refineries; sulfur and protein
Fluoride	Bones; teeth	Binds to magnesium, manganese, and other metals to interfere with endocrine function and enzymes; damage to calcium metabolism and pituitary water balance; dental and skeletal fluorosis and osteomalacia if calcium intake inadequate	Food and water; aluminum and other smelting
Asbestos	Pleura and peritoneum	Mesothelioma, rapidly fatal once symptomatic	Mining; brake linings; fireproofing; talcum powder; cement; ceiling tiles; clothing
Beryllium	Lungs	Sarcoidosis	Metal alloys for heat stress and coal burning

Note. Compiled from National Center for Environmental Health (1996).

cern. Of greatest concern, perhaps, are the increasing numbers of chlorinated hydrocarbons and organophosphates, many of which are known to be carcinogenic or teratogenic (causing malformation of the fetus). Many substances that are dangerous as pollutants are important economically. Lead is an important stabilizer, and is essential in many types of batteries. Polychlorinated biphenyls (PCBs) are noninflammable, have a high plasticizing ability, and have a high dielectric constant. They therefore are widely used in transformers and capacitors, as heat transfer and hydraulic fluids, as plasticizers in adhesives and sealants, and as anticorrosion coats for electric wires, lumber, and concrete. As PCBs leak, leach, and vaporize, however, they become air and water pollutants of great concern and occasional accidental polluters of food and feed. They are stored in fatty tissue, pass along the food chain, and persist for long periods in the environment. In addition to disinfecting water, chlorine and its compounds are used in the manufacture of pharmaceuticals and in their content. The organophosphates have become so useful that the world's food supply relies heavily on them.

Lead offers an excellent example of how our cultural capacity to alter the environment is outpacing our biological ability to adapt. Lead is common in the rocks on the earth's surface and therefore in its waters. It usually occurs at low levels, and in some places it probably has always posed a health hazard. Lead is a systemic poison that interacts with a range of body chemicals. Mainly it interferes in blood formation by retarding the maturation of red blood cells in bone marrow, but it is implicated in chronic nerve disease and brain damage because it affects copper metabolism, among other things. Lead accumulates in the bones, where it replaces calcium. Normally about twice as much lead is derived from food as from either air or water, and about 75% is excreted in the feces, a little is passed in urine, and a little more than 10% is stored in the bones. Up to 50% of the lead inhaled reaches the blood, whereas less than 10% of ingested lead does. Treating for chronic lead poisoning is difficult, because the process of chellation, by which a substance combines with the lead and causes it to be excreted from the body, can result in more lead being pulled out of the bone storage. This can precipitate an acute blood lead crisis that did not exist before treatment. Thus, prevention has to be given priority over approaches that emphasize treatment.

Outdoor Air Pollution

Air pollution may be loosely defined as the contamination of the atmosphere by a harmful level of toxic substances. The key words are "harmful level." The level of risk to any given individual is a product of both a substance's toxicity and the level of the individual's exposure. Virtually all substances are potentially harmful if present in sufficiently large quantities. The exact effects of air pollution on health are a function of dose delivered to the receptor and the ability of the receptor to cope with the resultant stress. In humans, the stress experienced by a critical organ or receptor tissue from particle inhalation depends on the properties of the particles. The delivered dose is a function of the anatomical features of the receptor as well as the manner of breathing, breathing rate, and the integrity of the body's defense systems. Some pollution-related diseases may take years, or even decades, to develop. It has proved difficult to connect specific types of air pollution with health hazards such as bronchitis or lung cancer in part because of the difficulties of valid sampling and appropriate scale. Researchers have often had to resort to classifications of urban or rural, for example, as surrogate measures for air pollution. These classifications, unfortunately, bring with them many confounding factors (see Chapter 12).

Atmospheric pollution is caused by a variety of substances, some gaseous and some solid. Here we focus on a few pollutants for which the Environmental Protection Agency (EPA) has established national air quality standards: carbon monoxide (CO), lead (Pb), nitrogen dioxide (NO_2), ozone (O_3), particulate matter whose aerodynamic size is less than or equal to 10 micronmeters (PM-10), and sulfur dioxide (SO_2). The EPA established limits for atmospheric concentrations of these pollutants in 1970, and these limits have been adjusted over time. Table 6-2 lists these pollutants and their quality standards as of 1995. According to the EPA, certain metropolitan regions in the United States have ambient levels of these criteria pollutants that exceed the established limits and thus may create health hazards where they are found (Figure 6-1).

The major source of CO is automobile exhaust. Although it can be a regional phenomenon, CO pollution is often localized, and occurs predominantly during cold weather. High concentrations may occur near areas of severe traffic congestion. In Tokyo, police directing automobiles at street intersections take frequent breaks during which they inhale pure oxygen to clear their lungs of pollutants. CO is the one pollutant that produces a change in human physiology that can be directly related to the concentration to which the subject was exposed. Death occurs in humans exposed to concentrations of around 1,000 parts per million, corresponding to blood levels of 60% blood carboxyhaemoglobin. Because CO blocks the transport of oxygen in the bloodstream, and those with certain heart diseases require a high oxygen supply, it is not unreasonable to draw the same parallel as has been made with cigarette smoking and heart disease and to suggest that CO is a contributing factor (Strauss & Mainwaring, 1984).

Although lead is also toxic to adults and affects virtually all organ systems, adverse effects on cognitive development and behavior in children up to the age of 6 are of special concern. In 1990, the Centers for Disease Control (CDC) estimated that about 3 million, or 15% of the under-6 population, had blood lead levels exceeding 10 micrograms per deciliter (μg/dL) of blood. This level is considered by the CDC as being high enough to trigger primary prevention campaigns in the local community. There are many sources of lead in the environment. Sewage sludge is commonly used as fertilizer in irrigation systems. Domestic sewage has almost everywhere been

TABLE 6–2. U.S. Environmental Protection Agency Criteria Air Pollutants and Health Effects

Pollutant	U.S. population potentially exposed (millions)[a]	Major sources[b]	Primary (health-related) standards[b]	Health effects
Carbon monoxide	89.1	Two-thirds of emissions from transportation sources	8-hour: 9 ppm; 1-hour: 35 ppm	Reduces oxygen delivery to body's organs and tissues; major threat to sufferers of cardiovascular disease
Lead	n/a	Lead gasoline additives, nonferrous smelters, and battery plants	Maximum quarterly average: 1.5 $\mu g/m^3$	May cause neurological impairment; fetuses and children may suffer from central nervous system damage
Nitrogen dioxide	12.1	Two main sources are transportation and stationary fuel combustion from electric utilities and industrial boilers	Annual arithmetic mean: .053 ppm	Lowers resistance to respiratory infections, especially in children
Ozone	126.8	Transportation and industry	Maximum daily 1-hour average: .12 ppm	Impairs lung function, especially among those with impaired respiratory systems
Particulates (diameter < 10 micrometers)	54.6	Industry, power plants, transportation, construction, fires, agriculture, mining	Annual arithmetic mean: 50 $\mu g/m^3$; 24-hour average: 150 $\mu g/m^3$	Impairs breathing; aggravates existing respiratory and cardiovascular diseases; may damage lung tissue
Sulphur dioxide	14.1	Coal and oil combustion; steel mills, refineries, pulp and paper mills; largest source: coal-burning electric power plants	Annual arithmetic mean: .030 ppm; 24-hour average: .14 ppm	Impairs breathing, aggravates respiratory and cardiovascular disease

[a]Data from American Lung Association (1996).
[b]Data from U.S. Environmental Protection Agency (1996).

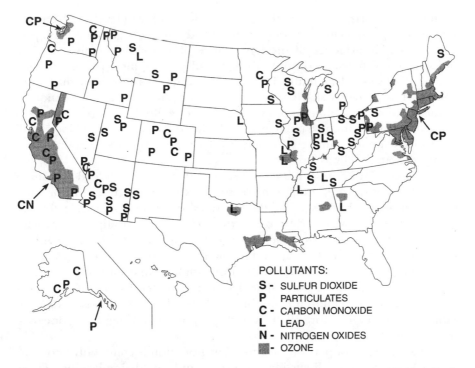

FIGURE 6-1. Air pollutant hazard regions in the United States for the EPA's criteria pollutants. Adapted from Doyle (1997, p. 27). Copyright 1997 by Rodger Doyle. Adapted by permission.

contaminated by industrial effluents, with the result that heavy metals such as lead and cadmium are present at relatively high levels. With repeated application of sewage, lead can quickly build up in the soil and thus pass into the human food chain.

The main source of lead exposure among lead-poisoned children in urban areas is lead-based paint in homes built before 1978. Although the use of lead-based paint in exterior and interior home surfaces was banned in 1978, the U.S. Department of Housing and Urban Development (USDHUD) estimates that 74% (57 million) of all private housing units built before 1980 contain lead-based paint (USDHUD, 1990). Children may ingest lead directly from paint chips, but an important route of exposure is the normal mouthing of hands or objects such as toys, resulting in the ingestion of small amounts of lead paint-contaminated housedust and soil.

Automobile emissions became the main focus of urban lead poisoning in the 1970s. Lead is used as a gasoline additive to improve the fuel's burning characteristics. It is emitted as a fine particulate in exhaust and settles in urban soils. There it is taken up by vegetation, including food crops in gardens, or children playing in or near streets are likely to ingest it as a result of breathing or handling food with soiled hands. The vertical (from the ground) and horizontal (from the road) gradients of lead levels in the air, as well as isotopic matching of local aerosol lead and local gasoline lead, provide irrefutable evidence of the importance of automobile emissions. The transportation network constitutes the broad geographical pattern of lead pollution. Levels of lead in the dirt of agricultural fields and in the dust of urban apartments decay sharply away from traffic. Since 1973, a reduction in tetraethyl lead in gasoline from over a gram per gallon to 0.1 grams per gallon was mandated in the United States. The incidence of elevated blood lead, particularly among inner-city minority (black and Hispanic) children, has dropped dramatically as a result.

Hunter's (1977) research demonstrated that childhood lead poisoning was a "summer disease," due to the seasonal exposure to gutter dirt or automobile emissions. Earickson and Billick (1988) described elevated lead levels in children in Louisville and Detroit in the 1970s, demonstrating statistical association between airborne lead and other pollutants and poor neighborhoods. Bailey, Sargent, Goodman, Freeman, and Brown (1994) investigated the geographic variation in lead poisoning among children living in Massachusetts in 1990. Their statistical analysis corroborated CDC (1992) reports that poor minority children living in female-headed households in deteriorating housing built before 1950 are at disproportionately high risk for excessive lead exposure.

One of the most pervasive forms of air pollution is commonly known as *smog* (smoke–fog). In discussing the policy and health implications of air pollution, one needs to distinguish between two quite different forms with different locational characteristics. The most serious air pollution episodes involve the *classical* or London smog so closely associated with England and the Appalachian region of the United States in the 19th and early 20th centuries. These episodes were characterized by high levels of sulfur dioxide and smoke particulate which build up under stagnant weather conditions lasting 3 days or more. In many industrial processes, sulfur is released during the burning of large quantities of coal and other fossil fuels. Combining with oxygen and eventually with water vapor, sulfur can become dilute sulfuric acid and damage buildings and cloth as well as human lung tissue (*Newsweek*, 1989).

Photochemical smog was first recognized as a problem in Los Angeles during World War II and has since been observed in and around many cities of the world (Stephens, 1987). In those early times in southern California, there was widespread awareness of an eye-burning haze, cracks in the sidewalls of rubber tires, and "bronzing" of sensitive vegetation. At first, this phenomenon was blamed on industry, then on the outdoor burning of trash. Only after exhaustive research did scientists become aware that the major source of these gas emissions was motor vehicles. Tropospheric (ground level) ozone (O_3) is the main constituent of Los Angeles smog. It is actually a *secondary pollutant* formed when hydrocarbons (HC), volatile organic compounds (VOCs), and oxides of nitrogen (NOx), known as *primary pollutants*, react in the presence of sunlight. Fuel combustion sources such as electric utilities and industrial boilers, as well as transportation vehicles, contribute to atmospheric O_3. Unlike carbon monoxide, ozone is worse during warm, sunny weather. Respiratory irritation and breathing problems can occur with chronic exposures to NO_2, particularly in people with asthma and bronchitis, at exposures as low as 100 parts per billion. Children also appear to be susceptible to bronchitis and breathing difficulties in the presence of low levels of nitrogen oxides.

Both forms of smog can be common health hazards in places characterized by frequent atmospheric *inversions*. Normally the temperature decreases with altitude up to 40,000 feet (12 kilometers). The regular rate of decrease is 3.5° F per 1,000 feet (6.50° C per kilometer) and is known as the adiabatic lapse rate. Because warm air rises, the polluted and heated air from the surface rises and is dispersed through atmospheric mixing. There are several ways, however, in which the air at lower altitude can become cooler than the air above it. Most frequently this can occur near a large body of water such as a large lake or the ocean. When the sun goes down in the evening and the land cools off, a light breeze can direct cool air off the lake or ocean onshore. This forms a cold layer under the warm one, which rises to cover the cold layer. This is called an "inversion" layer and will trap the body of air below it (Figure 6-2). In valleys between mountains, with steep sides, inversions occur as the morning or afternoon sun warms the upper layers of the air, while at the bottom the air is sheltered and remains cold or is cooled by a river flowing through the valley. An inversion at higher elevation can occur when there is atmospheric subsidence and divergence. Such upper-air inversions can occur under stagnating anticyclones, and they tend to occur in certain latitudinal zones where subsidence is common at least seasonally (see Vignette 3-1).

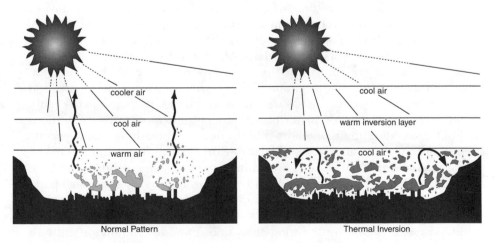

Normal Pattern   Thermal Inversion

FIGURE 6-2. The effect of a temperature inversion. The normal lapse rate may be reversed either near the ground or at high elevations.

Los Angeles became notorious for its smog not only because it has so many automobiles but because its location is characterized by onshore breezes; downhill air drainage; radiational cooling on clear, cloudless nights; lots of sunshine; and summertime atmospheric subsidence. Of all these factors, only the automobile emissions are subject to control.

Frequencies of inversions and the associated health hazards of smog vary greatly not only from place to place but seasonally. Industrial emissions and automobile emissions vary over the course of a week, as well as diurnally. Some pollutants persist for days and others for seconds or less. The various cycling times of years, seasons, weeks, days, hours, and minutes form a sampling nightmare for the researcher. Some particulate matter, such as lead, has a steep distance decay that may move from dangerous to inconsequential within 200 yards of an intersection; some gases, such as sulfur dioxide, may persist for thousands of miles. The several ways of modeling point sources of pollutants usually focus on mathematical models of plumes. Trigonometry can help predict where the pollutants will settle by calculating from the height of the ejection point (smokestack), wind speed, thermal stability, topography, and so forth. As numerous point sources merge into the areal base of a large metropolitan area, the dynamics of atmospheric mixing and movement become more relevant. The rate of emission is a major concern, of course, but so are wind speed and mixing height.

According to studies of U.S. metropolitan areas by Dockery and associates, the finest particles (smaller than 2.5 micrometers) of dust, soot, smoke, or tiny droplets of acid are believed to cost tens of thousands of lives each year in the United States (Dockery et al., 1993; Hilts, 1995). Their research found statistically significant and robust associations between fine-particulate pollutants and lung cancer and cardiopulmonary disease. Fine particles may be more dangerous than large ones because people can breathe them deeply into the lungs, where tissue damage can lead to breathing difficulties or worse. Dockery's research was important because the research design controlled for cigarette smoking and other risk factors. Figure 6.1 demonstrates that, in general, the worst fine-particle pollution is located in southern California and a belt stretching from the Gulf coast to the Great Lakes.

Sulfur dioxide (SO_2) is emitted largely from stationary source coal and oil combustion sources, such as steel mills, refineries, pulp and paper mills, and coal-burning electric power plants. Human exposure to concentrations of SO_2 exceeding the national standard can affect breathing and aggravate existing respiratory and cardiovascular disease. Sulfur is especially hazardous to asthmatics, individuals with bronchitis or emphysema, children, and the elderly. Smelting of ores and other industrial processes may emit small particles of heavy metals such as lead, iron, manganese, and titanium, but most particulates are commonly carbon, or soot, based. Mortality and respiratory illness increase significantly during heavy smog episodes. In London during a week in early December 1952, there were 3,500 to 4,000 more deaths than the expected average for that time of the year. The industrial valleys of Pennsylvania suffered a similar fate in 1948. Such dramatic events tend to raise public and official consciousness about air pollution.

There is another family of hazardous air pollutants, commonly referred to as *air toxics* that have been shown to cause cancer, poisoning, and immediate illness in humans (U.S. Environmental Protection Agency, 1996). Other less measurable effects include respiratory, immunological, neurological, reproductive, and developmental. Examples of air toxics include but are not restricted to dioxins, benzene, arsenic, beryllium, mercury and vinyl chloride. In fact, U.S. clean air legislation lists 189 pollutants as hazardous air pollutants (HAPs) and targets them for regulation. Air toxics emanate from both stationary and mobile sources. In 1988, manufacturers in the United States emitted an estimated 2.4 billion pounds of toxic pollutants into the atmosphere (Centers for Disease Control, 1991). Toxins may be inhaled directly or deposited onto soil or into water bodies, thereby indirectly affecting human health through ecological chains. Top consumers in the food web, usually consumers of fish, may accumulate chemical concentrations many millions of times greater than the concentrations present in the environment. As a result, fish consumption advisories have been issued in hundreds of water bodies in the United States, including the Great Lakes. The distribution of HAP emissions by state appears to correlate positively with the distribution of hazardous waste sites (U.S. Bureau of the Census, 1996, p. 238). The top 17 ranked states in terms of waste sites include 12 of the states in the highest HAP emissions category (more than 90,000 tons per year).

Hall and Kerr's (1992) *Green Index* features several maps that identify the regions of the United States that are responsible for high air and water pollution emissions. Based on the Resource Conservation and Recovery Act (RCRA) of 1976, the *Index* establishes a classification of toxins that cause cancer, birth defects, and/or nerve damage. Points are assigned to states according to the amount of health-hazard toxins produced there. The fewer the points, the better a state ranks on this classification. Figure 6-3 is a map of cumulative per capita weight of these toxic chemicals released to the environment. As may be seen, Indiana, Ohio, West Virginia, and the South lead the nation in RCRA toxins released, while such nonindustrial states as New Mexico, the Dakotas, Vermont, Idaho, Hawaii, and Alaska score best.

Cutter and Solecki (1989) and Cutter and Tiefenbacher (1991) also examined the spatial distribution of airborne releases of acutely toxic materials in the metropolitan United States throughout the 1980s and demonstrated through cartographic and statistical analyses that frequency of chemical firms and rail miles per state were good predictors of the number of incidents. Their study dispelled the notion that airborne releases of acutely toxic chemicals occur only at fixed sites or from spectacular rail accidents. The highest likelihood of toxic chemical incidents was associated with high concentrations of chemical manufacture and distribution facilities.

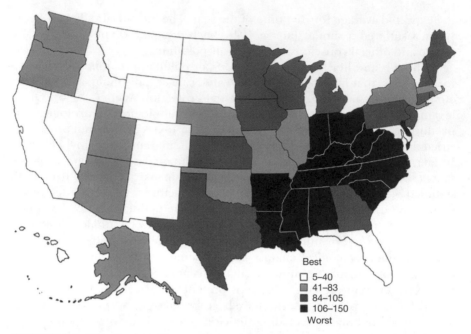

FIGURE 6-3. Distribution of per-capita toxic chemical releases in the United States.

Indoor Air Pollution

Recent research has added a new dimension to the air pollution picture. The startling finding, however, is that exposures to toxic chemicals are sometimes 70 times higher indoors than outdoors. This is partly because indoor air carries the double burden of outdoor pollutants brought inside as well as pollutants that are generated indoors. The CDC has classified indoor pollution as a factor of high environmental risk (Centers for Disease Control and Prevention, 1994). The largest burden of total indoor air pollutants is probably attributable to environmental tobacco smoke (ETS) both in the home and the workplace. The EPA estimates that this pollutant causes over 3,000 lung cancer deaths a year among nonsmokers and may be responsible for serious respiratory illness in hundreds of thousands of children (U.S. Environmental Protection Agency, 1992). As public awareness of the hazards of ETS exposure increases, businesses and communities throughout the United States are taking actions to prevent involuntary exposure. These actions range from prohibition of smoking indoors to limiting smoking to specially designated, separately ventilated smoking rooms.

A landmark study by the EPA in 1985 found it probable that such consumer products as paints, cleansers, propellants, plastics, and cosmetics as well as adhesives, fixers, resins, and building insulation materials were major sources of indoor pollution (Shabecoff, 1985). This study, which measured daily the chemicals in the participants' bodies, found significant correlation between blood levels of these chemicals and visits to gas stations and dry cleaners, use of paint or solvents at home, and smoking. Important studies of air pollution in domestic space are sure to follow, but the habitat dimension of pollution hazards has been interlocked again with the behavioral dimension of house type and clothing, hobbies, and customs of personal and domestic hygiene (see Chapter 2).

Modifications to the home environment in industrial countries has been linked with an increase in the prevalence of athsma (Jones, 1998). Modern homes are much better insulated than was previously the case. Many more homes now have central heating and sealed-unit double glazing. Fitted carpets have generally replaced loose rugs and advances in construction technology have led to a greater use of synthetic building materials. As a result, houses are warmer and more humid, lacking fresh air. In this environment, airborne contaminants are readily produced and build up to higher concentrations than are encountered out of doors. Various indoor exposures have been related to asthma, including house dust mites, molds and fungus, nitrogen dioxide from gas appliances, volatile organic compounds, and formaldehyde.

Researchers have been paying increased attention to the radioactive gas known as radon. Radon is an odorless, colorless gas that arises from the natural decay of radioactive elements commonly found in rocks and many types of soil. In tightly sealed masonry structures, radon gas can build up to hazardous levels. According to EPA surveys, the average radon level in U.S. homes is 1.25 picocuries per liter of air (see Table 6-3 for the definition of a curie). Almost all scientists agree that prolonged exposure to high levels (more than about 8 picocuries) of radon poses a genuine cancer hazard. The U.S. National Academy of Science estimates that radon is the cause of thousands of lung cancer deaths nationwide each year. Most of these deaths occur among people who smoke cigarettes. Other studies, however, show little evidence linking household exposure to cancer. In Winnipeg, for instance, researchers found that mean household exposures of 3.5 picocuries appeared to produce no increased risk for lung cancer. This raises questions about how much risk radon poses at low levels (Leary, 1994). In the United States, known radon concentrations are highest in western mountain states, the Midwest, and Appalachia.

Water Pollution

Several episodes have been responsible for attracting research attention and public interest to the hazards of water pollution. One of the first occurred in Minamata, Japan, during the 1950s, when more than 200 people died or suffered severe brain and nerve damage. The cause was methyl mercury polluting the water and being passed through the food chain in fish to the population.

TABLE 6-3. Measurable Units of Radioactivity

Unit	Abbreviation	Definition and application
Disintegrations per second	dps	A rate of radioactivity in which one nucleus disintegrates every second. The natural background radiation for a human body is about 2 to 3 dsp. This does not include "fallout" from man-made sources such as nuclear weapons.
Curie	Ci	Another measure of radioactivity. One Ci = 37 billions dps.
Picocurie	pCi	One-trillionth of a curie.
Roentgen	R	A measure of the intensity of X rays or gamma rays, in terms of the energy of such radiation absorbed by a body. (One R delivers 84 ergs of energy to 1 gram of air.) The roentgen may be considered a measure of the radioactive dose received by a body. The dose from natural radioactivity for a human is 5 R during the first 30 years of life. A single dental X-ray gives about 1 R, a full mouth X-ray series, about 15 R.
Rad		Another measure of radiation dosage, equivalent to the absorption of 100 ergs per gram of biological tissue.
Rem		A measure of the effect on humans of exposure to radiation. It takes into account both the radiation dosage and the potential for biological damage of the radiation. The damage potential is based on the following scale of factors:

$$\begin{array}{ll}\text{X rays, gamma rays, electrons:} & 1 \\ \text{neutrons, protons, alpha particles:} & 10 \\ \text{high-speed heavy nuclei:} & 20\end{array}$$

The rem is then defined by the relationship:

Rems = Rads H Biological damage factor

Therefore, 100 ergs per gram (X-rays) = 1 rad H 1 = 1 rem, but 100 ergs per gram (neutrons) = 1 rad H 10 = 10 rems

Note. Adapted from Blumenthal and Ruttenber (1995, p. 150). Copyright 1995 by Springer Publishing Co. Adapted by permission.

In the 1970s, Love Canal, near Niagara Falls, New York, focused national attention on the problems of hazardous waste disposal and the dangers of groundwater contamination. Hooker Chemicals and Plastics Corporation (now Occidental Chemical) purchased an uncompleted canal site, and between 1942 and 1953 disposed of about 22,000 tons of mixed chemical wastes into the ditch. Shortly after Hooker ceased use of the site, the land was sold to the Niagara Falls School Board for a price of $1. In the late 1950s, residential development of the area attracted 900 families and an elementary school was constructed on the property. Unusually heavy rain and snowfalls in 1975 and 1976 provided high groundwater levels in the Love Canal area. Portions of the Hooker landfill subsided and chemical residue surfaced, contaminating ponds and other surface waters. Basements began to ooze an oily residue, noxious chemical odors permeated the area, and chemical corrosion of subterranean pumps became apparent. In 1978 the New York Department of Health declared the Love Canal area a threat to human health and ordered the fencing of the landfill site. Later, the school was closed, and pregnant women and young children were evacuated from the site. Eventually, all the properties in Love Canal were purchased and a Federal Disaster Assistance Agency was created to assist the city of Niagara Falls to remediate the Love Canal site. Since then, gasoline leaks from underground tanks, PCB dumps into rivers and drains, and leakage from municipal landfills have poisoned the water supplies of scores of communities nationwide and forced Congress to create a Superfund program for toxic-waste cleanup (Zeigler, Johnson, & Brunn, 1983).

Ninety-five percent of all fresh water available on earth (exclusive of icecaps) comes from beneath the surface. Although most people in the world get their domestic water supply from surface water or shallow wells, about half of the population in the United States and large cities elsewhere tap groundwater sources. The purity of groundwater has long been held as sacrosanct; however, untreated contaminated water can carry many infectious agents. The EPA reports the leading sources and water pollutants in U.S. rivers, lakes, ponds, reservoirs, estuaries, and the Great Lakes (U.S. Environmental Protection Agency, 1994). Agriculture is the most widespread source of pollution in the nation's surveyed rivers. Bacteria from fecal contamination pollutes 34% of impaired river miles; excess nutrients, especially nitrogen and phosphorus compounds from agriculture, pollute 43% of lake acreage; and urban runoff and storm sewers are the most widespread source of pollution (nutrients and bacteria) in estuaries. The Great Lakes contain one-fifth of the world's fresh surface water and are polluted from both the air and surface runoff. In addition to nutrients from agriculture, toxic organic chemicals, primarily PCBs have been found in 98% of the samples taken. Air pollution from industry and pesticides from agriculture have been implicated.

Given the number of illnesses and deaths attributed globally to diarrhea, it seems fair to say that human feces remain one of the world's most hazardous water pollutants. A lack of access to clean water and sanitation still constitute two of the world's most serious health problems. In the developed world, these problems have been mitigated by providing indoor piped water and flush toilets to virtually all urban residents. The same is true for the wealthy in developing countries. For most developing nations, however, financially strapped governments can ill afford anything like complete coverage with indoor plumbing. Table 6-4 lists those developing nations that were worst off in terms of access to clean water and sanitation in the early 1990s.

In cities of the developing world, households without indoor piping often obtain their water from one of many sources, such as overcrowded or dis-

TABLE 6-4. Access to Safe Drinking Water and Sanitation, Selected Low-Income Nations, 1990

Country	Access to safe drinking water (%)		Access to sanitation (%)	
	Urban	Rural	Urban	Rural
Bangladesh	39	89	40	4
Burkina Faso	44	70	35	5
Central African Republic	19	26	45	46
China	87	68	100	81
Ethiopia	70	11	97	7
Guinea-Bissau	18	27	30	18
India	86	69	44	3
Indonesia	35	33	79	30
Mali	41	4	81	10
Mozambique	44	17	61	11
Myanmar	79	72	50	13

Note. Adapted from World Bank (1994). Copyright 1994 by Oxford University Press. Adapted by permission.

tant communal standpipes, expensive private water vendors, or heavily polluted shallow, hand-dug wells. Increasingly, developing countries are adopting bore-hole technology, where deep tubewells with engine-powered pumps are becoming important sources of uncontaminated domestic water. In countries where vector-borne disease is prevalent, for example, tubewells are providing parasite-free village water sources for bathing and laundry. Those without flush toilets may end up using pit latrines or latrines located over ponds, streams, drains, or open sewers—all of which demand far more rigorous hygiene behavior than is required for the standard technologies of the wealthy.

Figure 6-4 illustrates the strata of an artesian water source. Surface water percolates into the soil, eventually reaching the water table, or saturated zone of ground, above an impervious stratum of rock. This groundwater may also intersect depressions and form springs or help fill lakes. Below the stratum of impervious rock there often is another layer of pervious rocks, such as sandstone, and a layer of impervious rock below that. Most rock strata are tilted. Where the pervious layer has contact with the surface, precipitation percolates into it to form an *aquifer*. The source area of this precipitation may be many hundreds of miles from a desired well site, so aquifer water may be under pressure if the rock strata are even slightly tilted. An artesian well drilled through the rock cap into the aquifer may, if the location is right, flow under its own pressure. Although aquifers are filled by precipitation, in some places the water that originally filled the aquifer fell in other climatic periods and other continental locations.

There may be several layers of aquifers. Often the lowest one is saline. Injection wells are sometimes used to dispose of toxic wastes in saline

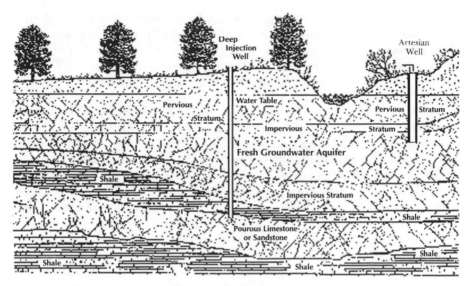

FIGURE 6-4. Groundwater strata.

aquifers. Under great pressure, and through wells constructed in layers and sealed to prevent leaching into higher strata, liquid wastes are injected into the saline aquifer. Overall, U.S. groundwater quality is considered "good quality," but some regions have experienced "significant ground water contamination." The most frequent sources of this contamination are leaking underground storage tanks, agriculture (pesticides and herbicides), Superfund sites, and domestic septic tanks (U.S. Environmental Protection Agency, 1994).

One of the most comprehensive recent studies of water pollution and human health effects was carried out in Puerto Rico by Hunter and Arboña (1995). Because of its historical linkages to the West and subsequent industrialization, the Commonwealth of Puerto Rico has pushed consumerism to levels comparable to those found in the United States. The result is an outpouring of sewage and solid waste that imperils this small, overcrowded tropical island that is dependent on groundwater. The sudden death of large numbers of fish has provided a sensitive biological indicator of environmental quality. The usual suspects include agricultural runoff and discharges from industry and municipal sewers. Here as elsewhere in the United States, water supplies are becoming increasingly polluted with toxins, yet water treatment techniques still primarily reflect concern with infectious diseases of the past rather than the carcinogenic pollutants of today's environment. It has been over two decades since the passage of the Safe Drinking Water Act, yet the gamut of toxic chemicals in the public water systems is broadening and threats to human health have increased rather than diminished. Concern about pollution of groundwater is growing. In the mid-1980s, the California Department of Health Service reported that one-fifth of the state's large drinking water wells fed by groundwater exceeded the state's pollution limits (Sun, 1986) Studies in two heavily populated counties in that state found high levels of trichloroethylene and dibromochloropropane, which pose reproductive and acute health risks, including stomach cancer and lymphatic leukemia (Kloos, 1995). Other studies, however, find no relationship between contaminants and disease. This is often the case when there is a failure to control for confounding factors or by basing conclusions about a population on samples obtained in small areas. This can lead to ecological fallacies, which have been mentioned elsewhere in this book. Pesticides have been detected in half of Iowa's city wells. More than 1,000 wells in Florida have been shut down because of contamination with EDB, a chemical used to kill soil nematodes. The common beliefs that pesticides would decompose in the soil and that nature would cleanse itself through percolation can no longer be accepted.

As with any pollution, the critical parameters are amount, mixing and dispersal, cleansing, and decay. The fate of chemicals in surface or groundwater is very different in these respects. Surface waters can be easily polluted, and the pollution can spread rapidly, be focused into high concentrations in time, and be flushed and removed. Large lakes and estuaries require a longer time to accumulate the pollutant, and perhaps decades to turn over and be cleansed. In contrast to these, groundwater quantities are enormous and spread over entire basins and even continents. The water is so slow moving that sometimes it is difficult to determine the direction of flow. It may take years for the pollutant to move more than a few feet from its source. It is difficult for pollutants to get access to groundwater because of filtration by the earth, but once contaminated groundwater is nearly impossible to cleanse and long periods (up to hundreds of thousands of years) may be required for its renewal. The actual size of the groundwater supply in the United States is not known because extensive mapping of the nation's aquifers has not been completed.

RADIOACTIVE POLLUTION

Nuclear and biological terrorism have become plausible contemporary threats to most nations. Besides the major nuclear powers, many smaller and less politically stable nations now possess the capacity to build nuclear devices. It is generally agreed that not only would outright nuclear war devastate specific target areas, but even a limited nuclear action could drastically affect the climate, ecosystem, and human genotype everywhere on earth (National Academy of Sciences & National Research Council, 1975). In this chapter, we address only the hazards of peaceful nuclear power.

Radiation Hazards

Naturally occurring radiation hazards are cosmic radiation and decay of radioactive elements. Cosmic sources provide a continuous background of eternal radiation with which all life has evolved. Today, about half of the radiation exposure to the average person in the United States is from the natural background. Another 40% is attributable to medicine in the form of diagnostic X rays and radiation therapy (Upton, 1982). Much of the natural radiation emanates from radioactive materials that have been around for some 4 billion years. Substances such as uranium 235 (U-235), uranium 238 (U-238), and thorium 232 have extremely long half-lives (the time required for a material's radioactivity to decrease by half). Knowledge of some of their decay sequences and byproducts helps in understanding the nature of certain environmental hazards.

In April 1986, a tremendous explosion from the reactor at the Chernobyl nuclear power plant sent a radioactive "plume" of radionuclides into the upper atmosphere, where they began to drift into northern and western Europe. Substantial areas throughout the continent were bombarded with different kinds of radioactive isotopes. From April 26 to 28, high atmostpheric pressure over northeastern Europe established a northerly air flow that carried the plume, at first affecting the former Soviet Union, then later northeast Poland and Scandinavia where radiation monitors in Sweden and Denmark indicated abnormally high readings. The triggering of these monitors was the first indication in western Europe that a significant nuclear accident had occurred (Gould, 1990). All territory within an 18-mile (30-kilometer) radius of the destroyed reactor had to be evacuated and remains uninhabited today. Radiation may have affected unborn fetuses near the site, but by the time the plume reached England, increases in perinatal mortality were insignificant (Bentham, 1991).

Chernobyl and other nuclear power plants use the fission power of U-235 and U-238. As U-238 decays it produces radon 222, an inert gas that diffuses into the atmosphere. Radon-222 is the source in turn of lead-210, a global constituent of atmospheric fallout. It decays to polonium-210. Among the radioactive daughter nuclei that result, cesium-137, iodine-131, and strontium-90 are particularly important because they accumulate within organisms. Cesium-137 has a half-life of 30 years and attacks the entire human body. Iodine-131, with a half-life of 8.1 days, collects in the thyroid gland. Strontium-90 is similar to calcium and becomes part of the bones, where it affects the production of red blood cells in the marrow. Bone marrow is essential for producing materials needed by the body's immune system.

Several radioactive gases are also produced by current nuclear technology and released to the atmosphere to become part of the background, or ambient, radioactivity. Principally these are the inert gas tritium and the isotopes krypton-85, xenon-133, and xenon-135. These do not enter into biological or chemical activity and so are not accumulated by organisms. The release of radioactive gases and other products is regulated to stay within limits of normal variation in background radiation. One often hears the reassurance after an unscheduled release of radiation that there is no more exposure for the population than getting a dental X ray. The exposure is, of course, in addition to the dental X ray.

Radiation can cause cancer and mutation. Damage to DNA may take generations to be expressed. As with any disease agent, some people will be affected at lower levels of radiation than others who remain apparently untouched. Little is known, however, of dose relationships either at the individual or the population levels. Is the relationship linear, the more radiation the more mutation? Is there a threshold level, below which the body usually can cope and above which damage begins? Are there different levels of tolerance, depending on whether the radiation is inhaled, ingested, or contacted?

There seems to be considerable variation among species in resistance to radiation. Much of our knowledge about what radiation does to the body has been provided by studying the effects of the atomic bombs dropped on Hiroshima and Nagasaki in 1945. Accidental and occupational exposures provide some data but generally about acute effects. The soldiers exposed to watching nuclear explosions in the early days of atmospheric testing have been claiming compensation for their cancers and reproductive problems, but it has proven difficult for all the experts in court to separate these problems from those occurring in the general population. If humans are exposed to a dose of between 100 and 250 rads (see Table 6-4 for the definition of a rad), they will develop fatigue, nausea, vomiting, diarrhea, and some loss of hair. However, most victims recover completely from the immediate illness. Doses of 400 to 500 rads, however, like strontium-90, impairs bone-marrow function. Fifty percent of those exposed in this dose range will die. A dose of 2,000 rads is almost always fatal within a few weeks of exposure (Turk, 1985).

Johnson (1981) investigated the case of the radiation hazard around Rocky Flats nuclear weapon plant near Denver, Colorado. He demarcated a region of hazard using the plutonium content of the soil for miles around the plant to measure cumulative exposure from 1953–1971. Figure 6-5 shows the results of calculating the relative risk of excess cancer deaths from 1969–1971. The cancers involved were those associated with Japanese survivors of the atomic bombs: leukemia; lymphoma; myeloma; and cancers of the lung, thyroid, breast, esophagus, stomach, and colon. The distance decay effect associated with plutonium released through the plant's smokestack (note the westerly wind direction configuration) clearly creates a hazardous region. The hazard zone was not perceived for two decades; otherwise the release of radionuclides might have been reduced or the population warned. Populations may be exposed to hazards without knowing it and may experience symptoms and not relate them to environmental conditions.

Since World War II, the dramatic growth in the use of electric and electronic devices has been accompanied by a parallel increase in human exposures to the electric and magnetic fields (EMFs) that these devices emit. Elec-

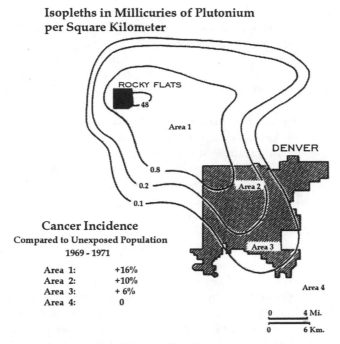

Isopleths in Millicuries of Plutonium per Square Kilometer

FIGURE 6-5. Cancer incidence around a nuclear weapons plant. An isoline map of plutonium that has accumulated in the soil provides a regionalization for exposure and correlation with cancer incidence. From Zeigler, Johnson, and Brunn (1983, p. 48). Copyright 1983 by Association of American Geographers. Reprinted by permission.

tric power and telecommunication systems, electric and electronic appliances, broadcast facilities, and radar systems have contributed to rising background levels of EMFs in living and work spaces in industrialized countries. We cannot deny the benefits of these technologies, yet they have raised concerns about whether exposure to typical levels of EMFs in the environment are harmful to health. In several compelling papers on the subject in *The New Yorker* magazine, Brodeur (1989, 1990) produced detailed descriptive accounts which he presented as circumstantial evidence that some cancer clusters were associated with chronic exposure to the magnetic fields that are given off by power lines carrying high current and high voltage to electric-power substations, which are not uncommonly located near residential areas. To support his case, he cited some two dozen epidemiological studies that had been conducted and published in the medical literature in the United States and elsewhere showing that children and workers exposed to power-line magnetic fields were developing leukemia, lymphoma, melanoma, brain tumors, and other cancers of the central nervous system. Such claims have been hotly contested by other epidemiologists. Florig (1992) concedes that

the scientific evidence about the healths risks of exposure to EMFs is "suggestive" of injurious health effects, but he notes that this evidence has thus far
not been compelling enough to trigger regulatory action by federal authorities. Because of possible confounders and biases in most of the epidemiological studies available at this writing, scientific opinion about whether the evidence from these studies represents a real EMF health effect varies
enormously.

The geographic scale of a research scheme can confuse resultant statistics. One example is provided in a study of child and young adult cancers in
New Jersey using surveillance at several scales—urban, suburban, rural
county, minor civil division, and individual communities (Schneider,
Greenberg, Donaldson, & Choi, 1993). If one compared New Jersey's pediatric cancer incidence with that of other states, that state's cancer rate appeared to be on the increase. Surveillance at a finer scale, however, showed
no statistically significant pattern of excess cases. Yet another level of surveillance suggested that pediatric cancer does cluster statewide, and that
clustering is strongest among white cases in specific age groups with specific cancer types. A final examination of individual cases yielded information
that clusters were exemplified by very few cases and very few small political
divisions. Thus, although clustering may exist at the state scale, few smaller
jurisdictions have enough cases to support expensive epidemiologic studies
that might yield fruitful results. Knowing this information at the outset
counterbalances political pressures for government action that emanate
from concerned local populations.

Political responses to community health concerns have had the effect of
delaying the siting and licensing of new power lines, radar systems, and communications antennas, and numerous court cases have arisen in which plain-
tiffs claimed impaired health due to exposure to EMFs. Hundreds of millions
of dollars have been spent in the United States alone on behalf of government and industry to investigate the biological effects of EMFs. Because the
scientific evidence on EMF bioeffects is both complicated and contradictory,
regulatory bodies and organizations concerned with scientific standards have
been unable to reach a consensus on prescriptive approaches to EMF risk
management (Flynn, Kasperson, Kunreuther, & Slovik, 1997). Rerouting of
power lines, repacking of wires, moving of office spaces to distance workers
from power sources, and increasing the shielding of emissions from electrical
appliances are some of the possible ways to ameliorate exposures. All of this
is obviously expensive and raises economic issues, such as whether mitigation
costs balance out potential health benefits, or whether any party bears an un-
fair burden of potential risk. Like other environmental issues, the EMF controversy is as much about sociopolitical and ethical concerns as it is about
health risk. There is a fertile field here for geographers to investigate not
only the deleterious health effects in proximity to EMF sources but also the
perceptual context (Sooman & Macintyre, 1995).

Other Sources of Radiation Hazards

The hazards associated with nuclear power plants and nuclear weapons have been emphasized previously, but there are other sources of hazard. One is the use of radiation in hospitals and research laboratories and the disposal of the low-level radioactive wastes they produce. Another is the mining of uranium and the manufacture of nuclear fuel. Yet another is the transport and storage of all the used material.

Uranium ore typically contains 2 to 5 pounds of uranium oxide per ton. After uranium is mined, therefore, large piles of waste and tailings remain. Efforts have been made to grade the slag heaps and stabilize them with vegetation, but in the Colorado River basin alone they cover several thousand acres and contain tens of millions of tons. From the heaps thorium 232, U-238, and radon can be leached by rainfall and eroded into water systems. The occupational exposure of the miners and subsequent processors has to be carefully controlled. The ore is crushed, ground, and leached with acid, and uranium is recovered from the leached liquid by such procedures as ion exchange and solvent extraction. Radioactive wastes are produced with each step.

The need to transport radioactive material creates linear hazard zones. Uranium from the mines must be transported to enrichment and fuel fabrication facilities. The fuel must be transported to nuclear reactor sites. Spent fuel must be transported to storage sites. Most nuclear power plants in the United States are east of the 100th meridian, in the more densely populated parts of the country. The linear hazards of transport are not going to diminish as the amount of spent fuel from later generation plants increases and as the older plants themselves begin to be dismantled and transported for storage. Dry-cask storage enables these wastes to be stored for a century or more at existing power plants and storage sites; however, permanent repositories which may be considered "safe" for more than 10,000 years are needed. U.S. energy agencies began a search in 1975 for such a site in the states of Michigan, Ohio, New York, Utah, Texas, Louisiana, Mississippi, Washington, and Nevada. In 1982, Congress passed the Nuclear Waste Policy Act (NWPA), which designated that two repositories would be constructed, one in the western half of the nation, the other in the eastern half. Considerable political opposition from targeted states ensued, and in 1987, the NWPA was amended and Yucca Mountain, Nevada, was named as the only repository site to be studied. This project has been stalled by unexpected scientific, management, intergovernmental, cost, public opposition, schedule, and regulatory compliance problems. As of this writing, the state of Nevada remains opposed to this repository, and although development of the site proceeds, it is not a certainty that all high-level nuclear waste in the nation will ultimately reside there (Flynn et al., 1997).

The health consequences of nuclear power are difficult to assess and easy to exaggerate. Clearly, however, the spread of nuclear power for the generation of electricity to low-income countries that, because of lack of money and skilled personnel, are less able to regulate it and maintain the highest standards of safety practice is a matter of concern. It necessarily involves greater international shipment of nuclear fuel and, because of efforts to control the general availability of plutonium, which can be used for nuclear weapons, the return shipment of spent nuclear fuel. We are now well into the nuclear age.

Risk Assessment and Prevention

With more than 3 million chemicals registered, 70,000 chemicals in general use, and new ones appearing at a rate of more than 1,000 a year, it is not surprising that the environment in the industrialized countries has become contaminated. Exposure to pollutants can be either acute or chronic. A person may be exposed once for a few minutes at work to a leakage or spill or consume over a lifetime undetectable levels of contaminant in food or water. Toxic waste from a dump may contaminate a nearby residential water supply to very high levels, or low levels of benzene may be breathed throughout a lifetime in the ambient air of an urban area. Even for most of the chemicals thought to be hazardous, little is known of threshold levels or dosage effects. Threshold limit values (TLV) for major chemicals have been announced by government agencies responsible for protecting workers. These values establish time-weighted average concentrations that are acceptable for occupational exposure, in the same way that standards have been set for exposure to radiation, noise, and airborne dust. Few standards have been estimated for nonoccupational exposures. Research is complicated because reliable, subnational-scale data do not exist for etiological study. There are, for example, no microarea data for industrial exposures, cigarette or alcohol consumption, or dietary composition. One must work between small, local surveys of specific points and broad, socioeconomic classification of national associations and trends. It is not surprising that point and area data often are improperly mixed, that researchers generalize across scale, or that spatial autocorrelation is ignored (see Vignette 3-1 for an explanation of this). The personal monitors, currently being tested, that identified indoor pollution may, in the future, provide reliable data for researchers interested in studying microscale exposure through daily and weekly activity patterns. For now, most studies rely on surrogate but measurable variables, such as substituting ethnicity for diet.

One of the clearest and most concise explanations of the measurement and uncertainties associated with risk estimation was written by Talcott (1992), who claims that sizable uncertainties are associated with quantitative environmental risk assessments. Risk estimates incorporate the following questions: What is the probability that release of a substance will occur? What quantity of this substance will be released? How will the concentration of this substance change as it disperses from the point of release? How many people or other organisms in the environment will be exposed to this substance? How much of the delivered dose of this substance will be taken up by organisms? And what will be the relationship between a particular dose of this substance and an organism's response—that is, how will the toxic effects of this substance increase with increased dose? From the point of view of environmental justice, this last question has deadlocked many a jury. The toxicity of a particular dose of a substance varies not only across species but among individuals of the same species. Sex, age, size, diet, and the geography of exposure to a substance, among other confounders, affect how toxic increased doses of a substance are to organisms.

One way the EPA assesses population at risk is by using the tools of geographic information systems to identify the buffer zones around hazardous sources such as dumps or nuclear power plants. Complicating factors include prevailing wind direction, changes in humidity, local turbulence and mixing, air drainage, frequency of inversion, and differences in soil, rock, and topography. Underground movement of water causes a population situated upflow to be at higher risk from the hazard location than a population situated downflow a little further away. The transportation system and routing, labor circulation, or seasonal changes in population density or industrial production also affect risk. Studies by political scientists, sociologists, and geographers have shown that often the most critical locational determinant for siting a hazardous facility is the political weakness of the local population (Greenberg & Schneider, 1996).

Geographers can help in the detection of old waste disposal sites, the planning of new sites, and the etiological analysis of diseases in developed economies. Processes of siting, transporting, storing, processing, concentrating, or dispersing occur in a differentiated environment of short-term micrometeorology, local geomorphology, transportation systems, settlement patterns, and economic and social activity. Risk assessment of population exposure to known and unknown hazards is a multiscale and complicated business of intrinsic geographic interest, but there has been limited geographic contribution thus far.

GLOBALIZATION AND THE PERCEPTION OF HEALTH HAZARDS

Pollution flows without regard to international boundaries. Acid rain, the greenhouse effect of increasing levels of carbon dioxide, and the fallout of strontium-90 as a result of atmospheric nuclear testing are problems shared by humans in general, regardless of the sources. There has been a less generally recognized but concomitant diffusion of the useful technology that produces hazardous by-products. Among the most sought after industrial capacities are petroleum refineries, the manufacture of plastics and synthetic materials, electronics, pharmaceuticals, and the production of fertilizers and insecticides. Mining and smelting are being extended into previously undeveloped areas. Agriculture is being intensified through application of more chemicals. Research is progressing into such useful areas as recombinant DNA and the capacity to produce strains of food crops resistant to fungi and insects—without consideration of what effects the "naturally occurring" plant chemicals that produce resistance will have on human health.

Chlorofluorocarbons (CFCs) emitted into the atmosphere, because of their extraordinary chemical stability, reach the stratosphere where they release chlorine by photolysis. This free chlorine scavenges ozone and destroys it (Lindley, 1988). Release of CFCs occurs through industrial activity, equipment leakage, or the disposal of old refrigeration and air-conditioning units, as well as by use of aerosol cans using CFCs as propellants. Even some members of the health profession use CFCs as a diluent for ethylene oxide in cold sterilization procedures in hospitals, clinics, and the manufacture of health-related devices. Whereas CFCs are the most voluminous ozone depleters, there are several other ozone-depleting substances in use, including carbon tetrachloride, hydrochlorofluorocarbons, halons, methyl bromide, and methyl chloroform.

The ozone layer was observed to be thinning over Antarctica in the late 1970s. Repeated observations have confirmed the attenuation and charted its progress (Stolarsky, 1988). There is some attenuation in the Northern Hemisphere as well, but at about 60° north, not over the pole. On average, the global stratospheric ozone layer declined by 2–4% between 1980 and 1988 (Last & Guidotti, 1991). Between 1988 and 1995, global production of CFCs dropped 76%, due mainly to a reduction in use of ozone-depleting substances in industrial nations.

There has been a noticeable increased human exposure to ultraviolet (UV) light in recent years. Ozone in the stratosphere absorbs much of the UV light that would otherwise reach the earth's surface. It has been estimated that a 1% reduction in the ozone shield would result in a 2% increase in the UV light reaching the surface. The human health effects of increased UV irradiation due to ozone depletion include higher risks of nonmelanoma skin cancer, malignant melanoma, cataract and retinal degeneration, and possible impaired immunological responses that increase risks of other conditions, including systemic malignancies. Even at high northern latitudes, exposure to sunlight is the principal determining factor for nonmelanoma skin cancer (MacKie & Rycroft, 1988). Oddly, the amplification factor appears to decrease with increasing latitude, which means that residents in the highest latitudes of North America may be at less increased risk for the carcinogenic effect of increased UV penetration than those at lower latitudes where most of Canada's population lives. There have been successful attempts to curb CFC generation and release (French, 1997). On January 1, 1996, production of CFCs was to have ceased in developed countries under the provisions of the Montreal Protocol of the Vienna Framework Convention on Ozone-Degrading Substances. However, given that developing countries have until 2010 to phase out use of these chemicals, and the long half-life of CFCs (75 years or more), ozone-depleting activity is expected to persist at significant levels well into the 21st century. Consumption is rising rapidly in some countries with large populations, including China, India, and the Philippines. Also, there is a black market in smuggled CFCs in Eastern Europe that threatens to undermine the phaseout in industrial countries.

The experience gained by industrial nations as they passed through their technological transition should have been of great preventive value to poor developing nations, but there is little evidence of its application. Modern health hazards are diffusing rapidly. Most developing countries perceive the immediate benefits of technology more acutely than they see the distant, nebulous hazards. Their national budgets are stretched thinly to cover the needs of education, health, and infrastructural development. Civil servants with the education and skills required to inspect and regulate plants that use advanced chemical technology are in limited supply. The general populace is usually uninformed and naive about modern chemicals. Farmers, for example, commonly contract urticaria and more severe poisoning from handling insecticides and herbicides, and they sometimes rinse their equipment in streams that provide water for drinking and washing. If they are illiterate, they cannot read labels. Farmers in Southeast Asia have been known to dump insecticide in streams to kill fish for harvest, as they used to do with native plant toxins. Chemical and drug manufacturers have been known to export to developing nations poisons and other substances that have been banned for use in developed countries. Herbicides similar to Agent Orange, used in the Vietnam War, have been marketed to countries such as Colombia, resulting in reports of miscarriages and birth defects. The attitude in developed countries is often that other countries must regulate themselves but seldom are the expert knowledge and resources available in the developing world.

The Geometry of Hazards, Power, and Policy

There are many spatial dimensions to environmental health hazards. Atmospheric and water pollution constitute areal hazards; mines, manufacturing sites, refineries, and waste and storage dumps constitute point hazards; and the roads and sealanes of transportation constitute linear hazards. Each is of concern at a different scale and involves different kinds of regulatory and preventive policies and different levels of government. Technology control and alternatives must be carefully considered in terms of social justice and compensation, private investment, and tax costs. Geographically, the costs and benefits may or may not coincide in one place. In the case of automobile accidents or pharmaceutical side effects, for example, the zone of maximum benefits from the technology and the zone of maximum risk of its hazards coincide.

Zones at risk from atmospheric or water pollution usually contain, but extend well beyond, the place that economically benefits from production.

In contrast, the hazards of agricultural technology are usually felt most by farmworkers, but the benefits extend to a much wider area. Toxic wastes, radioactive wastes of all kinds, and their transportation form a class by themselves, because the maximum risk is usually borne by a place far removed from the zone of maximum benefit. For example, malfunctions at the Chernobyl nuclear power plant endangered the local populations as far north as Scandinavia, and most of the chemical industry that fills South Carolina's major toxic waste dump is located in and benefits other states.

Whether the noxious facility at issue is the permanent, national, high-level radioactive waste dump or a mental hospital, they must be located somewhere (Elliott & Taylor, 1996). One research question asks, How do people perceive the risk of noxious facilities and react to them? A team of geographers and others at McMaster University in Canada (Eyles, Taylor, Johnson, & Baxter, 1993; Elliott et al., 1993) discovered that Canadians residing in southern Ontario took for granted proximate solid waste disposal facilities ("just a part of the landscape") because these sites had existed for an extended time without incident. It is not that people were unconcerned about risks to safety and property value. Indeed, across the three sites studied by this research team, levels of reported concern ranged from a low of 28% (existing solid waste incinerator) to 67% (existing solid waste landfill) to 74% (proposed solid waste landfill). However, those interviewed perceived that risks were beyond their control: "uncertain, perhaps invisible, sometimes stigmatizing impacts of social and environmental change" (p. 811).

A longitudinal analysis of one of the original sites studied by the Canadian research team confirmed these earlier findings (Elliott et al., 1997). While levels of reported concern around a *proposed* solid waste disposal facility were relatively high (74% of residents within 4.5 km of the site), levels of reported concern decreased significantly over time (measured at the time of landfill construction and 2½ years after operation began) while levels of unsolicited "dislike" increased significantly. It would appear, therefore, that residents in close proximity to the site have learned how to cope with the existing landfill in their midst. This in no way implies that area residents are happy about the situation. As one respondent put it: "It's not because you like it any better. When there's nothing you can do about it, you just accept it and go on."

At what scale should democratic control of technology be exercised? Noxious facilities are usually located where people have the least political power. For urban facilities, this usually means areas where ethnic minorities or the poor live, rather than the upper-class suburbs. It makes sense to locate hazardous facilities in areas of sparse population, if the geology is compatible. The sparseness of population, however, also means that there are fewer people to oppose the will of the numerous people elsewhere who have reaped the benefits.

Eyles (1997) sets out a critical and theoretical environmental health research agenda, which includes the language and perception of environmental risk in everyday life, concepts of structure and power, consensus and conflict in environmental health policy, and questions about definitions of environmental quality. This agenda has a sociopolitical dimension because it pits property owners, workers, consumers, and others concerned about health risk against economic entities and government agencies. It has an ethical dimension because it involves balancing individuals desires to eliminate involuntarily imposed risks (however small) with society's need to have reliable technology at an affordable price. Geographic research cannot afford to ignore these sociopolitical and ethical concerns.

CONCLUSION

The hazards faced by urban and rural areas, or by old industrial and newly developing places, are converging as technologies and pollution spread. As many industries decentralize and spread to other countries, so do certain hazardous occupational exposures. As trucks and automobiles, insecticides and herbicides, radios and air conditioners become universal, so do the products of their manufacture. Less than a decade after the 1978 declaration in the United States of the first national emergency due to technological, and not natural, causes (at Love Canal) came the disasters of thousands of deaths from the release of poisonous gas by a pesticide plant in Bhopal, India, in 1985, and the catastrophe at Chernobyl in Ukraine, in 1986. Agricultural intensification, proliferation of industrial occupations, production of toxic and radioactive wastes, and consumption of petrochemicals, pharmaceuticals, synthetic textiles, electronics, glues, and paints are now almost universal. The scale of environmental change does not match the scale of contemporary regulation and control.

The ultimate causes of our environmental problems are those of population numbers, inequalities and diminishing natural resources. As humans multiply, they seem to be oblivious to the fact that resources are finite, and that everything on earth has not been placed here explicitly for their benefit. Human gains have been achieved at the cost of material resource depletion and extinction of many other forms of life. The greatest "gains" have accrued disproportionately to the wealthy nations and industrial organizations, who have been best able to marshall technology. Tropical populations, though not wealthy by Western standards, have also exacted their cost on the environment. Over the past few decades, intensive logging and burning of forests worldwide, partly to open up land for agriculture, has contributed to air pollution and microclimatic change. Unfortunately, technology has not been employed as effectively as it might have been to reduce pollution of the environment. To effectively reduce emissions, nations must adopt policy measures such as energy or fuel-efficiency standards for appliances and transport vehicles and eliminate market distortions such as low, subsidized energy prices that reduce the economic benefit to the consumer of saving energy (World Resources Institute, 1996, pp. 315–338).

REFERENCES

Abelson, P. (1994). Chlorine and organochlorine compounds. *Science, 265,* 1155.

American Lung Association. (1996). *Health effects of outdoor air pollution.* Washington, DC: Author.

Bailey, A. J., Sargent, J. D., Goodman, D. C., Freeman, J., & Brown, M. J. (1994). Poisoned landscapes: the epidemiology of environmental lead exposure in Massachusetts children 1990–1991. *Social Science and Medicine, 39,* 757–766.

Bentham, G. (1991). Chernobyl fallout and perinatal mortality in England and Wales. *Social Science and Medicine, 33,*429–434.

Blumenthal, D. S., & Ruttenber, A. J. (1995). *Introduction to Environmental Health* (2nd ed.). New York: Springer.

Brodeur, P. (1989, June 12, 19, 26). Annals of radiation: The hazards of electromagnetic fields. *New Yorker,* pp. 51–89; 47–73; 39–68.

Brodeur, P. (1990, November 19). Department of amplification. *New Yorker,* pp. 135–150.

Centers for Disease Control. (1991). Toxic air pollutants and noncancer health risks—United States. *Morbidity and Mortality Weekly Report, 40.*

Centers for Disease Control. (1992). Reports on human lead exposure. *Morbidity and Mortality Weekly Report, 41.*

Centers for Disease Control and Prevention. (1994). *National Health and Nutrition Examination Survey (NHANES III).* Atlanta: U.S. Department of Health and Human Services.

Cutter, S. L., & Solecki, W. D. (1989). The national pattern of airborne toxic releases. *Professional Geographer, 41,* 149–161.

Cutter, S. L., & Tiefenbacher, J. (1991). Chemical hazards in urban America. *Urban Geography, 12,* 417–430.

Dockery, D. W., Arden Pope, C., III, Xu, X., Spengler, J. D., Ware, J. H., Fay, M. C., Ferris, B. G., Jr., & Speizer, F. E. (1993). An association between air pollution and mortality in six U.S. Cities. *New England Journal of Medicine, 329,* 1753–1759.

Doyle, R. (1997). Air pollution in the United States. *Scientific American, 276,* 27.

Dubos, R. (1965). *Man adapting.* New Haven, CT: Yale University Press.

Earickson, R. J., & Billick, I. H. (1988). The areal association of urban air pollutants and residential characteristics: Louisville and Detroit. *Applied Geography, 8,* 5–23.

Elliott, S. J., Taylor, S. M., Walter, S., Stieb, D., Frank, J., & Eyles, J. (1993). Modelling psychosocial effects of exposure to solid waste facilities. *Social Science and Medicine, 37,* 791–804.

Elliott S. J., & Taylor, S. M. (1996). Worrying about waste: Diagnosis and prescription. In: D. Munton (Ed.), *Hazardous waste siting and democratic choice: The NIMBY phenomenon and approaches to facility siting* (pp. 290–318). Washington, DC: Georgetown University Press.

Elliott, S. J., Taylor, S. M., Hampson, C., Dunn, J., Eyles, J., Walter, S., & Streiner, D. (1997). "It's not because you like it any better. . .": Residents' reappraisal of a landfill site. *Journal of Environmental Psychology, 17,* 229–241.

Eyles, J., Taylor, S. M., Johnson, N., & Baxter, J. (1993). Worrying about waste: Living close to solid waste disposal facilities in southern Ontario. *Social Science and Medicine, 37,* 805–812.

Eyles, J. (1997). Environmental health research: Setting an agenda by spinning our wheels or climbing the mountain. *Health and Place, 3,* 1–13.

Florig, H. K. (1992). The potential health effects of electric and magnetic fields. *Science, 257,* 468.

Flynn, J., Kasperson, R. E., Kunreuther, H., & Slovic, P. (1997). Overcoming tunnel vision: Redirecting the U.S. high-level nuclear waste program. *Environment, 39,* 6.

French, H. F. (1997). Learning from the ozone experience. In L. R. Brown et al. (Eds.), *State of the World, 1997.* New York: Norton.

Gould, P. R. (1990). *Fire in the rain.* Baltimore: Johns Hopkins University Press.

Greenberg, M. R., & Schneider, D. (1996). *Environmentally devastated neighborhoods.* New Brunswick, NJ: Rutgers University Press.

Hall, B., & Kerr, M. L. (1992). *1991–1992 Green index: A state-by-state guide to the nation's environmental health.* Washington, DC: Island Press.

Hilts, P. J. (1995, March 10). Deadly toll is found in dirty-air cities. *New York Times,* p. A1.

Hunter, J. M. (1977). The summer disease: An integrative model of the seasonality aspects of childhood lead poisoning. *Social Science and Medicine, 11,* 691–703.

Hunter, J. M., & Arboña, S. (1995). Paradise lost: An introduction to the geography of water pollution in Puerto Rico. *Social Science and Medicine, 40,* 1331–1355.

Johnson, C. J. (1981). Cancer incidence in an area contaminated with radionuclides near a nuclear installation. *Ambio, 10,* 176–182.

Jones, A. P. (1998). Asthma and domestic air quality. *Social Science and Medicine, 47,* 755–764.

Kloos, H. (1995). Chemical contaminants in public drinking water wells in California. In S. K. Majumdar, E. W. Miller, & Fred J. Brenner (Eds.), *Environmental contaminants, ecosystems and human health* (pp. 30–43). University Park: Pennsylvania Academy of Science.

Last, J., & Guidotti, T. L. (1991). Implications for human health of global ecological changes. *Public Health Review, 18,* 49–67.

Leary, W. E. (1994, September 6). Studies raise doubts about need to lower home radon levels. *New York Times,* p. B-7.

Lindley, D. (1988). CFCs cause part of global ozone decline. *Nature, 323,* 293.

MacKie, R., & Rycroft, M. J. (1988). Health and the ozone layer. *British Medical Journal, 297,* 369–370.

National Academy of Sciences National Research Council. (1975). *Long-term worldwide effects of multiple nuclear-weapons detonations.* Washington, DC: National Academy of Sciences.

National Center for Environmental Health. (1996). *1995 Year in Review.* Washington, DC: U.S. Department of Health and Human Services.

Newsweek. (1989, June 12). Our dirty air. p. 49.

Schneider, D., Greenberg, M. R., Donaldson, M. H., & Choi, D. (1993). Cancer clusters: the importance of monitoring multiple geographic scales. *Social Science and Medicine, 37,* 753–759.

Shabecoff, P. (1985, June 11). U.S. calls eleven toxic air pollutants bigger threat indoors than out. *New York Times,* p. A1.

Sooman, A., & Macintyre, S. (1995). Health and perceptions of the local environment in socially contrasting neighbourhoods in Glasgow. *Health and Place, 1,* 15–26.

Stephens, E. R. (1987, February 17). Smog studies of the 1950s. *Eos,* pp. 1–5.

Stolarsky, R. (1988). The Antarctic ozone hole. *Scientific American, 258,* 30–36.

Sun, M. (1986). Ground water ills: Many diagnoses, few remedies. *Science, 232,* 1490–1493.

Talcott, F. W. (1993, Winter). How certain is that environmental risk estimate? *Resources, 107,* 10–15.

Upton, A. (1982). The biological effects of low-level ionizing radiation. *Scientific American, 246*, 41–49.

U.S. Bureau of the Census. (1996). *Statistical abstract of the United States: 1996* (116th ed.). Washington, DC: U.S. Government Printing Office.

U.S. Department of Housing and Urban Development. (1990). Comprehensive and workable plan for the abatement of lead-based paint in privately owned housing: Report to Congress. Washington, DC: Author.

U.S. Environmental Protection Agency. (1992). *Respiratory health effects of passive smoking.* Washington, DC: Author.

U.S. Environmental Protection Agency. (1994). *National water quality inventory, 1994 report to Congress.* Research Triangle Park, NC: Author.

U.S. Environmental Protection Agency. (1996). *National air quality and emissions trends report, 1995.* Research Triangle Park, NC: Author.

World Bank. (1994). *World development report.* New York: Oxford University Press.

World Resources Institute. (1994). *World resources 1994–95.* New York: Oxford University Press.

World Resources Institute. (1996). *World resources 1996–97.* New York: Oxford University Press.

Zeigler, D. J., Johnson, J. H., & Brunn, S. D. (1983). *Technological Hazards.* Washington, DC: Association of American Geographers.

FURTHER READING

Briggs, D. J., & Elliott, P. (1995). The use of geographical information systems in studies on environment and health. *World Health Statistics Quarterly, 48*, 85–94.

Brown, L. R., et al. (Eds.). (1999). *State of the world.* Washington, DC: Worldwatch Institute.

Burton, I., Kates, R. W., & White, G. F. (1993). *The environment as hazard.* New York: Guilford Press.

Croner, C. M., Sperling, J., & Broome, F. (1996). Geographic information systems: New perspectives in understanding human health and environmental relationships. *Statistics in Medicine, 15*, 1961–1977.

Hester, R. E., & Harrison, R. M. (1998). *Air pollution and health. London: Royal Society of Chemistry.*

Monmonier, M. (1997) *Cartographies of danger: Mapping hazards in America.* Chicago: University of Chicago Press.

Platts-Mills, T. (Ed.). (1999). *Asthma: Causes and mechanisms of this epidemic inflammatory disease.* Cleveland, OH: CRC Press.

Pollock, S. T. (1993). *The atlas of endangered places (environmental atlas).* New York: Facts on File.

Strauss, W., & Mainwaring, S. J. (1984). *Air pollution.* London: Edward Arnold.

Waller, L. A. (1996). Geographic information stystems and environmental health. *Health and Environment Digest, 9*, 85–88.

7

Geographies of Disease in Economically Developed Areas

conomically developed countries have reached the end of the classic
mortality transition, when death is caused mainly by degenerative and
chronic diseases such as heart disease, stroke, and cancer (Chapter 4).
Death in childhood is unusual and there is a long life expectancy; therefore,
the population is older than in less developed countries. Conditions in the
equivalent stage of the mobility transition include high-population circulation rates and active urban–urban migration. Much of the research literature
in medical geography, and some of its most sophisticated methodology, is
concerned with the patterns of health conditions and disease etiology in
North America, Europe, and Japan. These patterns are increasingly shared
by recently industrialized countries, especially in Asia. Economically developed places also have the trained human resources and the financial capacity
to investigate the distribution, causation, treatment, and prevention of the
technopathogenic complexes described in Chapter 6.

Table 7-1 compares some of the causes of death in developed countries
for Japan, the United States, and Russia. The last year currently available for
which mortality data including the Russian Federation, newly devolved from
the Soviet Union, can be examined on a valid and comparative basis is 1993.
The chaos in health care delivery, the failure of vaccination and resultant
outbreak of diphtheria and other epidemics, the crisis in alcoholism, with
heart attacks for men and fetal alcohol syndrome for new borns, probably the
cancer consequences of the terribly polluted industrial environment, along
with the dramatic decline in status and other such factors, have resulted in a
mortality increase never imagined for a developed country. In Japan there
have also been changes. Strokes are no longer more important than heart
disease, although they are still twice as important as in the United States.
Heart disease is still the number one killer, but the heart disease "epidemic"

TABLE 7-1. Comparative Death in Three Developed Countries

	Japan (1992)		United States (1993)		Russian Federation (1993)	
	Male	Female	Male	Female	Male	Female
Life expectancy (years)	76.3	83.0	72.2	78.5	58.9	71.9
Mortality rate, 1991 (per 100,000)	803.0	463.3	998.8	612.5	2128.0	1041.0
Infant mortality, 1991	4.5		8.4		21.8	
Heart disease	157.9	104.8	325.7	191.6	576.2	296.4
Cancer	228.2	113.7	248.9	163.5	322.4	143.2
Stroke	101.4	73.7	51.2	45.4	328.7	248.5
Chronic lung disease	20.1	7.3	44.6	24.7	78.6	20.8
Vehicular accidents	16.4	5.7	22.1	9.6	40.7	11.0
Diabetes	8.0	5.9	19.4	17.4	?	?
Suicide	20.7	10.3	19.9	4.6	68.9	12.1

Note. Life expectancy and death rates per 100,000 for Japan, the United States, and the Russian Federation in the latest year of comparable data. The deterioration of health and soaring death rates of Russians, especially men, has never before been observed in a developed country. Data from Centers for Disease Control and Prevention (*www.cdc.gov/nchswww/fastats/*).

of just 10 years ago seems to be over. The population age-adjusted death rates have been brought down to 134.5 as this century ends. On the other hand, diabetes has become worse (21.3 men, 25.0 women) and chronic lung disease, mostly emphysema, had improved somewhat for men (42.0) but gotten worse for women (38.0), trailing the change in smoking behavior. Vignette 7-1 presents more of these changes by gender.

Population–behavior–habitat interactions provide a framework that can integrate and support many research directions. Genetic susceptibility and resistance, for example, affect the results of many exposures to carcinogens. Probably no area of medical research has advanced as much in the past decade as knowledge of genetics at the molecular level. These advances have implications for screening for risk, for developing DNA vaccinations, and for gene therapy of inherited diseases. Diet can be both the cause of disease and the treatment for it. The sophistication and technology of health care systems, part of social organization but in the habitat, are critical to resulting patterns of mortality. For the health of people living in industrialized societies, the built environment (and the pollution syndrome it includes) is the main habitat of exposure. The social environment has proved to be important both for maintaining high levels of health and for recovering from such treatments for disease as surgery or chemotherapy.

Infectious agents of disease are having an emergence even in consideration of these supposedly noncommunicable diseases. Most convincingly, a species of bacteria, *Helicobacter pylori*, has been shown to be the agent of chronic gastritis and ulcers. Thriving in the acid of the stomach, the bacteria infects 20–50% of people in developed countries and higher proportions in developing ones, yet most people remain without symptoms even when infected from childhood. It would appear that the stresses that have been associated as causes of ulcers again act through the endocrine and immune system to reduce health (Chapter 2). It now seems likely that bacteria in the circulatory system determine where the plaques of cholesterol that narrow arteries and cause artherosclerosis will form. A major new center combining the medical schools of the University of North Carolina and Duke University has just been established to investigate the role of dental ecology and hygiene in the introduction of such systemic bacteria, as through gum disease. Finally, not even helminths are out of consideration in chronic diseases. One new research direction is developing the hypothesis that the intestinal helminths that have been part of us for hundreds of thousands of years may now cause imbalance in our immune system by their absence, and imbalance expressed as autoimmune diseases such as inflammatory bowel disease or Crohn's disease.

The older age structure and long-standing mobility of the population mean that exposures to hazards are difficult to trace or determine. Often exposure occurred in a place different than where the disease becomes manifest. Most of the diseases become manifest a long time after the susceptible person is exposed to the risk (insult). Trying to understand the spatial pattern of chronic and degenerative diseases is thus very difficult. Some of the studies described in this chapter use statistics with which the reader may not be familiar. We have tried to present them so that the substance is understandable, even if the precise methodology or significance may be obscure. Statistical approaches are introduced in vignettes for classes that use them: chi square (Vignette 12-2) and correlation/regression (Vignette 12-3).

Degenerative and chronic diseases have multiple causes. Often a single cause has multiple effects. Careful research design, based on knowledge of the biological disease process as well as the spatial relationships of the units of observation, is absolutely essential in geographic research on these complex disease patterns. Nonsense correlations occur frequently with multiple variables and large data sets: There must be a plausible biological pathway for cause to have effect. Categories of chronic and degenerative diseases are often hard to define precisely. Sophisticated radiology and laboratory procedures may not be available for diagnosis. Terminology fads mean that definitions change. The latency of these diseases may last decades. Cause is often difficult to determine because we do not know whether there is a dose or a threshold relationship between disease expression and original hazards. There are many epistemological and methodological problems with scale of analysis, units used as observations, spatial autocorrelation, confounding, and other issues discussed in Chapters 12 and 13 (this volume).

This chapter describes and puts into context some of the major disease processes of the economically developed world and reviews some of the most basic and innovative geographic research.

THE POVERTY SYNDROME

Many diseases seem to occur consistently more often among the poor than among the affluent. There seems to be a sociopathological complex made up in large part of stress, lifestyle, diet, housing, polluted air, old paint, and old pipes. Physical, social, and mental diseases have similar patterns within urban areas. Some diseases, such as tuberculosis are traditionally associated with the poor. Others, such as breast cancer, have more often afflicted the affluent. And some, such as lung cancer, have recently decreased at high socioeconomic status (SES) and increased at lower.

Many of the associations of health problems with poverty occur throughout the world. As Harpham, Lusty, and Vaughan (1988) model them, a wide range of the diseases of the poor have universal associations characterized as direct, environmental, or psychosocial. Their direct factor would list unemployment, low income, limited education, inadequate diet, prostitution. Their environmental factor is composed of water quality. sanitation, overcrowding, poor housing–rubbish accumulation, lack of garden land, traffic, industrial hazards, pollution, accidents. Their psychosocial one includes stress, alienation, insecurity, depression, smoking, alcoholism, drugs, abandoned children. These characteristic associations occur from the slums of Bombay (Mumbai) to London.

There is a higher-order causality to these associations, a political economy, which in geography includes study of the relations of societal process with spatial form. Dear and Wolch (1987) describe how "landscapes of despair" were formed when mentally ill people and others were "deinstitutionalized" in the late 1970s and released into unprepared and largely unfunded communities for service and support. Turn-of-the-19th-century human services policy was spatially expressed in the location of public asylums in major cities. As the cities grew into industrial centers, the growth of downtown areas and suburbanization of people working there led to clear identity of central business district–fringe zone as one of dependence that housed noninstitutionalized dependent populations (e.g., blocks of single-room-occupancy hotels in which the elderly poor, alcoholics, transients, and others congregated). The general philosophy of treatment and care of service-dependent and institutionalized people had become a "specifically urban phenomenon" across North America, a social construction of "the service-dependent ghetto." In the United States, in the early 1980s, community building, housing subsidy, and welfare funds were substantially reduced. People deinstitutionalized who did not return home to supportive families, churches, or other social groups gravitated toward "inner-city landscapes where increasing demand for assistance were met by diminished capacity to supply both shelter and services" (p. 199). Similar and related changes in urban landscapes and conditions are presented by Wallace (Wallace, Huang, Gould, & Wallace, 1997) with regard to AIDS in Chapter 8.

Homelessness, people having not even shelter, is a process affected by global and local economic, social, and political forces that gets localized in specific places. People can become homeless because they lose a job and thereby ability to pay rent, flee physical abuse, have a supportive relative who dies or is imprisoned, become incapacitated by substance abuse, and for many other reasons. Some people are homeless for only short periods; some cyclically find and lose jobs/apartments/families; some become chronically homeless. Wolch and Dear (1993) describe the following dualism that results in poverty, with overwhelming health risks around the world. On one hand, there is rising economic marginality of persons or groups that results from economic restructuring, welfare state restructuring, and demographic change. One the other side, there is decreased affordable shelter because of national housing policy, urban housing markets, and loss of affordable units. In the United States, policies of "rolling back the welfare state" through reduced eligibility for benefits, the new federalism of "devolving" authority to local and state level to support, and privatization of services has meant at least in the short run more children in deeper poverty (p. 11).

Housing itself is probably the easiest part of the sociopathological complex to understand. The poor are often overcrowded. Older residences have often been subdivided into apartments for numerous families and individuals. Larger families mean that small children add to the high room-density measure frequently associated with influenza, bronchitis, and tuberculosis. Old pipes may have lead solder and occasionally are composed of lead; they tend to be made of metals whose cadmium and other trace elements are easily eroded. Although lead is no longer allowed in house paint in the United States, older buildings still have lead paint dust. Usually considered a Northern inner-city problem, in the rapidly growing South lead may be more of a rural risk (Hanchette, 1998). Exposed asbestos is a more recently recognized hazard. Central heating systems frequently are obsolete or in poor repair. In Britain the poor frequently live with dampness, fungi, and drafts. Dark interiors are suitable to tubercle bacilli, which may be concentrated because of crowding and poor ventilation.

A diet high in starchy foods, sugar, and fat seems in international comparisons to contribute to a greater tendency toward diabetes and coronary heart disease. There is, however, remarkably little small area-based dietary information or longitudinal studies with which to confirm or study relationships. Obesity is even more frequent among black females than other segments of the U.S. population and more frequent among poor whites than among rich ones. The role of diet is closely tied to lifestyle factors. When people in the United States started jogging and aerobic dancing for health reasons, these cultural practices, like most others, diffused down the socioeconomic scale from people with higher levels of access to information to those more tied to traditional ways.

Usually an innovation, or fad, diffuses from metropolitan areas in California and New York to other urban centers and out to small towns and rural areas. Diffusion also occurs among neighborhoods of a city and blocks within neighborhoods. Knowledge about the benefits of steaming vegetables instead of overboiling them; the hazards of bacon fat, whole milk, salt, or beef; or the uses of exotic substitutes such as tofu spreads slowly. A new definition of a healthy diet seemed to appear among the educated just when dietary behavioral patterns once associated with the well-off became widely practiced among the poorly educated.

There are also socioeconomic impediments to change of lifestyle. Health spas, gyms, and safe jogging paths are not readily available to the poor. Night shifts, double jobs, and lack of child care impede many changes. Crime and fear of it can lead to deprivation of social life, especially for the elderly (see heat waves, Chapter 5). Stress also results from anxiety over jobs, fear of inscrutable institutional policies, insecurity over social security or aid to dependent children payments and medical care/insurance coverage, and hassles with landlords.

One way of viewing the whole sociopathological complex is in terms of the accumulation of insults to health (Chapter 2). Some people with high levels of health can cope with the insults and emerge stronger and more creative for the struggle. Others, their health depressed by psychological and social insults, are unable to rally from infectious, chemical, or further mental insults. They become part of that small percentage of the population that accounts for a large percentage of illness and repeated health care needs.

ISSUES OF RACE IN THE STUDY OF HEALTH RISKS

Shifting in scale from universality to the particular case of the United States, one additional factor needs to be addressed: race, especially black and white. Race is a genetic classification that has limited relevance to disease etiology (Chapter 2, this volume). Some diseases are genetically caused, such as sickle-cell anemia or Huntington's chorea. In some diseases a special susceptibility seems to be involved, such as "essential hypertension" in blacks. In others, such as prostate cancer, genetic susceptibility may be part of the etiological puzzle. Too often, however, automatic separation into racial categories masks a superficial socioeconomic, or class, analysis that could be more etiologically significant.

African Americans are a heterogeneous population, and they are a minority of less than 13% of the U.S. population. This means that although a higher proportion of blacks are in poverty, on welfare, are single mothers, unemployed teenagers, high school dropouts, and so forth, substantially larger numbers of people who are in these categories are white. Millions of African Americans are college-educated professionals leading the lifestyles of the affluent. However, if even college-educated black women have lower-weight babies, is there a role of genetics aside from lower access to adequate prenatal care? Or, if race is taken as a social construction, a category that affects the behavior of people both within and outside it, is there another kind of cause? The work of Evans (1994) and those who have followed him, for example, strongly indicates that it is not absolute deprivation but relative status which affects health (as discussed in Chapter 2).

The main groups of Americans who are in poverty are single mothers, the disabled, the aged, and children. There has been a long trend of deterioration in the relative health circumstances of the poor versus the rich, uneducated versus the educated, and black versus white expressed as increasing socioeconomic inequalities in mortality. Demographic projections make obvious that there will be a future increase in the proportion old, disabled, minority (not just black), and probably single mothers (not just never married, but divorced, abandoned, and widowed), and in the proportion of children living in poverty. The withdrawal and reduction of benefit levels will have an adverse impact on the health status of the most disadvantaged. The structure and pattern of these relations are complicated by their strong spatial variation, with concentrations differing among states, counties within states, and neighborhood within cities and counties. Scales of analysis addressing "population" without place can easily miss the significant associations or opportunities for intervention.

The well-recognized inverse gradient of socioeconomic status and mortality (see inverse care law, Chapter 12) is in part causation and risk from environment or behavior, in part public health prevention (or lack thereof), and in part health service: early detection, access to care, aggressive treatment, social support. Besides genetic susceptibilities and socioeconomic associations there are also cultural differences in such things as perception of symptoms, compliance with medical regime, and family networking. Not only the patient but also health care provider can be influenced by belief systems and perception in ways that effect early detection, aggressive treatment, or simply recognition of problem. Separating the racial, socioeconomic, cultural, and institutional/policy components of the mortality differential is not simple.

Table 7.2 reflects both the dimension of inequality in mortality and the complexity of its causation. In the study outlined in this table, the population in four poor areas and four nonpoor areas for whites and blacks, respectively (i.e. a total of 16 groups) was analyzed for 1989–1991 using demographic methods. The dimensions of inequality are shocking: Whereas the overall difference in the standardized mortality ratio (see Chapter 12) is almost 1.9:1, black males in Watts and black females in Harlem die at about three times the national white rate. Put another way, the probability of a 15-year-old black male in Harlem surviving to 65 is only 37%, whereas that of a white female in Sterling Heights, near Detroit, is 93%. Poor white men in Detroit die at twice the national rate. For both sexes, the death rate in each poverty area is excessive. But the differences in the patterns of excess mortality also emphasize the importance of other social factors than measurement of socioeconomic status. As the study authors note, the black belt in Alabama has the highest rate of poverty but the lowest excess mortality; Harlem has the lowest rate of poverty but the highest excess mortality. The social, economic, cultural, racial, and regional geography of mortality in the United States is *very* complex.

CANCER

Cancer is a family of diseases. There is no one cause or one cure for cancer; there are only multiple effects of multiple treatments and outcomes. Our knowledge and classification of cancer is analogous to our knowledge of infectious disease in the early 19th century. Then, cholera was not differentiated from yellow fever or typhoid from diphtheria. There was only fever, "flux," vomiting, rash, flatulence, cramps, and so forth. The best doctors of the day could write of malaria "becoming typhous in its course." It was only after germ theory gave us a microbe for each disease that the separate entities were classified and causation and treatment defined appropriately. Classification of cancer by the site of occurrence is similar to classification of "fever" in the 19th century. For example, if stomach cancer and cancer of the pancreas are both caused by a certain chemical, they are classified as different diseases; but pancreatic cancers that are caused (for all we know) by minerals or viruses are lumped together by organ in spite of their different disease agents. As we learn more of the different causes and of appropriate prevention and treatment, our classification scheme is bound to change.

The long latency of the disease has bedeviled etiological research because of the many changes over time and space that occur. Geographers, whose study usually encompasses areas large enough to have significant population mobility, need to appreciate these time-exposure processes. A new synthesis in cancer research presents a model of cancer causation. Figure 7-1 illustrates why it takes cancer so long to develop. When a carcinogen enters the body, it is usually detoxified by enzymes, broken down, and excreted. Occasionally, these enzymes and related processes can activate the carcinogen and enable it to enter a cell. If it binds to anything in the cell except the DNA, it can only affect that individual cell. If it binds to the DNA, many repair mechanisms attack it. The bonds between the carcinogen and the DNA are broken, and the carcinogen is broken up, transported, and excreted. Only if the DNA is replicated before the carcinogen is removed can the carcinogen affect the new cell information, creating a cancer gene. The evidence clearly indicates that one altered gene is usually not enough to cause cancer. The process must be repeated, seemingly against all odds, by another carcinogen in a cell that already has the altered genetic material. The odds are changed if substances known as "promoters" (sometimes metal elements, fractions of hydrocarbon chains, fatty acids, or substances such as saccharin)

TABLE 7-2. Measures of Mortality among Blacks and Whites 15 to 64 Years Old in Selected Populations, According to Sex, 1989–1991

Group	Annual death rate	Total No. of deaths	Annual excess-death rate	Standardized mortality ratio (95% confidence interval)	Probability of survival from the age of 15 to the age of 65
U.S. male population					
Whites	417	—	0	1.00	0.77
Blacks	791	—	374	1.90	0.62
Black men					
Poor populations					
Harlem	1713	1600	1296	4.11 (3.91–4.32)	0.37
Central Detroit	1163	1881	746	2.79 (2.67–2.92)	0.50
Watts	1216	1449	799	2.92 (2.77–3.07)	0.50
Black Belt Alabama	755	516	338	1.81 (1.66–1.97)	0.63
Comparison populations					
Queens–Bronx	491	822	74	1.18 (1.10–1.26)	0.75
Northwest Detroit	691	1101	274	1.66 (1.56–1.76)	0.66
Crenshaw–Baldwin Hills	781	871	364	1.87 (1.75–2.00)	0.63
Northern Alabama	728	697	311	1.75 (1.62–1.88)	0.64
White men					
Poor populations					
Lower East Side, New York City	625	782	208	1.50 (1.40–1.61)	0.69
Detroit	838	898	421	2.01 (1.88–2.15)	0.60
Appalachia	574	602	157	1.38 (127–1.49)	0.70
Northeast Alabama	544	968	127	1.30 (1.22–1.39)	0.71
Comparison populations					
Queens	363	521	−54	0.87 (0.80–0.95)	0.80
Sterling Heights	172	192	−245	0.41 (0.36–0.47)	0.89
Western Kentucky	360	418	−57	0.86 (0.78–0.95)	0.80
Southwest Alabama	462	512	−46	1.11 (1.02–1.21)	0.75
U.S. female population					
Whites	225	—	0	1.00	0.87
Blacks	439	—	214	1.95	0.77
Black women					
Poor populations					
Harlem	759	803	535	3.38 (3.15–3.62)	0.65
Central Detroit	580	960	355	2.58 (2.42–2.75)	0.71
Watts	584	795	359	2.60 (2.43–2.79)	0.71
Black Belt Alabama	425	342	201	1.89 (1.70–2.10)	0.77
Comparison populations					
Queens–Bronx	242	456	18	1.08 (0.98–1.18)	0.87
Northwest Detroit	335	572	110	1.49 (1.37–1.62)	0.82
Crenshaw–Baldwin Hills	347	447	122	1.54 (1.41–1.69)	0.81
Northern Alabama	470	469	246	2.09 (1.91–2.29)	0.75
White women					
Poor populations					
Lower East Side, New York City	250	268	26	1.14 (0.99–1.26)	0.86
Detroit	428	440	203	1.90 (1.73–2.09)	0.77
Appalachia	311	321	87	1.39 (1.24–1.55)	0.82
NortheastAlabama	283	508	58	1.26 (1.15–1.37)	0.84
Comparison populations					
Queens	90	315	−35	0.84 (0.76–0.94)	0.89
Sterling Heights	121	126	−104	0.54 (0.45–0.64)	0.93
Western Kentucky	203	240	−21	0.91 (0.80–1.03)	0.88
Southwest Alabama	197	222	−27	0.88 (0.77–1.00)	0.88

Note. The annual death rates shown are per 100,000 members of the population, after standardization for age based on the distribution of whites. From Geronimus, Bound, Waidmann, Hillemeier, and Burns (1996, p. 1554).

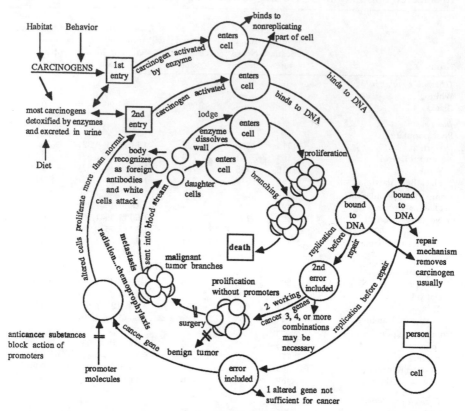

FIGURE 7-1. Cancer causation. Repeated alteration of genetic material is usually required to cause cancer, and the generally low probability that the necessary alteration will be repeated is affected by the presence of "promoter" substances and the dosage and duration of carcinogens, as well as the presence of protective nutrients for repair and buffering mechanisms.

encourage the altered cells to proliferate faster than normal cells. This process creates an increasing number of targets for another carcinogen to enter. The rare chance that such a contact will occur, among all the normal cells of the body, helps to explain why decades may elapse before expression of the disease. It also explains why cancer is most common in tissues with normally high rates of proliferation, such as skin or the lining of the intestines and uterus, and rare in nonproliferating tissues such as nerves. Proliferation increases the number of cells containing the altered genetic information. Every time a carcinogen enters the body, the whole chain of chance events must repeat. In 1999, scientists succeeded in turning normal human cells into cancerous ones by altering four genes. They turned on an oncogene to make the cell multiply quickly, shut off a tumor-suppressor gene that limited replication, disabled a gene that caused abnormal cells to self-destruct, and turned on a gene to rebuild the telomere caps on chromosome ends that normally shorten and age with each division. It took these four changes in one cell to create a cancer. A benign, noninvasive tumor can be removed by surgery. If the tumor sends out branches and envelops other tissue, it is cancer. The malignant tumor can send "daughter" cells into the bloodstream, an event known as metastasis. The daughter cells drift with the bloodstream, in danger of being recognized as foreign and attacked by the body's antibodies and white cells, until they lodge. They produce an enzyme that dissolves the blood vessel wall, which allows them to enter normal tissue and begin proliferation and invasive branching in the new site. Eventually vital tissues and processes are involved, and death results.

Cancer's need for repeated defiance of the odds in an orderly but improbable sequence of events explains the long latency period. The need for separate carcinogens, promoters, and overcoming of at least four defense mechanisms of the body explains the often baffling etiology and outcome. The adequacy of vitamins (and other antioxidants) in the diet is important for the body's ability to detoxify the carcinogen, especially after it has bonded within a cell. The status of the immune system is critical because it must identify cells with altered genetic information as foreign and destroy them. All the interactions and balances of this complex process change over time.

The Genetic Base

Some kinds of cancer have long been suspected of being genetically linked. There is evidence that some cancers affect men more than women when there has been equal exposure. Others are common in some population groups (e.g., nasopharyngeal cancer among the southern Chinese) and rare in others. Some cancers are more common in a family than in the general population. It is for these "familial" cancers that genetic markers are most likely to be found. As is true with Parkinson's and Alzheimer's diseases, the specific genes involved in familial disease may not be involved at all in the "sporadics," or cases that occur without an apparent hereditary role.

Cells must divide and replicate if tissue is to grow and maintain health. Each replication involves the exact reproduction of their DNA. Accidents happen. The four bases of the DNA may spell out G,C,A,T for example. In replication G matches with C, and A with T, to form a three-dimensional molecular structure that locks with a specific enzyme. If during replication somehow G matches with T, an error of mismatch has occurred. Alternatively, radiation may knock a proton off, changing G, and causing an error of excision. Genetic excision or damage may eliminate the ability to receive and regulate a chemical, as when a damaged cell without ability to respond by negating a cell growth signal turns cancerous. In either case, proteins patrolling the DNA have to recognize the damage and call in repairs. Figure 7-1 implies several mechanisms of genetic involvement.

The importance of genetically given damage recognition and enzyme combinations in DNA repair and carcinogen detoxification makes it plausi-ble that genetic differences may make people more susceptible (Haac, 1995). A variant of the p450-gene enzyme that is poor at metabolizing a certain car-cinogen, for example, may increase a person's susceptibility to the toxic ef-fects of cigarette smoke. People suffering from a rare disease called xeroder-ma pigmentosum, for another example, have been found to have a mutation that results in a lack of the enzymes necessary to break the abnormal bonds formed among subunits of a gene under ultraviolet light. They have high rates of skin cancer. There is growing evidence that men may be more sus-ceptible to many mutagenic agents because they bind more carcinogen to their chromosomes. This has been most studied with regard to lung cancer and carcinogens and promoters in cigarette smoke. Men have been found to have greater stimulation of DNA repair synthesis, resulting from the increas-ing amount of damage. Damage and repair activities increase with age for both sexes but are higher at all ages for men.

The best single example of the processes above lies with *Science*'s 1993 "Molecule of the Year," P53, which is resident on chromosome 17. When it was first found that P53 was involved in 60% of cancers, and even 80% of colon cancers, it was implicated as a carcinogen. Advancing research, howev-er, demonstrated that P53's role is to halt the replication of any cell with DNA damage, thus stopping abnormal growth processes. It is a tumor killer. Damage to P53 itself, however, can sabotage this critical control and defense system. It is now the gene scientists turn off when they are studying the process of carcinogenesis discussed previously.

One of the most active areas of cancer research concerns oncogenes and the breaking of chromosomes. Molecular biologists have identified more than 20 of these mysterious genes, which normally are inactive. They are found in such diverse organisms as flies, fish, mammals, and yeast. Thus, al-though their functions are unknown, they are presumed to be vital because they have been so carefully conserved throughout evolution. Oncogenes seem to be found consistently in tumorous cells, often in multiple copies. Sometimes they are involved in turning on growth genes, and possibly in chromosome breaking. It seems clear that chromosomes have a propensity to break in certain places. Genetic control of these places may be involved in susceptibility to cancer.

The Behavioral Base

Cultural risk factors for cancer involve a variety of customs and practices as well as economic goods and occupations. Given that solar radiation and ge-netic susceptibility by population group have not changed, the propensity of modern youth to sunbathe aggravates risk of skin cancer, compared to earli-er practices of wearing long sleeves and broad hats and modestly covering the body. Tobacco smoking is the most obvious endangering behavior, but mouth cancer has also been linked to chewing betel. Diet may be endangering: A diet poor in fiber means that undigested food passes too slowly through the intestines. It is thought that this allows toxic bacterial products to become concentrated and risks increase for colon cancer. Fatty acids may be a risk factor for breast cancer. The hydrocarbons and nitrosamines of smoked fish (and presumably other smoked products) and charred meat seem to be risk factors for stomach cancer. Diet may also be preventive: Carotenoids from green and yellow vegetables serve as antioxidants to protect cell walls. The vitamin E in fish skin or the antioxidants in green tea may do the same. The human diet contains a variety of natural carcinogens, promoters, antimutagens, and anticarcinogens. Science has barely begun to address the relative risk or protection of the enormous variety of dietary habits around the world.

The behavioral base in economic structure, occupation, industrial processes, and regulatory control has dominated risk assessment. Workers exposed to asbestos, to the manufacture or use of industrial chemicals, to agricultural sprays, or to the other multiform dusts and radiations connected with earning a livelihood in an industrialized society have long served as the guinea pigs for most of our threshold and effect data. The larger-scale behavior of locating certain enterprises, such as oil refineries, nuclear power plants, or toxic waste incinerators, in certain populous areas and not others, has rarely been evaluated from such an experimental perspective. An increasing concern for issues of environmental racism, highlighted by geographers and other social scientists, has directed such research by the Environmental Protection Agency.

Patterns and Change

There is amazing geographical variation in the occurrence of cancer. For decades it has been recognized that differences of incidence rates, not only between men and women but also between urban and rural populations and among countries, hold etiological clues. The highest female cancer rate by country is far less than the top 10 male rates. Japan has the highest stomach cancer rates but is not ranked in the top 10 for lung, breast, or rectal cancer. Given the country's biometeorology, the population's genetics, and such behavioral patterns as ranching and surfing, one can suggest reasons why Australia is the highest ranked in skin cancer, but why should countries as diverse as Uruguay, France, and Singapore be ranked so highly for esophageal cancer? Furthermore, within each country, urban and rural rates can differ as greatly as international rates.

The extraordinary data richness at microscale in China was published as an atlas which portrayed the most dramatic spatial patterns of concentration (Editorial Committee, 1979). Not only was nasopharyngeal cancer concentrated among Cantonese on the Guangdong plateau, but there were extremely high foci of esophageal cancer west of the Taihang Shan in Shanxi and liver cancer around the mouth of the Yangtze and southeastern coast. At the national level, these cancers, which are almost unknown in the United States, have been the major cause of death. With economic liberalization in the late 1970s to the 1980s, cigarette smoking reached prodigious levels, however, and the familiar consequence of lung cancer has built to a wave that is breaking now.

The pattern of cancer incidence has changed over time. Lilienfeld and Lilienfeld (1980) outlined several possible reasons. The changes may be artifactual; that is, they may result from errors due to changes in the recognition, classification, or reporting of the disease or from errors in enumerating the population. Real changes may result because the age structure of the population has changed, because people survive diseases that were once incurable and thereby live long enough for cancer to become manifest, or because genetic or environmental factors have changed. (As epidemiologists, the Lilienfelds include behavioral changes under environmental factors.)

Greenberg (1983b) found a spatial convergence of cancer mortality in the United States between 1950 and 1975. He divided counties into those that were strongly urban (10%), moderately urban, and rural (69%). (Elsewhere, Greenberg, 1980, presents his method for allocating components of the incidence changes to county, regional, and national scales, building on scale differences in variance, as discussed in Chapter 13.) The strongly urban–rural ratio for cancers of the bladder, kidney, larynx, esophagus, lung, tongue, rectum, and large intestine in the 1950s was 1.9 overall, and locally as high as 2.4. By the early 1970s, the ratio was only 1.2 overall and lower for white females. There were other important changes as well. Rates for some sites of cancer increased, especially lymphoma, multiple myeloma, and melanoma, and connective tissue, lung, brain, pancreas, and central nervous system cancers. Other types decreased greatly, including five that had been among the most important: stomach, rectum, liver, cervix uteri, and corpus uteri. Females had the least increase and greatest decrease, so that the gap between males and females widened. Nonwhite males had a trend opposite to white females. In 1950–1955, white males had a cancer rate 7% higher than nonwhite males and 18% higher than white females. By 1970–1975, nonwhite male cancer rates were 22% higher than white male rates, 65% higher than nonwhite female, and 86% higher than white female cancer rates. There was a strong parallel trend for most types of cancer. Cancer rates diverged by sex and race subgroups of the population but converged geographically.

Greenberg contends that this spatial convergence of cancer mortality, (i.e., development of a homogeneous pattern), in the United States and other industrialized countries was caused by change in the geography of risk factors associated with the diffusion of urban culture. These risk factors include air and water pollution, cigarette smoking, alcohol consumption, diet, occupation, socioeconomic status, stress, and medical practices. These changes have not, however, affected everyone equally. Greenberg (1989) refers to cancer in black males as "a slow-motion health disaster." By 1981, the black male death rate from cancer was already 41% higher than the white male rate; there was a 60% excess of cancer mortality among black males 70 years old or younger. Some of the increase was due to improvements in diagnosis, treatment, and certification of death cause. Continuing inadequacy in early detection and treatment, however, also contributed to higher death outcomes. Black females, for example, in the mid-1990s had lower rates of incidence of breast cancer than did white females but much higher mortality rates from their cancer. Greenberg contended that practical known measures were capable of preventing roughly half the cancer. Probably in part as a result of such efforts, by 1996 cancer rates (not death rates) for white males were 8.9% higher than for black males, 43% higher than for black females, but only 11.9% higher than for white females (National Center for Health Statistics, 1998). Much of the increase in white female cancer was due to lung cancer (Plate 7-1B).

Because most forms of cancer are relatively rare, most data have been mapped at national or international scales. Small numbers of deaths tend to fluctuate randomly and give misleading associations (Chapter 13). The National Cancer Institute (Mason, McKay, Hoover, Blot, & Fraumeni, 1975) first published an atlas of cancer mortality at the county level by aggregating cases over 20 years. The scale at which to map cancer comparatively has been especially problematic. Rare cancers, such as brain, have a low range of rates compared to common cancers, such as colon. The distribution of the African American population varies greatly across the United States, leaving regions of counties with almost no population denominator when cancer deaths are broken down by age and gender. One solution, which this atlas and also a more recent cancer atlas by the U.S. Environmental Protection Agency (1987) used, is to map white rates at county level and black rates at the scale of state economic areas, which aggregate counties into clusters. The recent *Atlas of U.S. Mortality* used health service areas as the scale of aggregation for all its disease maps (National Center for Health Statistics, 1997). Plate 7-1 (following page 246) illustrates some of these. The rates are age-adjusted and mapped as mortality ratios compared to U.S. national rates, and the distribution of death rates by health service areas is presented in a graph (see Chapter 13 for discussion of these issues of mapping). Hatching indicates where the data are sparse, mostly because of small populations at risk.

The map of all cancers for black females (Plate 7-1A) shows that the highest rates, based on substantial data, occur in and around the metropolitan centers of Chicago and southern Lake Michigan, New Orleans and the mouth of the Mississippi, and Washington, DC, and surrounding parts of Delaware, Maryland, and Pennsylvania. The lowest rates, based on substantial data, occur on the southern coastal plain where population concentrations are greatest and of longest standing and also still the most rural. Plate 7-1B presents the example of white female lung cancer mortality. The concentration of lung cancer along the coast of the Gulf of Mexico follows the pattern established in the National Cancer Institutes' previous atlas, though the high rates of the Georgia and Florida Atlantic coasts are new. The high rates in the coal-mining country of Kentucky and West Virginia are not unexpected. The high rates, with substantial data, of the Pacific Coast and Southwest are astonishing. White male lung cancer does not occur that way, nor does black female or other white female cancers. The text of the atlas points out, with following maps, that the mortality rates are concentrated in an age group or population cohort. The interpretation given is that large numbers of white females first began to smoke cigarettes in the West, and that white females in that region were the first to stop smoking cigarettes.

Some Studies of Cancer

Geographers have studied spatial patterns to identify risk factors. Often the research questions and methodology involve determining regions and investigating common or different factors (Chapter 12 describes such causal reasoning and analog area analysis). For example, several regions can be identified in which stomach cancer has a high incidence. Iceland, Japan, and northern Minnesota and Wisconsin are three such regions. Copper seems to be unusually concentrated in the soils of one of these—is it also high in the others? People in Iceland eat smoked and salted fish and are of Scandinavian descent. Do people in Japan eat salted and smoked fish, and do people of Scandinavian descent in Minnesota and Wisconsin continue ethnic dietary practices? Some people in eastern Africa have a high incidence of esophageal cancer in a culture area in which home-distilled alcohol is made. People outside that culture area have lower cancer rates: Perhaps the alcohol or method of its production is involved. The region around the Caspian Sea in Iran, however, has some of the world's highest rates of esophageal cancer, and people there do not consume alcohol. Research suggests that the Iranian risk area is characterized by nutrient-deficient saline soil, halophytic vegetation, and poor crops. Alcohol could easily absorb elements from the pottery and cans in which it is distilled. Could trace element deficiency or toxicity be common to both regions?

Geographers in Japan, Europe, and North America have analyzed the pattern of cancer occurrence in relation to environmental, socioeconomic, and demographic factors by means of multivariate statistical procedures. The Japanese have found associations of lung cancer with air pollution, urbanization, and living in fishing ports and near refineries and mines. A cartographic analysis of cancer mortality in the British Isles also identified the urban affinity of lung cancer (Howe, 1981). However, it did not support the epidemiological hypotheses that mortality from cancer of the large intestine and rectum is related to a carbohydrate-rich diet, or that risk of gastric cancer is associated with blood group (genetic heritage). Others, struggling to relate aggregate data to exposure patterns and microenvironments, have inconclusively studied the relationship of various classifications of cancer to hardness and trace elements of water in Quebec (Thouez, Beauchamp, & Simard,

1981). Several geographers have analyzed the way various sites of cancer (cancer of the stomach, pancreas, esophagus, lungs, blood, etc.) form groups when their patterns of spatial distribution are compared. Types of cancer having the same pattern of spatial distribution may share a common etiological factor.

Studies that are based on general populations, that do not select disease categories for research carefully and deliberately or target fortuitous places, may run into many data and methodological problems. They so often suffer from the ecological fallacy (Chapter 13) that ecological studies as a whole have earned a reputation for scientific weakness. Such multifactor, population-based studies are, however, a powerful means for choosing places for case-control and other detailed studies. An important research question regarding disease distribution concerns the degree of spatial clustering. Does clustering occur at the county scale or at the household scale? If three cases of leukemia occur on a city block, is that more than could occur by chance? If there are inimical effects from a chemical factory or a power line, at what scale would the health consequences cluster around it? Map patterns alone cannot eliminate chance in clustering, but observed patterns can be compared to randomized ones using stochastic approaches and chi-square tests.

The study of microscale mobility and exposure to different environments can be used to identify possible etiological factors and for new hypotheses. Armstrong (1976, 1978) studied nasopharyngeal cancer, a disease of unknown etiology, among the Chinese in Malaysia. Using a case-control method (Chapter 12), he compared the exposure patterns of people with the disease and of controls, people without the disease, to what he called self-specific environments. He measured how much time was spent daily in agricultural areas, in squatter housing or middle-class housing, in shop workplaces, factories, shopping on the street, in various means of transportation, in public places, and so forth, and also how much time was spent in smoky places, crowded places, around chemicals, and under conditions of bad air pollution. He examined such indices of traditional or modern/assimilated cultural patterns as having an altar in the house and eating meals in a formal manner, as well as details of what people ate and how they prepared it. He found that among genetically susceptible Chinese, important stimuli are associated with industrial or trade occupations, smoky workplaces, poorer housing, traditional lifestyle, a diet with less variety of foods, and childhood consumption of salted fish. This methodology can be extended to many searches for unknown causes of disease (see cardiovascular disease in Savannah, Chapter 13, this volume).

A different approach was taken by Glick. He opened up a new methodology by regarding spatial autocorrelation as an etiological tool instead of a statistical nuisance (Vignette 13-1). Spatial autocorrelation is the association between a variable's values taken from two adjacent places. What Glick did was use the scale and intensity of that association to test etiological hypotheses.

Glick (1979a, 1979b, 1980, 1982) used east–west and north–south tran-

sects across dozens of counties of the United States and the spatial relationships of cities and industries among states to study the spatial organization of
cancer rates. Because different cancer-inducing processes act most strongly at
different scales, knowledge of the relationship of scale and cancer variation
can help identify the process. Glick started with theoretical models of carcinogenesis and inferred the spatial relationships.

There are two major classes of skin cancer. Basal or squamous cell carci-
nomas are fairly common and relatively innocuous because they can be successfully treated without hospitalization. Malignant melanoma, a rare form of
skin cancer, is often fatal. Glick (1979a) had data from four special surveys of
skin cancer. He used regression techniques to estimate the effects of age and
of ultraviolet radiation levels and found that nonmelanoma skin cancer has a
strong age effect, as one would expect if the carcinogenesis process required
repeated exposures and alterations of the cell (as illustrated in Figure 7-1).
Glick reasoned that because nonmelanoma skin cancer involves more stages
of exposure, it should have a steeper spatial gradient of mortality. Indeed, he
found that the gradient in mortality rate for a transect (line) through Minnesota–Iowa–Missouri–Arkansas–Louisiana was very steep and constant for
nonmelanoma skin cancer, going from about 1.0 to 2.6 per 100,000, whereas
mortality from melanoma ranged from 1.1 in Minnesota to 1.8 in Louisiana,
with a less constant gradient.

Figure 7-2 presents a spatial correlogram for two types of cancer that illustrates the spatial pattern of point and area exposure to risk. Across the X-
axis are the spatial lags in association. For example, at lag 1 the average autocorrelation of each county in the state with adjacent counties is expressed,
whereas at lag 5 the autocorrelation is with five counties away. The autocorrelation is expressed as a normal (Z) score on the Y-axis. The farther away from
zero, either positively or negatively, the stronger the association among counties. The line that shows point exposure has a steep distance decay in autocorrelation from high positive (similar to adjacent county) to high negative
(different from nearby county). It represents a spatial pattern of isolated foci
of incidence, such as might result from contagious disease occurring in large
cities but not yet diffused across the county, or from behavior limited to ethnic enclaves. Stomach cancer in Pennsylvania shows such a pattern, whereas
bladder cancer is characterized by a nearly horizontal correlogram for lags
1–3 (Glick, 1980). Such a pattern, as illustrated, portrays a large region of
similar rates and suggests an environmental carcinogen found over large
areas, such as water catchment basins, rather than a diffusion process.

Prostate cancer is one of the most prevalent in the United States, with especially high rates among African Americans. It is of unknown etiology. As
discussed in Chapter 13 (see Figure 13-11), Hanchette used regression and
trend surface analysis to draw out the association of ultraviolet light, prostate
cancer, and a possible role of vitamin D and its associated enzymes
(Hanchette & Schwartz 1992). The strong north–south gradient of this disease is also correlated with colon cancer, as well as with multiple sclerosis.

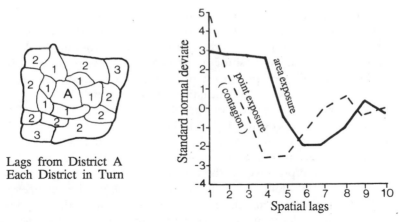

FIGURE 7-2. Spatial correlograms. Point and areal (regional) sources of exposure are reflected in different levels of correlation between spatial units when thge units are lagged incrementally.

Population migration, if large well-defined streams can be identified and followed, can be used analytically to separate the role of environment, cultural behavior, and even genetics. The argument is that a sudden change in disease incidence upon migration would be due to some environmental factor, failure to change at all would suggest genetic disposition, and change over decades or generations would suggest behavioral roles and exposures. The classic epidemiological example was of breast cancer among Japanese in Hawaii. The United States has among the world's highest rates for breast cancer and Japan among the lowest. Rates did not change for Japanese women who migrated. Third-generation Americans, however, did not have the low rates of their ancestral (and genetic) homeland but intermediary rates between Japanese and white American women. In an updated study of women in Hawaii and California, among 597 cases and 966 controls there was a six-fold gradient in breast cancer risk by migration pattern (Ziegler et al., 1993). Asian American women born in the United States had a 60% higher risk than those born in Asia. Among those born in the United States, the risk was determined by the number of grandparents born in the United States Among Asian Americans born in Asia, the risk was 30% higher if prior community was urban, and 80% higher if they had lived in the United States over 10 years. Such evidence strongly suggests the importance of American lifestyles.

CARDIOVASCULAR DISEASE

The group of diseases known as *cardiovascular disease* (CVD) constitutes the major cause of death in economically developed countries (Figure 4-2). It includes ischemic heart disease (heart tissue damage because of obstruction of blood flow to heart muscle itself), cerebrovascular disease (blood vessels supplying brain), atherosclerosis (an arteriosclerosis, or hardening of the arteries, characterized by fatty deposition and fibrosis of the inner lining), hypertension (high arterial blood pressure), and rheumatic heart disease (reduced function because of heart inflammation and scarring due to previous rheumatic fever). The resistance of the blood vessels to the flow of blood through them is blood pressure. This is affected by the volume and composition of the blood, by the dilation and constriction of blood vessels, and by narrowing of the arteries caused by the buildup of fatty deposits. Systolic blood pressure is the pressure on the arteries when the heart contracts and pumps out a surge of blood; diastolic blood pressure is the pressure on the arteries between contractions, the minimum pressure that the arteries feel continuously. High blood pressure for which the cause is unknown is referred to as essential hypertension. When the heart's blood supply is drastically affected, a myocardial infarction (heart attack) occurs. If the blood supply is only partially restricted, a chronic coronary thrombosis usually results. When the blood supply to the brain is blocked, a stroke results (apoplexy).

CVD is the overwhelming cause of death in developed countries. Just arteriosclerosis causes one-half of all the deaths in the United States among persons ages 35 to 65. It is the major cause of permanent disability. It accounts for more hospitalizations than any other illness. Cardiovascular disease is the greatest contributor to excess mortality among African Americans today, an excess increasing partly because of less rapid decline of heart disease (Vignette 7-1, Table 3). It has been declining since the 1960s, especially among white males.

These diseases all have a wide variation geographically. Age-specific rates of ischemic heart disease, for example, vary more than 500-fold among nations. The etiology of cardiovascular disease rests on the familiar triangle of population–behavior–habitat interactions.

The Population Base

A wide range of genetic factors is involved in cardiovascular disease. Several kinds of congenital defects may be involved, such as improperly closed heart valves. Genetic controls on metabolism are also important: People process, store, and remove fats in different ways. There may be genetic predisposition to hypertension, acting through the renal enzymes that control fluid volume and excretion. Individuals react differently to chemicals (in drugs and foods) that promote vasodilation. The facility with which blood clots form has a strong genetic component. One of the most marked genetic differences is expressed in the lower incidence of ischemic heart disease among premenopausal women as compared with men, a protection that diminishes with the loss of estrogen (see Vignette 7-1). Sex hormones influence how the body metabolizes and stores cholesterol and other fats. The level and composition of hormones differ not only between males and females but also among individuals and from family to family.

Personality is also partly based on genetic combinations, although it has a behavioral expression and environmental impress. It forms one of the bridges from genetic to behavioral considerations. There have been many intervention studies designed upon the distinction of type A and type B personalities. Type A personality involves aggressiveness, excessive drive, compulsive behavior, competitiveness, impatience, and insecurity. It is considered a coronary risk factor, and intervention programs try to get people to slow down and relax. Numerous studies have suggested that it is the dimension of hostility and anger that is most destructive in the type A personality syndrome.

The Behavioral Base

The behavioral base for cardiovascular disease involves cigarette smoking, drinking alcohol, diet, exercise, occupation, psychosocial insults, stress, and stress management. Cigarette smoking is clearly a risk factor. The cadmium in cigarettes raises blood pressure, and chemicals they introduce to the blood circulation affect vasodilation. A little alcohol consumption is protective; apparently it favorably affects cholesterol balance. Heavy alcohol consumption interacts with nutrition, weight, and exercise to constitute a risk factor. Many dietary factors in cardiovascular disease are still unknown. The high potassium levels found in some vegetables may be protective, for example, and calcium may be more important than previously recognized. Two dietary hazards hazards have been clear: high salt consumption and cholesterol. Given the different kinds of cholesterol, the fact that the body makes its own, and the role of exercise, alcohol, and dietary combinations, today even the cholesterol in eggs no longer seems so important.

The role of cholesterol and other blood lipids (fats) is complicated by the fact that the liver makes some cholesterol itself, regardless of diet, and by the need to differentiate subcategories of lipids. High-density lipid cholesterol (HDL) acts to transport fats and clean out the circulatory system. It is the "good cholesterol." Low-density lipid cholesterol (LDL) builds up in deposits. It is bad. The metabolic changes associated with exercise, with a little consumption of alcohol, and with some drugs increase the ratio of the protective HDL to the endangering LDL and so lower the risk of atherosclerosis. Exercise, then, has the dual impact of increasing the capacity of the circulatory system to pump blood so that it can better cope with sudden demands on it and inducing a more favorable lipid balance through metabolic changes.

Stress is a rubric that covers many evils. The connections between stress and the body are through the immune and endocrine systems (Chapter 2 "The Social Environment"). Psychosocial insults come from situations as diverse as occupation and working conditions, neighborhood blight, domestic problems with spouse or children, and prolonged fear and anxiety. Many studies have found sudden myocardial infarction to be the illness most related to life-event stress. Loss of job, upward mobility, marriage, divorce, death of a spouse, change of residence, and trouble with children characteristically are common for heart attack patients (see also Figure 2-1 and Audy's levels of health). Similarly, the important occupational characteristic seems not to be specific job categories as much as lack of control, repetitiveness, inability to use one's skills, and similar frustrations in one's work. This seems related to the work of Evans, Barer, and Marmor (1994) and Marmot and Theorell (1988) that not simple deprivation but relative status and hierarchy are involved in cardiovascular disease etiology. Marmot and Mustard (1994) consider the improvement in Japanese health, and especially the change from stroke as the leading cause of death to cardiovascular disease, both at lower levels than in the United States.

All the stresses related to the poverty syndrome are especially relevant to cardiovascular disease. Numerous studies within industrialized countries have shown a positive health effect from a prosperous and growing economy. Times of recession and unemployment add tremendously to life stresses and to mortality. There is, however, a rather complicated relationship with socioeconomic change in the Third World. Cross-cultural studies have found that increased hypertension is often related to greater participation in the money economy. This generally entails major changes in diet, occupation, mobility, and other conditions. Economic change and loss of traditions add to stress, and economic growth and upward mobility are associated with increased risk of cardiovascular disease. Not just the social organization and technology parts of the behavior vertex are involved here, but, importantly, beliefs and values. As Corin (1994) put it: "The impact of changing conditions varies according to the significance attached to traditional ways of life" (p. 105).

Our knowledge of just how socioeconomic status relates to biology, behavior, and social factors on one hand and CVD morbidity and mortality trends on the other, especially with regard to minorities, remains limited. There is agreement about the need to improve our understanding of the concept of SES and the ways in which it reflects the conditions of everyday life to people of various economic strata (Lenfant, 1996). We know that there are strong, consistent inverse relationships: lower SES means higher CVD risk factors (varying by age, sex, ethnicity) such as smoking and obesity. The relations are weaker and less consistent with serum cholesterol, deliberate exercise, and lifestyle, all of which have poor national data. Psychosocial variables for SES groups of various ethnic backgrounds especially need research: how is the import of job change, unemployment, economic instability, social support perceived?

Complications of race cut across all the SES and behavioral components. It seems, for example, that not just race or SES but also place of birth matters (Fang, Madhavan, & Alderman 1996). When CVD of blacks was compared with that of whites in New York City but linked by census records (PUMS) to birth in the Northeast, the South, or the Caribbean, black mortality overall was indeed greater than white. But blacks born in the Northeast had almost the same death rates (per 100,000) as whites (white males, 285/black males, 299; white females, 155/black females, 165). Caribbean-born blacks had lower rates of death from heart disease than even Northeast-born whites in all age groups. Black males 25–44 years old who were born in the South had a 30% higher heart disease mortality rate than did black males born in the Northeast. Strokes to males ages 45 to 64 were a little less dramatically matched (white males, 25.3/black males, Northeast, 74.0/black males, South, 102.9), but the pattern is clear. Geographers cannot help remarking that, of course, there is spatial variation and regionalization of socioeconomic conditions, discrimination and opportunity, and health care, as well as cultural factors such as religion. The United States is big and diverse in culture, people, and environment; it is not at all a uniform surface with an undifferentiated national population well studied by national sampling. More research needs to be done at varying scales. Such studies of race, SES, and place led Gillum (1996) to editorialize that the public health response and understanding had neglected the dynamic aspects of the problem and especially the heterogeneity of rates among blacks. He hypothesized factors associated in six stages: precolonial Africa, modern urban Africa, modern black populations in the West Indies, rural populations in the southern United States (similar to West Indies), poor in the inner-city United States, and affluent in the new suburbs.

The effects of stress on health have illuminated the importance of stress management. Intervention programs are being implemented to teach people how to relax, to use exercise as a stress release, to engage in meditation, and to soothe themselves by caressing pets and taking time to smell the roses. The role of social support and close relationships in coping with stress has come to the fore.

The Habitat Base

There are three important components of the habitat vertex of cardiovascular diseases. Available health services are especially important. The detection, treatment, and control of hypertension are among medical science's greatest interventions. The development of emergency medical systems and of cardiopulmonary resuscitation techniques has been important for heart attacks. The other two critical aspects of the habitat are weather and geochemistry.

Several physical mechanisms of acclimatization and adaptation to changes in pressure and temperature were discussed in Chapter 5. Cardiovascular disease has a peak occurrence during periods of cold weather. Incidence seems to be responsive to the passage of fronts and other meteorological events. Because of physiological conditions of vasodilation and vasoconstriction, peripheral capillary networks for heat dissipation or conservation, and changes in the composition and thickness of blood, it is also likely that different climatic circumstances have something to do with the wide range of disease incidence.

An active area of research concerns the etiological significance of trace elements. These elements occur in such small amounts that only recently have scientists been able to measure them accurately, in parts per billion. The study of trace elements is further complicated by the constant interaction among them. Zinc, for example, is important to tissue healing. After a heart attack, most of the body's zinc is concentrated in the heart, and it seems reasonable that deficiency in zinc may play a role in fatal outcome. Zinc, however, is blocked by copper, so that the adequacy of zinc in the diet cannot be studied separately. Cadmium, a heavy metal and systemic poison like lead, is known to raise blood pressure in laboratory animals when they are constantly fed minute amounts of the metal. It might well be important in essential hypertension. Selenium, however, seems to block the action of cadmium and is a constituent of blood enzymes important for blood clotting and cholesterol metabolism. Selenium could be measured only recently, by expensive techniques of nuclear absorption. Similarly, lead, nickel, chromium, manganese, lithium, potassium, sulfur, cobalt, and iron are variously involved in nerve transmission to the heart, muscle healing, cholesterol metabolism, blood clotting, and hypertension. They all combine, enhance, block, and precipitate each other in various combinations. In addition, abundant elements such as calcium and magnesium are important electrolytes and have been implicated in arrhythmia's and sudden death.

A geographer has to be concerned about the pathways that these elements can take to the individuals at risk. The *water factor* has been implicated in many studies. More than a score of international studies have found water hardness to be inversely related to cardiovascular disease mortality. Hardness is usually based on the amount of calcium carbonate, but sometimes other minerals are included. The suggestion is that soft water has a different composition of trace elements than does hard water (Gardner, 1976). Only some elements, however, can be consumed in water in sufficient quantity to make any difference. Thus, water may be a significant source of copper, but thousands of gallons would have to be consumed daily to obtain significant nutritional input of iron or potassium. Food is a much more concentrated source of most elements. Further complications can result from using analysis of surface water for populations which drink from artesian sources, or from water supply altered by treatment plants (e.g., softening) and passed through municipal pipes.

Figure 7-3 illustrates some of the geochemical pathways that trace elements take from the environment to humans. The original rock is very important. Limestones are high in calcium and magnesium and are accompanied usually by strontium, phosphorus, and zinc, and sometimes by cadmium and lead. Shales are high in aluminum silicates and, locally, in molybdenum, vanadium, and uranium. Sandstone is rich in silica, but it is usually leached of trace elements. Serpentine rock is high in iron and magnesium, and often

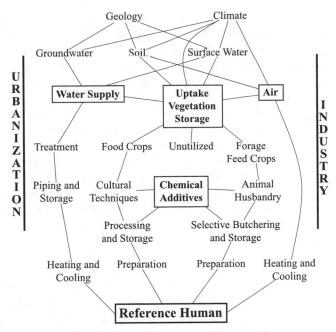

FIGURE 7-3. Geochemical pathways. Human consumption of trace elements is strongly influenced by the complex steps of processing and distributing of soil or water.

in chromium, nickel, and manganese. How these elements become bound and available depends on temperature, other minerals available, and groundwater and surface water supplies. The uptake of these elements by vegetation may be controlled by the plant's metabolism, regardless of soil concentration, and the elements may be stored in plant parts that humans do not consume. Heating often causes the elements to combine and precipitate, while the passage of time during food processing and water piping permits them to absorb and bind to other elements. Herbicides, insecticides, fungicides, and preservatives, which usually derive much of their potency from metals such as mercury or selenium, add to the concentrations of elements associated with the original soil or river water. After all these sources have contributed, the elements ingested by humans are still measured in parts per billion. It is no wonder that the effects of water hardness and various trace elements remain a controversial subject (Meade, 1980).

Patterns and Analysis

The high prevalence of cardiovascular disease in industrialized countries is a basic component of the mortality transition (Chapter 4). This generality, however, obscures important variation among places. Most geographers studying cardiovascular disease have been concerned with mapping it and modeling its spatial variation. The identification of patterns of clustering and the changing associations at different scales has attracted considerable study. Ziegenfus and Gesler (1984), for example, identified incidence of major cardiovascular, acute ischemic, chronic ischemic, and cerebrovascular disease in four distinct clusters of counties in the urban corridor from New York through New Jersey to Philadelphia (see Vignette 13-1). Multivariate statistics have been used to analyze associations of CVD with measures of housing, income, ethnicity, and variables that make up the poverty syndrome. At a microscale, many of the risk factors have become well established. In an impressive demonstration, Brenner and Mooney (1982) developed a model, including variables of long-term economic growth, deleterious behavioral risk factors, economic instability related to unemployment and income loss, health care, and very cold temperatures, that closely predicts the trend and fluctuations in male and female cardiovascular disease in England, Wales, and Scotland from 1955–1976.

The element most related to cardiovascular disease in British water studies is calcium. In Britain as well as Ontario, Canada, calcium has been associated with sudden death due to arrhythmia, which results from imbalance in the electrical activity of the heart. There is a strong north–south gradation of cardiovascular disease in the United Kingdom (West, 1977). The death rates of Scotland have been long recognized as mysteriously high. There has been great interest, therefore, in the inverse association with water hardness. The lower southeastern incidence coincides with the hard waters of Tertiary and Cretaceous formations, the higher northwestern incidence with the soft waters of Precambrian rock formations. West and Lowe (1976), however, also found the same northwest–southeast gradient for temperature and rainfall. Others have suggested the importance of genetic distribution (marked by blood types) in Britain, due to its invasion and settlement history (Howe, 1972). More plausibly, it has been noted that the industrial revolution began in the regions with soft water partly because of the water quality. Early urbanization and industrialization might involve confounding factors. The pattern persists, however, even without the industrial cities. Jones and Moon (1987) point out that studies of the water hardness factor offer good examples of the Modifiable areal-unit problem (Chapter 13, Figure 13-1). In Canada, the inverse relationship exists for all Canadian municipalities together, but it becomes positive when analyzed separately for British Colombia and the Maritime and Prairie Provinces.

Cardiovascular disease in the United States also has a strong regional pattern (Plate 7-1C and D). Schroeder (1966) was the first to study cardiovascular disease and the water factor there, using data on finished water supplies in 1,300 municipalities across the country. At the national scale, significant inverse relationship was found for male and female deaths and water hardness. Cerebrovascular disease is strongly clustered in the southeastern counties along the coastal plain of Georgia and South Carolina, a region sometimes referred to as the *enigma area* (Meade, 1979). Again, the water factor has been implicated, as well as the deficiency of certain trace elements, such as selenium, in the soil and water. Temperature, population settlement and inheritance, agricultural patterns, poverty, late urbanization, and dietary factors may all be related as well.

The spatial correlation of a geochemical factor and cardiovascular disease would be most convincing if it held consistently at several scales and for all subgroups of the population. It would be further strengthened if geochemicals as etiological agents could be plausibly connected with a biophysical mechanism. Researchers have noted that the more rigorous the study and the more focused the study area, the weaker and more contradictory the geological connection (raising geographical questions about appropriate scale). The relationship may be weak, or it may turn upon some factor that has not been identified (e.g., the water factor). As Comstock (1979) noted, however, associations may be spurious, coincidental, or casual, and the association of a geochemical factor with cardiovascular disease is not spurious. Many independent studies in many countries have found statistically significant correlations. Comstock further laments that most studies have relied on correlation coefficients (scatter around the line) rather than regression coefficients (slope of the line) which indicate strength of relationship (see Vignette 12-3). Using those that did publish regression coefficients, he estimated the relative risk at 1.25. This would certainly be low for, say, and occupational exposure; but water affects the entire population and such risk would not be unimportant to public health.

Most of the regionalization of cardiovascular disease within countries remains unexplained. A microscale approach through study of population mobility may allow the identification of new environmental risk factors. The high death rates from cardiovascular disease on the southeastern coastal plain of the United States, mentioned previously, cluster in a way that cannot be explained by the conventional risk factors. Counties of the southeastern coastal plain cluster for both stroke and heart disease, for whites and blacks and males and females (Plate 7-1C and D). The lower Mississippi Valley has high rates and, for whites, the poor region of Appalachian Mountains. Are these associations of SES? The maps from the *Atlas of United States Mortality* of correlates (see Vignette 12-2) include Plate 7-1E and F, in which poverty seems to covary spatially positively and college education somewhat negatively at the county scale. Cigarette smoking is supposed to affect heart disease, but apparently the two do not covary at state scale (Plate 7-1G), although sedentary lifestyle (Plate 7-1H) seems related to both poverty and white male heart disease.

Analyzing the associated distribution and covariation of CVD with a series of overlays of geochemistry, agriculture, economics, ethnicity, industry, age of building construction, and various sources of water might suggest some new hypotheses. Meade (1983) selected census tracts within the city of Savannah, Georgia, on the basis of socioeconomic variables that predict stroke and blood pressure. Tracts that are well predicted serve as controls for those where stroke is significantly higher than predicted. Interviews ascertained the population's exposure to habitats within the city and defined the water and food pathways of trace elements from the local environment. Chapter 13 presents analysis of some of the differences in environmental exposures and behavioral patterns (Figures 13-13, 14, 15, and 16).

Japan has a geographical variation in CVD and in cancer that has attracted geographical and epidemiological study. The incidence of stroke is especially high in the northeastern parts of the main island of Honshu, the region of Tohoku, but lower around the Inland Sea. Takahashi (1981) found that salt consumption was higher in Tohoku and the water hardness ratio was low in Tohoku and high in the Inland Sea area. Kagami (1991) especially has sought to elucidate regional variation of disease in Japan as a geographical phenomenon at various scales. He examined regional variation down to prefecture level in cause of death through the demographic transition, from Meiji, Japan in 1899 to 1985. Among the factors he considered, using statistical analysis, trend surface, and mapping, were earned income, occupation, labor, animal protein and salt in diet, agricultural cropping and land use, temperature, patient–doctor ratios, migration, and socioeconomic factors of industrial structure, population structure, and lifestyle. He observed that through time, national diversity between urbanized and rural regions reflected on the dominant diseases in each prefecture: tuberculosis urbanized, gastroenteritis and cerebrovascular disease rural. Regional variation of cerebrovascular disease was described using trend surface as low in the southwestern plateau and high in the northeastern basins differentiated by lower winter temperatures, mountainous terrain, and later industrialization. Within the northeastern region, Yamagata Prefecture was analyzed by its regional divisions using multiregression analysis and factor analysis. The highest mortality was characterized at division level by rice cultivation as the major industry, labor migration to the cities in winter, insufficient medical service and underdeveloped infrastructure, deficiency of animal protein and fat, and high intake of salt from winter consumption of pickled vegetables. Kagami concludes that previous studies have considered only main factors of diseases and have given little attention to the regional character as a complex of various scales.

MENTAL ILLNESS

Mental illness is certainly not limited to industrialized societies. Various forms of it are common in isolated, pastoral, and rural areas. Because of rapid social change and urbanization, mental illness is common in developing countries. The fact that it is treated in traditional medical systems suggests that all societies are familiar with mental illness. The opposition in health studies between social and biomedical models is especially sharp and clear on the subject of mental illness. On one hand, it is clear that a biochemical disorder within the brain underlies most mental illnesses. Furthermore, there is a genetic component to some kinds of illness, clearly: when people diagnosed with schizophrenia have an identical twin, even reared apart under different conditions, more than half the time the twin has already been diagnosed, too. The biochemical approach results in new technologies, psychoactive drugs to treat schizophrenia, depression, and other serious illnesses. It has successfully put people back in their families, back at work, relieved of depression, and in control of manic–depression. Counterposed to this approach are numerous psychological models that draw on theories of individual behavior and how people adapt their behavior to their surroundings and others, efforts to determine normal and deviational in social context, and social models that are concerned with how society conceptualizes the individual and how labels are used for social control. In industrialized countries there are demographic and social processes that have hampered the ability of society to absorb and cope with affected individuals. The need to cope with technological society may, through stress, isolation, and lack of emotional support, itself induce certain forms of mental illness.

Many forms of mental illness seem to be organically based, perhaps resulting from genetics, alcoholism, syphilis, or senility. In what is possibly a momentous breakthrough, recent advances in genetics have identified genetic risk factors for late-onset Alzheimer's (the most common form). The gene for Apolipi-protein E (ApoE), which ferries cholesterol in the bloodstream, occurs in three known alleles. One gene for ApoE3 occurs in 90% of the population, and both genes in over 60%. Having two genes for a less common form, ApoE4, is associated with a risk of Alzheimer's eight times greater than for having no genes for that form. It is found almost universally in familial cases, and in two-thirds of sporadic cases. It binds to B-amyloid, a peptide found at high levels in the plaques that pervade Alzheimer's brains. It also binds to the tau proteins of the neurofibrillary tangles found in diseased brains. Although there may be little geographical input into causation of the disease, the impact of Alzheimer's on health service facilities and personnel and on economics is enormous, and so will be any breakthroughs in pharmaceutical treatment or public health prevention of it.

Some believe that alcoholism, suicide, and such social pathology as homicide are mental illnesses. Some mental illness has long been regarded as functional, meaning that the familial and social environment have had a role in its development. Even that illness may develop only in susceptible individuals. The forms of mental illness illustrate levels of health struggling under the barrage of new insults (Chapter 2). For example, McNeil says,

> The form and frequency of mental derangement has a host of correlations with other life circumstances and we cannot attribute causation exclusively to any one of these. . . . In this welter of discrete items related to psychosis must be

hidden a single overriding factor that can connect all the disparate parts into a meaningful whole. Being white, having a stable marriage, being gainfully employed, being educated, and being intelligent may all summate to a condition called security and freedom from anxiety. Having all these "advantages" may be the critical factor in determining how easily and successfully one copes with the tasks of living. The absence of any one of these conditions may diminish the human capacity to adjust. The absence of a great number of them may spell psychosis. (in Giggs, 1973, p. 71)

Studies of Mental Health

Social science studies of mental health are increasingly informed by social theory and concerned with higher political and economic structuring of causation than individual-level etiology. Geographers have made limited contributions to etiological studies of mental health. Most of these have related to urban spatial structure and its development and effects.

Schizophrenia is a common (in some estimates, it affects 1% of the population), chronic, serious psychosis that can produce lifelong invalidism. It usually strikes young people: 75% of schizophrenics have a first attack before age 25. There are problems with subdiagnosis, but it is one of the most replicable classifications of mental illness. There is strong seasonality of birth for individuals with schizophrenia (Chapter 5).

One of the classic ecological studies of schizophrenia related its incidence in Chicago to the then newly developed Burgess model of urban structure, which identified concentric rings of land use and development history (types of industry, residential density, business, decay, and transition, etc.). Faris and Dunham (1965) regionalized 120 sub communities of Chicago into 11 types of milieus. They related paranoid schizophrenia, for example, to patient origins in rooming house districts of the city. These stretched along the main transportation arterials and housed single, white-collar workers who commuted to the central business district. They noted the transient nature of the neighborhoods and suggested that the isolation and lack of communication might precipitate the psychosis.

Schizophrenia has been studied by Giggs (1973, 1983). He addressed the same questions of urban structure in Nottingham, England, using more contemporary methodology. He used factor analysis to determine 10 components of the city's ecological structure. One dimension, for example, he interpreted as "social and material resources," another as "urbanism/familism," and a third as "family life-cycle axis." Using Poisson probability, he tested the incidence of schizophrenia in 15 areas in Nottingham based on the ecological structure of the city. He demonstrated that the distribution of patient origins was very localized and that there were strong and statistically significant links between his characteristics of schizophrenic patients, such as age, sex, marital status, and birthplace, and the five leading components of the city's structure.

Smith (1977) addressed the neighborhood environment context of mental health. He and other geographers were concerned with the deinstitutionalization of mental patients, which started in the 1970s and spread quickly in the United States. They are particularly concerned about the location of community mental health facilities. Smith identified several relevant dimensions of neighborhood environments by studying the incidence of recidivism (return to the mental hospital) among deinstitutionalized patients.

Smith found a spatial dimension and landscape expression to community mental health. Landmarks and the layout or spatial design of a community provide orientation and facilitate a sense of identity. Facilities such as community centers, places for parties, churches, and libraries promote rootedness and provide means to transcend the daily conditions of life. People can be separated from noise, vehicular traffic, and pollution.

By considering such environmental characteristics, Smith thought he could identify how neighborhoods function as therapeutic communities. Living in commercial and industrial areas, characterized by high traffic and industrial buildings, was a good marker for recidivism. Being old and living alone, however, was not as reliably associated with recidivism. He suggested that neighborhoods that offer many patients a familiar setting and a place to be alone are therapeutic. Overall, it was easier to predict nonreturn on the basis of positive neighborhood characteristics than to predict return on the basis of negative ones. People seemed able to tune out what they did not want to see.

Depression is beginning to attract attention as a geographical subject (Moore, Rosenberg, & McGuinness, 1997). Social support and contacts for those living alone, for immigrants, for those of different classes and ethnicity and gender, all have expression in space and place. Loss of a spouse seems to have harsher consequences for men than women, who are thought to maintain more of their social supports and activities. As numbers of people living alone and single mothers and elderly people increase the need for home contact and institutional supports increases.

Neighborhood studies have moved into another dimension. Dear and others (Dear, Taylor, & Hall, 1980; Dear & Willis, 1980; Isaak, Taylor, & Dear, 1980) have investigated community attitudes toward mental health facilities and patients and the fit between community characteristics and type of facilities. He has developed methodology for investigating mental health service delivery and has connected medical geography to geographic studies on location of noxious facilities and on cognition and perception of environments. Dear and Wolch's (1987) and Wolch and Dear's (1993) work on deinstitutionalization of the mentally ill and community care, homelessness, and place has had a strong impact on mental health community. The historical context of the location of mental hospitals, changes in urban structure, aspects of the political economy of the deinstitutionalization of patients, and their drift to socially structured, service-dependent ghettoes are described in this chapter in the section "The Poverty Syndrome." The work of Dear and

Wolch has also connected medical geography with the movement in social science away from positivist epistemology and toward greater social phenomenology.

UNKNOWN ETIOLOGY AND OTHER QUESTIONS

A geographic perspective on a disease can result in discovering patterns of association. Developing etiological hypotheses for diseases of unknown cause is potentially a fruitful, but perilous, endeavor. Mayer (1981), for example, has focused attention on the dramatic geographic pattern of multiple sclerosis (MS). The disease has a latitudinal gradient from high northern rates to low southern ones in Europe and North America. Only Japan is anomalous, having very low rates even at high latitudes. The low incidence in Japan and among people of Asian descent in the United States suggests a lack of genetic susceptibility. Studies of population migration, which results in differential exposure to risks in separate places, provide some of the best analytic frameworks for addressing the etiology of MS (Williams, Jones, & McKeran, 1991).

The most obvious latitudinal environmental factor is solar radiation, but it may be spurious. Less obvious variations north to south in both Europe and North America include agricultural crops, development of industry, level of urbanization, and economic standards. Migration streams to Israel from MS high-rate areas of Europe and low-rate areas of Africa have been studied for MS incidence later in life. Childhood exposure to some unknown factor is important: Adults who migrate have the risk of their place of origin, whereas small children take on the risk of their destination. The new generation of native Israelis, surprisingly, has high MS rates despite low latitude, implying that some environmental conditions associated with industrialization and developed economies are important (Lowis, 1986). In the United States, however, California, though more industrial, has lower MS rates than Washington State. Migrants from the low-rate South and high-rate North to California and Washington have been studied. Children assume the high or low rates of their destination, as in the Israeli study. Adult migrants from the South to Washington have higher MS rates than in their birthplace but lower than for native Washingtonians. This implies that some protective factor may continue to shield the migrants in the presence of greater environmental hazard. In the absence of a U.S. registration system, however, it is difficult and expensive to get a large enough stream of migrants to be able to analyze rare diseases.

Rheumatic diseases, responsible for widespread suffering and loss of work time, have received little attention from geographers. Rheumatic diseases include degenerative conditions such as osteoarthritis, rheumatoid arthritis, spinal disk degeneration, gout, ankylosing spondylitis, and disease of the connective tissue, such as lupus. Etiological hypotheses in the general

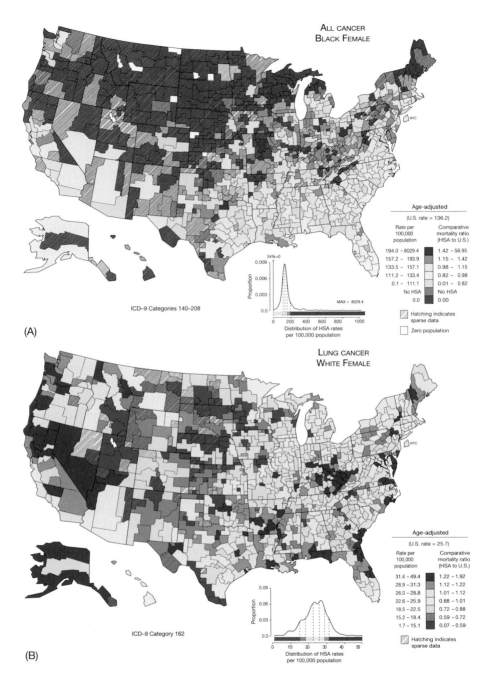

ALL CANCER
BLACK FEMALE

Age-adjusted

(U.S. rate = 136.2)

Rate per 100,000 population	Comparative mortality ratio (HSA to U.S.)
194.0 – 8029.4	1.42 – 58.95
157.2 – 193.9	1.15 – 1.42
133.5 – 157.1	0.98 – 1.15
111.2 – 133.4	0.82 – 0.98
0.1 – 111.1	0.01 – 0.82
No HSA	No HSA
0.0	0.00

Hatching indicates sparse data

Zero population

ICD–9 Categories 140–208

24%=0

Proportion

MAX = 8029.4

Distribution of HSA rates per 100,000 population

(A)

LUNG CANCER
WHITE FEMALE

Age-adjusted

(U.S. rate = 25.7)

Rate per 100,000 population	Comparative mortality ratio (HSA to U.S.)
31.4 – 49.4	1.22 – 1.92
28.9 – 31.3	1.12 – 1.22
26.0 – 28.8	1.01 – 1.12
22.6 – 25.9	0.88 – 1.01
18.5 – 22.5	0.72 – 0.88
15.2 – 18.4	0.59 – 0.72
1.7 – 15.1	0.07 – 0.59

Hatching indicates sparse data

ICD–9 Category 162

Proportion

Distribution of HSA rates per 100,000 population

(B)

PLATE 7-1. Selected causes of death, United States, 1988–1992, and selected measures for correlation. Mortality maps (A, B, C, D) are of age-adjusted rates by health service areas (HSAs). Graphs show the range and proportion, or frequency, of rates. Keys show the map mortality categories expressed both as rate per 100,000 population and as a comparative mortality ratio of HSA to the entire United States. Maps of variables for examination of correlation (E, F, G, H) are at two scales of analysis. (A) All cancer, black females. (B) Lung cancer, white females. (C) Heart disease, white males. (D) Stroke, black males. (E) Percentage of population below poverty level at county scale. (F) Percentage of population completing college education at county scale. (G) Percentage of population smoking tobacco at state scale. (H) Percentage of population leading sedentary lifestyle at state scale. From National Center for Health Statistics (1997).

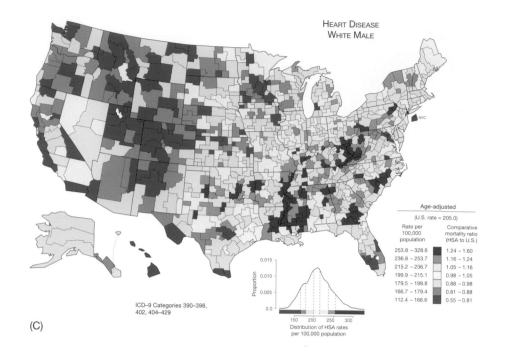

HEART DISEASE
WHITE MALE

Age-adjusted

(U.S. rate = 205.0)

Rate per 100,000 population	Comparative mortality ratio (HSA to U.S.)
253.8 – 328.6	1.24 – 1.60
236.8 – 253.7	1.16 – 1.24
215.2 – 236.7	1.05 – 1.16
199.9 – 215.1	0.98 – 1.05
179.5 – 199.8	0.88 – 0.98
166.7 – 179.4	0.81 – 0.88
112.4 – 166.6	0.55 – 0.81

ICD–9 Categories 390–398, 402, 404–429

Distribution of HSA rates per 100,000 population

(C)

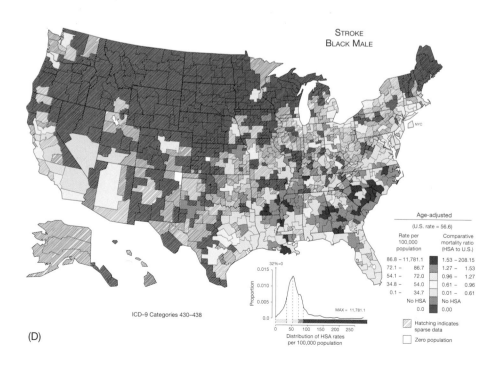

STROKE
BLACK MALE

Age-adjusted

(U.S. rate = 56.6)

Rate per 100,000 population	Comparative mortality ratio (HSA to U.S.)
86.8 – 11,781.1	1.53 – 208.15
72.1 – 86.7	1.27 – 1.53
54.1 – 72.0	0.96 – 1.27
34.8 – 54.0	0.61 – 0.96
0.1 – 34.7	0.01 – 0.61
No HSA	No HSA
0.0	0.00

Hatching indicates sparse data

Zero population

ICD–9 Categories 430–438

32%=0

MAX = 11,781.1

Distribution of HSA rates per 100,000 population

(D)

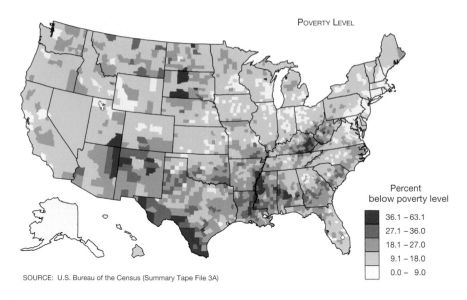

POVERTY LEVEL

Percent
below poverty level

■	36.1 – 63.1
	27.1 – 36.0
	18.1 – 27.0
	9.1 – 18.0
	0.0 – 9.0

SOURCE: U.S. Bureau of the Census (Summary Tape File 3A)

(E)

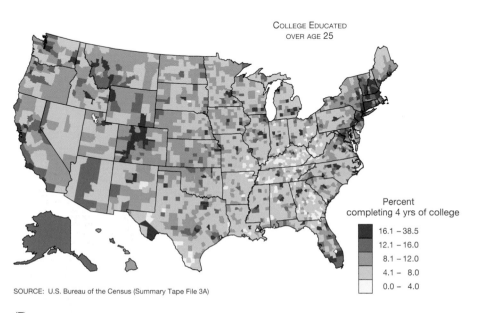

COLLEGE EDUCATED
OVER AGE 25

Percent
completing 4 yrs of college

■	16.1 – 38.5
	12.1 – 16.0
	8.1 – 12.0
	4.1 – 8.0
	0.0 – 4.0

SOURCE: U.S. Bureau of the Census (Summary Tape File 3A)

(F)

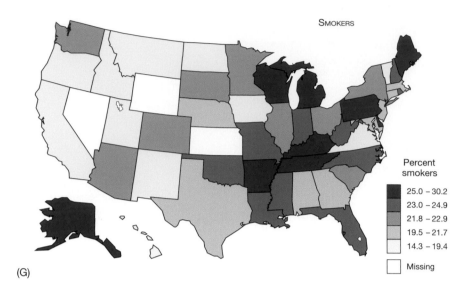

(G)

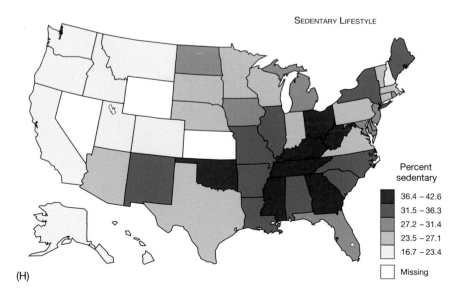

(H)

literature include the causal impact of wear and tear, calcium deficiency, metabolic deficiency in regulating blood uric acid levels, infectious agents, "bad" water, diet, occupation, and emotional stress. Genetic heritage has often been implicated, but the best designed studies have found the least evidence for familial clustering. The rheumatic diseases are notoriously difficult to confirm or detect in any repeatable manner, especially at subclinical levels. Even the blood serum test for rheumatoid factor (anti-gamma globulin) is know to flip capriciously across the arbitrary border that separates positive and negative results. It is often difficult to know what to look for without knowledge of etiology.

Another geographically neglected disease is Parkinson's disease (paralysis agitans), which affects millions of people, mostly over age 60. It is due to degeneration and death of cells in one region of the brain (substantia nigra). The dysfunction of these cells results in a loss of the dopamine they produce, resulting in blocked nerve impulses in the basal ganglia of the brain. Semiautomatic movements (such as movement of the tongue while speaking or swing of the arms while walking) become difficult, while involuntary movements (tremors) become common. Balance is disturbed, stiffness occurs, paralysis develops, and the disease progresses slowly but inexorably as regional brain cells continue to die. The reason those particular brain cells die is unknown. An accidental discovery showed that a toxin (MPTP), a by-product of the manufacture of illicit drugs, produces a Parkinsonism-like disease, even in young people (Lewin, 1984). Furthermore, MPTP can induce the symptoms in monkeys and so has created the first animal model for studying the disease and its treatment. This discovery strongly implies that exposure to one or more unknown environmental toxins may cause the disease.

Factors thought to be associated with increased risk of Parkinson's disease include aging, white race, male gender, trauma (as from boxing), shy personality, environmental exposures (to, variously, manganese, iron, drinking well water, farming, rural residence, herbicide and pesticides, wood pulp mills, steel alloy industry, and swine flu 1918 epidemic). There is a lot of confounding here from cohort experience. There was Parkinsonism long before there were chemical pesticides, and the 70- and 80-year-olds who have the disease now mostly grew up in a rural America. Familial inheritance as a risk factor affects only a small portion of those who develop the disease, especially the variety with early onset. Recent identification of a genetic marker has created a lot of excitement about development of new treatments, but that chromosome is involved only with the familial, and not the sporadic cases, which are more common. Treatment possibilities for Parkinsonism are advancing quickly. Not only are there new drugs being added to the current treatment, dopamine replacement, but there are also new types of brain surgery to eliminate some symptoms, as well as implantation of a variety of dopamine-producing cells from human fetuses and even xenografts from pigs. All these are being tested for long-term relief. None of this progress, however, has advanced knowledge of causation and prevention very much.

Incidence data for Parkinsonism are hard to get. In the early stages, it often is not diagnosed properly. As for its morbidity, it is reported less as a cause of death than it should be. It is a cause of death, but because it progresses slowly, mortality statistics are difficult because other causes of death commonly intervene first. Mainly because of the difficulty of getting any geographically based data on prevalence, there has been little geographic analysis of the spatial distribution and environmental circumstances of this serious disease.

CONCLUSION

This chapter has reviewed some of the geographic research on diseases of primary importance in the economically developed countries. As the mortality, fertility, and mobility transitions continue and the world's population urbanizes and ages, the etiology, prevention, and treatment of degenerative diseases is increasingly dominating world health concerns.

The spatial patterns, causal relationships, and time and scale parameters of these diseases are complex matters. If hypotheses are to have value, the geographic researcher needs to understand the disease processes as founded in the population's biology and its interaction with habitat and behavior. The complexities of spatial pattern and disease etiology demand competence in statistics and demography. On this foundation rests the ability to project population health needs, as distinct from economic demand, and to plan for the delivery of appropriate health services.

REFERENCES

Ames, B. N. (1983). Dietary carcinogens and anticarcinogens. *Science, 221,* 1256–1264.

Armstrong, R. W. (1971). Medical geography and its geologic substrate. *Geological Society of America Memoir, 123,* 211–219.

Armstrong, R. W. (1976). The geography of specific environments of patients and non-patients in cancer studies, with a Malaysian example. *Economic Geography, 52,* 161–170.

Armstrong, R. W. (1978). Self-specific environments associated with naso-pharyngeal carcinoma in Selangor, Malaysia. *Social Science and Medicine, 12D,* 149–156.

Brenner, M. H., & Mooney, A. (1982). Economic change and sex-specific cardiovascular mortality in Britain 1955–76. *Social Science and Medicine, 16,* 431–442.

Calabrese, E. J. (1985). *Sex differences in response to toxic substances.* New York: Wiley.

Chesney, M. A., & Rosenman, R. H. (Eds.). (1985). *Anger and hostility in cardiovascular and behavioral disorders.* Washington: Hemisphere.

Comstock, G. W. (1979). The association of water hardness and cardiovascular disease: An epidemiological review and critique. In U.S. National Committee for Geochemistry, *Geochemistry of water in relation to cardiovascular disease* (pp. 46–68). Washington, DC: National Academy of Sciences.

Corin, E. (1994). The social and cultural matrix of health and disease. In R. G. Evans,

M. L. Barer, & T. R. Marmor (Eds.), *Why are some people healthy and others not?* New York: Aldine de Gruyter.

Dear, M., Taylor, S. M., & Hall, G. G. (1980). Attitudes toward the mentally ill and reactions to mental health facilities. *Social Science and Medicine, 14D,* 281–290.

Dear, M., & Willis, T. (1980). The geography of community mental health care. In M. S. Meade (Ed.), *Conceptual and methodological issues in medical geography* (pp. 263–281). Chapel Hill: University of North Carolina, Department of Geography.

Dear, M. J., & Wolch, J. (1987). *Landscapes of despair: From deinstitutionalization to homelessness.* Princeton, NJ: Princeton University Press.

Doyal, L. (1995). *What makes women sick? Gender and the political economy of health.* New Brunswick, NJ: Rutgers University Press.

Editorial Committee for the Atlas of Cancer Mortality in the People's Republic of China. (1979). *Atlas of cancer mortality in the People's Republic of China.* Shanghai: China Map Press.

Evans, R. G., Barer, M. L., & Marmor, T. R. (1994). *Why are some people healthy and others not?* New York: Aldine de Gruyter.

Fang, J., Madhavan, S., & Alderman, M. H. (1996). The association between birthplace and mortality from cardiovascular causes among black and white residents of New York City. *New England Journal of Medicine, 335,* 1545–1551.

Faris, R. E. L., & Dunham, H. W. (1965). *Mental disorders in urban areas: An ecological study of schizophrenia and other psychoses.* Chicago: University of Chicago Press.

Gardner, M. (1976). Soft water and heart disease. In J. Leniham & W. W. Fletcher (Eds.), *Health and the environment* (pp. 116–135). New York: Academic Press.

Geronimus, A. T., Bound, J., Waidmann, T. A., Hillemeier, M. M., & Burns, P. B. (1996). Excess mortality among blacks and whites in the United States. *New England Journal of Medicine, 335,* 1552–1558.

Giggs, J. A. (1973). The distribution of schizophrenics in Nottingham. *Transactions of the Institute of British Geographers, 59,* 55–76.

Giggs, J. A. (1983). Schizophrenia and ecological structure in Nottingham. In N. D. McGlashan & J. R. Blunden (Eds.), *Geographical aspects of health* (pp. 197–222). London: Academic Press.

Gillum, R. F. (1996). The epidemiology of cardiovascular disease in black Americans [editorial]. *New England Journal of Medicine, 335,* 1597–1599.

Glick, B. J. (1979a). Distance relationships in theoretical models of carcinogenesis. *Social Science and Medicine, 13D,* 253–256.

Glick, B. J. (1979b). The spatial autocorrelation of cancer mortality. *Social Science and Medicine, 13D,* 123–130.

Glick, B. J. (1980). The geographic analysis of cancer occurrence: Past progress and future directions. In M. S. Meade (Ed.), *Conceptual and methodological issues in medical geography* (pp. 170–193). Chapel Hill: University of North Carolina, Department of Geography.

Glick, B. J. (1982). The spatial organization of cancer mortality. *Annals of the Association of American Geographers, 72,* 471–481.

Greenberg, M. R. (1980). A method to separate the geographical components of temporal change in cancer mortality rates. *Carcinogenesis, 1,* 553–557.

Greenberg, M. R. (1983b). *Urbanization and cancer mortality: The United States experience, 1950–1975.* New York: Oxford University Press.

Greenberg, M. R. (1989). Black male cancer and American urban health policy. *Journal of Urban Affairs, 11,* 113–130.

Haac, L. (1995). DNA repair: Mapping cancer's origins. *Cancer Lines 6*, 1–4.

Hanchette, C. L. (1998). *The geographic modeling of lead poisoning risk in North Carolina.* Unpublished doctoral dissertation, Department of Geography, University of North Carolina at Chapel Hill.

Hanchette, C. L., & Schwartz, G. G. (1992). Geographic patterns of prostate cancer mortality. *Cancer, 70,* 2861–2869.

Harpham, T., Lusty, T., & Vaughan, P. (Eds). (1988). *In the shadow of the city. Community health and the urban poor.* New York: Oxford University Press.

Howe, G. M. (1972). *Man, environment, and disease in Britain.* New York: Barnes & Noble.

Howe, G. M. (1981). Mortality from selected malignant neoplasms in the British Isles: The spatial perspective. *Social Science and Medicine, 15D,* 199–211.

Isaak, S., Taylor, M., & Dear, M. (1980). Community mental health facilities in residential neighbourhoods. In F. A. Barrett (Ed.), *Canadian studies in medical geography* (pp. 231–256). Downsview, Ontario, Canada: York University, Department of Geography.

Jones, K. & Moon, G. (1987). *Health, Disease and Society: An Introduction to Medical Geography.* London: Routledge.

Kagami, M. (1991). A geographical study on regional variations of disease mortality. *Science Report Institute of Geoscience, University Tsukuba, 12*(sect. A), 65–89.

King, P. E. (1979). Problems of spatial analysis in geographical epidemiology. *Social Science and Medicine, 13D,* 249–252.

Koblinsky, M., Timyan, J., & Gay, J. (Eds.). (1993). *The health of women in global perspective.* Boulder, CO: Westview Press.

Lenfant, C. (1996). Conference on socioeconomic status and cardiovascular health and disease. *Circulation, 94,* 2041–2044.

Lewin, R. (1984). Trail of ironies to Parkinson's disease, *Science, 224,* 1083–1085.

Lilienfeld, A. M., & Lilienfeld, D. E. (1980). *Foundations of epidemiology* (2nd ed.). New York: Oxford University Press.

Lowis, G. W. (1986). Sociocultural and demographic factors in the epidemiology of multiple sclerosis: An annotated selected bibliography. *International Journal of Environmental Studies, 26,* 295–320.

Marmot, M. G., & Mustard, J. F. (1994). Coronary heart disease from a population perspective. In R. G. Evans, M. L. Barer, & T. R. Marmor (Eds.), *Why are some people healthy and others not?* (pp. 189–214). New York: Aldine de Gruyter.

Marmot, M. G. and Theorell, T. (1988). Social class and cardiovascular disease: the contribution of work. *International Journal of Health Services, 18,* 659–674.

Mason, T. J., McKay, F. W., Hoover, R., Blot, W. J., & Fraumeni, J. F., Jr. (1975). *Atlas of cancer mortality for U.S. counties: 1950–1969.* Washington, DC: U.S. Department of Health, Education, and Welfare, Epidemiology Branch, National Cancer Institute.

Mason, T. J., McKay, F. W., Hoover, R., Blot, W. J., & Fraumeni, J. F., Jr. (1976). *Atlas of cancer mortality among U.S. nonwhites: 1950–69.* Washington, DC: U.S. Department of Health, Education, and Welfare, Epidemiology Branch, National Cancer Institute.

Mayer, J. D. (1981). Problems of spatial analysis in geographical epidemiology. *Social Science and Medicine, 13D,* 249–252.

McGlashan, N. D. (1972). Food contaminants and oesophageal cancer. In N. D. Mc-

Glashan (Ed.), *Medical geography: Techniques and field studies* (pp. 247–257). London: Methuen.

Meade, M. S. (1979) Cardiovascular mortality in the southeastern United States: The Coastal Plain enigma," *Social Science and Medicine, 13D,* 257–265.

Meade, M. S. (1980). An interactive framework for geochemistry and cardiovascular disease. In M. S. Meade (Ed.), *Conceptual and methodological issues in medical geography* (pp. 194–221). Chapel Hill: University of North Carolina, Department of Geography.

Meade, M. S. (1983). Cardiovascular disease in Savannah, Georgia. In N. D. McGlashan & J. R. Bluden (Eds.), *Geographical aspects of health* (pp. 175–196). London: Academic Press.

Minowa, M., Shigematsu, I., Nagai, M., & Fukutomi, K. (1981). Geographical distribution of lung cancer mortality and environmental factors in Japan. *Social Science and Medicine, 15D,* 225–231.

Moore, E. G., Rosenberg, M. W., & McGuinness, D. L. (1997). *Growing old in Canada: Demographic and geographic perspectives* [Census Analytic Monograph]. Ottawa: Statistics Canada and Nelson.

National Center for Health Statistics. (1997). *Atlas of United States mortality.* Washington, DC: U.S. Government Printing Office.

National Center for Health Statistics. (1998). Table 8: Deaths and death rates for the 10 leading causes of death in specified age groups, by race and sex: United States, 1996. *National Vital Statistics Report, 47,* 26–36.

Ohno, Y., & Aoki, K. (1981). Cancer death by city and county in Japan, 1969–1971: A test of significance for geographical clusters of disease. *Social Science and Medicine, 15D,* 251–258.

Schroeder, H. A. (1966). Municipal drinking water and cardiovascular death rates. *Journal of the American Medical Association, 195,* 81–85.

Smith, C. J. (1977). *Geography and mental health.* Washington, DC: Association of American Geographers.

Takahashi, E. (1981). Geographic distribution of cerebrovascular disease and environmental factors in Japan. *Social Science and Medicine, 15D,* 153–172.

Thouez, J. P., Beauchamp, Y., & Simard, A. (1981). Cancer and the physicochemical quality of drinking water in Quebec. *Social Science and Medicine, 15D,* 213–223.

Travis, J. (1993). New piece in Alzheimer's puzzle. *Science, 261,* 828–829.

U.S. Environmental Protection Agency. (1987). *The United States cancer mortality rates and trends 1950–1979: Vol. 4. Atlas.* Washington, DC: U.S. Government Printing Office.

Wallace, R., Huang, Y. -S., Gould, P., & Wallace, D. (1997). The hierarchical diffusion of AIDS and violent crime among U.S. metropolitan regions: Inner-city decay, stochastic resonance and reversal of the mortality transition. *Social Science and Medicine, 44,* 935–947.

West, R. R. (1977). Geographic variation in mortality from ischaemic heart disease in England and Wales. *British Journal of Preventive and Social Medicine, 31,* 245–250.

West, R. R., & Lowe, C. R. (1976). Mortality from ischaemic heart disease—Inter-town variation and its association with climate in England and Wales. *International Journal of Epidemiology, 5,* 195–201.

Williams, E. D., Jones, D. R., & McKeran, R. O. (1991). Mortality rates from multiple sclerosis: geographical and temporal variations revisisited. *Journal Neurology, Neurosurgery & Psychiatry, 54,* 104–109.

Wolch, J., & Dear, M. (1993). *Malign neglect: Homelessness in an American city.* San Francisco: Jossey-Bass.

World Health Organization. (1999). *The world health report 1999.* Geneva: Author.

Ziegenfus, R. C., & Gesler, W. M. (1984). Geographical patterns of heart disease in the northeastern United States. *Social Science and Medicine, 18,* 63–72.

Ziegler, R. G., Hoover, R. N., Pike, M. C., Hildesheim, A., Nomura, A. M. Y., West, D. W., Wu-Williams, A. H., Kolonel, L. N., Horn-Ross, P. L., Rosenthal, J. F., & Hyer, M. B. (1993). Migration patterns and breast cancer risk in Asian-American women. *Journal of the National Cancer Institute, 85,* 1819–1827.

FURTHER READING

Anderson, R. (1984). Temporal trends of cancer mortality in eastern New England compared to the nation, 1950–1975. *Social Science and Medicine, 19,* 749–757.

Andrews, H. F. (1985). The ecology of risk and the geography of intervention: From research to practice for the health and well-being of urban children. *Annals of the Association of American Geographers, 75,* 370–382.

Burbank, F. (1972). A sequential space-time cluster analysis of cancer mortality in the United States: Etiological implications. *American Journal of Epidemiology, 95,* 393–417.

Cleek, R. K. (1979). Cancer and the environment: The effect of scale. *Social Science and Medicine, 13D,* 241–247.

Eyles, J. & Woods, K. J. (Eds.). (1983). *The social geography of medicine and health.* New York: St. Martin's Press.

Gardner, M. J., Winter, P. D., & Acheson, E. D. (1982). Variations in cancer mortality areas in England and Wales: Relation with environmental factors and search for cause. *British Medical Journal, 284,* 284–287.

Greenberg, M. R. (1983a). Environmental toxicology in the United States. In N. D. McGlashan & J. R. Blunden (Eds.), *Geographical aspects of health* (pp. 157–174). London: Academic Press.

Howe, G. M., Burgess, L., & Gatenby, P. (1977). Cardiovascular disease. In G. M. Howe (Ed.), *A world geography of human diseases* (pp. 431–476). London: Academic Press.

Isaak, S., Taylor, M., & Dear, M. (1980). Community mental health facilities in residential neighbourhoods. In F. A. Barrett (Ed.), *Canadian studies in medical geography* (pp. 231–256). Downsview, Ontario, Canada: York University, Department of Geography.

Lewis, N. (1998). Intellectual intersection: Gender and health in the Pacific. *Social Science and Medicine, 46,* 641–659.

Lux, W. E., & Kurtzke, J. F. (1987). Is Parkinson's disease acquired? Evidence from a geographic comparison with multiple sclerosis. *Neurology, 37,* 467–471.

McLafferty, S., & Tempalski, B. (1995). Restructuring and women's reproductive health: implications for low birthweight in New York City. *Geoforum, 26,* 309–323.

Momsen, J. (1991). *Women and development in the Third World.* New York: Routledge.

Pyle, G. F. (1971). *Heart disease, cancer, and stroke in Chicago* (Research Paper No. 134). Chicago: University of Chicago, Department of Geography.

Pyle, G. F. (1979). *Applied medical geography.* New York: Wiley.

Robinson, V. B. (1978). Modeling spatial variations in heart disease mortality: Implications of the variable subset selection process. *Social Science and Medicine, 12D,* 165–172.

Shigematsu, I. (1981). *National atlas of major disease mortality in Japan.* Tokyo: Japan Health Promotion Foundation.

Waterhouse, J., Correa, P., Muir, C., & Powell, J. (Eds.). (1976). Cancer incidence in five continents. Lyon, France: International Agency for Research on Cancer.

Weinstein, M. S. (1980). *Health in the city: environmental and behavioral influences.* New York: Pergamon Press.

VIGNETTE 7-1.   Women's Health

Women's health has become a focus of interest because in the past it was buried in the totality of health and disease, so that little was learned about it. Sometimes men's health was considered synonymous with human health: Clinical trials of the efficacy of pharmaceutical drugs were conducted only on men but assumed valid for all. Sometimes studies of causation, prevention, and treatment of a major disease, such as heart disease, were focused on men because they had higher rates of that disease and the economy suffered great loss. Although such studies were cost-effective and the results clearer and stronger precisely because the variability and confounding posed by including women's differences were avoided, nevertheless the results were considered applicable to the general population across all differences. Women are both the same and different than other people: Differentials in health or treatment of disease are not simply due to money, power, and social construction of interpretation. Examples involving women's health have been used throughout this text, from ascaris to AIDS. This vignette focuses on how the concepts and approaches of this text are all relevant to women through the integrative framework of the triangle of health ecology (Figure 2-2), with its three vertices of interactions among population, habitat, and behavior.

POPULATION

Gender, genetics, and age are felted and printed with immunological and nutritional status. The genetics of being female results in a few gender-specific diseases, especially those of the sexual organs. Female hormones are genetically given, of course, as well as the elaborately orchestrated capacity for pregnancy and lactation. Several genetic conditions are gender-linked at the chromosome level. For example, genes that cause a serious condition, hemophilia, and those that cause a mild condition, color blindness, both occur predominantly in males because their short chromosome contains no countergene to repress such recessive characteristics when they are carried on the female chromosome. The full luxuriance of the felt, however, is pressed through the life cycle.

The sex ratio of humans at birth is about 105 males for every 100 females. This ratio is assumed to be an evolutionary adaptation reflecting the fact that from fetus to centenarian, males die at a higher rate than females (Vignette 7-1, Table 1). This very statement, however, is an expression of the world view of economically developed countries. Historically, women died at high rates from the rigors and cumulative risks of pregnancy and childbirth, and it has been the recent reduction of fertility which has most spared their lives. When, as in India and China, young girls die at a higher rate than boys, it is usually taken as prima

VIGNETTE 7-1, TABLE 1. Gender Differences in Death Probability

	Probability of dying <5 (per 1,000 births), 1998		Maternal mortality ratio (maternal deaths/ 100,000 live births), 1990
	Males	Females	
More developed countries			
Russian Federation	25	19	75
Canada	8	6	6
Germany	7	6	22
Japan	6	5	18
Less developed countries			
India	82	97	570
Indonesia	69	56	650
China	43	54	95
Thailand	37	33	200
Haiti	112	97	1,000
Brazil	51	41	220
Mexico	41	34	110
Cuba			
Mali	244	227	1,200
Ethiopia	193	174	1,400
Kenya	107	101	650
Egypt	65	64	170

Note. Data from World Health Organization (1999).

facie evidence of severe discrimination in nourishment, nurturance, and care, which on occasion even results in female infanticide.

Between menarche and menopause, women are biologically vulnerable to a range of insults associated with their reproductive role. These include such things as infection of the urinary (kidney) tract, scarring, and infertility resulting from sexually transmitted disease, and nutritional shortages of iron, vitamin A, calcium, and so on (Koblinsky, Timyan, & Gay, 1993). Besides blood lost to menstruation, malaria and intestinal parasites, nutritional deficiencies are made worse by pregnancy, and greatly depleted by multiple ones. More than half the pregnant women in tropical Africa and Asia are anemic (which in addition to the usual energy and health complications can result in oxygen crisis for mother and child at birth). Advanced vitamin A deficiency is usually monitored as xerophthalmia, but depleted by recurrent pregnancy, lower levels of deficiency pass unnoticed while they damage the immune system. In developed countries, despite good nutrition and prenatal care, most embryos do not survive to become fetuses. Nevertheless, in the developing world, crude and septic induced abortions are a significant cause of maternal mortality for women without means of birth control. The high rates of maternal mortality evident in Vignette 7-1, Table 1 the general association with infant mortality that reflects nutritional stress, disease, complications of pregnancy, and lack of medical care. They also are reminders of the large number of children rendered motherless by the lack of birth control.

Cyclic exposure to estrogen seems to affect cholesterol metabolism and act protectively against heart disease. On the other hand, cumulative estrogen exposure is one of the clearest insults increasing the risk of breast cancer. Hormonal fluctuation can affect mental health, especially postpartum depression, and be a risk factor for suicide.

In the developed world, more than two-fifths of a woman's life is lived after menopause. Fertility rates of fewer than two children per couple also mean that most of a woman's life is not engaged in reproduction. Medicine and health research in general has been so preoccupied with women's reproductive processes, reproductive organs, and their infections and diseases that little has been learned about the health of women. Even clinical trials of drugs were carried out only on men, because of the expressed fear that a fetus might be harmed (some would say a construction of the value of a woman's life). It has recently been learned that women's hearts, women's bones and calcium metabolism, and women's patterns of fat deposition are different from men's, and that so are the effects of relevant drugs. Several large longitudinal studies, such as the Nurses' Study and the Women's Health Initiative, are currently under way to research the effects of estrogen supplementation, calcium supplementation, various exercise regimes and diets, and common drugs such as aspirin, on women.

There are notable interactions of population with habitat and behavior. Customs about the seclusion of women and definitions of modesty affect diffusion of contagion, exposure to vectored disease, and even biometeorological influences: Rickets in Saudi Arabia, for example, is purely a cultural artifact of purdah. Cultural beliefs determine at what age marriage is suitable, and such things as the degree of inbreeding to cousins or outbreeding to other ethnic groups is tolerated. Values about desired family size, use of contraception, provision of medical services, accessibility of education to girls, job opportunities, and status/financial contribution from outside the home for women have all changed enormously, as expressed at the 1994 International Population and Development Conference in Cairo. Increases in income, trade, and agricultural production as well as the technology of food preservation, storage, shipment and marketing have changed nutrition enormously. One consequence in the developed world of continually abundant, high-protein and fatty food has been the lowering of the age of menarche. It used to be 16 or more rather universally, but now in places it occurs at 11 and younger, with consequences for reproductive behavior and attendant risks even as age of marriage has been culturally raised to more than 20 in much of the world. Probably the most notorious cultural control on nutrition is the widespread custom of husband eating first and then children. When at last the woman eats the leftovers, the most nutritious foods are gone and adequate calories may not remain. In the developing world, when mother's milk is changed to a bottled substitute, baby's antibodies to disease and exposure to diarrheal agents also may change. On the other side of the world, more open advertisement about new products for menstruation created and spread a new toxic shock syndrome almost overnight.

HABITAT

The natural, built, and social components of human habitat affect women's health in ways already described for people and yet somewhat differently than men's. Of course, this is the least studied and understood aspect. There is different exposure to insults because of different roles. In the Malaysian land development impact on disease ecology, for example (Vignette 3-2), women were exposed to scrub typhus from rat mites on settlement pathways, whereas men were out tending their tree crops before dawn, when *Anopheles* mosquitoes were still biting. Mobility, jobs, and relationships are among the behavioral components which structure the exposure to habitat conditions.

Radon and other radiation occur naturally in many environments but may be a greater hazard for a fetus. Women suffer more from hay fever and chronic sinusitis (see Vignette 7-1, Table 2) from natural allergens. The chlorinated hydrocarbons and polychlorinated biphenyls distributed in the environment have an affinity for storage in fatty tissue, which puts women's bodily deposits, especially breast tissue, especially at risk (Calabrese, 1985).

The greatest risk factor of the built environment for women is simply that generally they spend so much time at home. The exposure to ascaris and other infectious agents of children is predominantly at home. Whatever the insults from cleaning agents, formaldehyde, or household allergens, they especially affect women. To the extent that women have different types of factory or office jobs than men, the insults of the workplace environment would also differ, but this has been little studied. The built environment includes the presence or absence of such facilities as health clinics and family planning centers, day-care facilities, schools, nursing homes, and hospitals.

The most obvious habitat differences for women are social: Activity spaces, mobility patterns, isolation, or social contact mediate exposures to such things as air pollution, cigarette smoke, motor vehicle accidents, contagious disease, fresh air, and social support or stimulation, to name a few.

VIGNETTE 7-1, TABLE 2. U.S. Reported Chronic Conditions, 1994

Condition	Per 1,000 ages 45–65		
	Female	Male	F/M
Arthritis	297.0	176.5	1.7
Chronic sinusitis	210.2	147.5	1.4
Hay fever	133.4	107.3	1.2
Heart disease	111.0	162.0	0.7
Chronic bronchitis	82.7	43.8	1.9
Back impairment	109.6	94.5	1.2
Hearing impairment	87.5	191.9	0.5

Note. Data from Centers for Disease Control and Prevention (*www.nytimes.com/specials/women/data/chronic.htm*).

BEHAVIOR

The most complex and yet clearest interactions for women's health fall in the behavior vertex of beliefs, social organization, and technology. Indeed, most of the approaches to health promotion informed by social theory focus on this vertex alone (Koblinsky et al., 1993; Doyal, 1995). The multiple social roles of women—child nurturer, caregiver, homemaker, wage earner, career professional, community organizer, lifelong learner—lie here. Should the woman do the infant's toiletry (and get worms), tend the child's fever (and catch it), deal emotionally with the elder's deterioration and needs, and wash the cadaver (and get cholera)? Has the woman any control over whether to have five children or two or none? Must she cope with full-time job demands, whether law clerking or gutting chickens on a conveyor, as well as the domestic chores and parenting and connubial relationship? What are these relationships and duties, and how are they determined and by whom anyway?

Cultures have strong belief systems about everything from what foods are taboo for pregnant women to how thin or plump women should be; from what sick role is allowed women to what home remedies mothers should use; from what exercise is appropriate for women to how much domestic violence must be tolerated. Should menstruating women be shut away in separate buildings? Should postpartum women be "roasted" daily in overheated rooms, as is done in some places, to reduce the womb? Should female genitals be mutilated so husbands can know their spouses will be pure and uninterested in sex? Should women burn themselves alive on their husband's funeral pyre, or are widows allowed to remarry, if only to be able to care for their children? Is it appropriate for women to expose themselves to the sun? Is it appropriate for them to smoke cigarettes? The behaviors that result from such cultural beliefs have fundamental implications for health. As can be seen from Vignette 7-1, Table 3, the beliefs can sometimes, perhaps unexpectedly, be strong cultural buffers against harm.

Social organization that affects women's health can be as personal as customs of polygamy or monogamy sanctioned by religious systems, or as bureaucratic as welfare aid to homeless women with dependent children. Broad social structure and institutions affect women's health: child-care services; programs of higher education and of job training; and programs for health care, vaccination, life enrichment for senior centers, nursing home pet visitation. Legal structures—work laws, minimum wage, safety regulations, antidiscrimination and affirmative action laws—channel health effects. There is a lifetime of social science research to be done in political economy about such relations.

The complexities of interaction even within just this behavioral vertex are inscrutable when the context of major concerns, such as mental health, is addressed. Consider simply the dimension of substance abuse. Women have the same range of alcohol metabolisms that men do, although their generally lower body weight gives them generally less capacity for absorption. Under the influence of alcohol, women are especially susceptible to rape and to physical abuse.

VIGNETTE 7-1, TABLE 3. 1998 Deaths Attributed to Tobacco

	Female (000)	Male (000)	F/M
All member states[a]	782	3241	0.24
Africa	13	112	0.12
Eastern Mediterranean	22	160	0.14
Low- and middle-income Americas	38	130	0.29
Low- and middle-income Europe	94	641	0.15
Low- and middle-income Southeast Asia	.24	173	0.14
Low- and middle-income West Pacific	8	56	0.14
India	51	332	0.15
China	130	783	0.17
High-income Americas	262	342	0.77
High-income Europe	113	425	0.27
High-income Pacific	28	88	0.32

Note. Data from Statistical Annex, World Health Organization (1999).
[a]Regions are those of the World Health Organization.

Women tend to drink for different reasons than men do, for different emotional needs, and to escape different problems. More important, they generally drink alone—probably because society has in the past thought women drinking alcohol at all to be unacceptable, let alone in public. Because they are not social drinkers, they are hidden drinkers. They are less prone to drunk driving manslaughter, and they are less subject to social intervention or the concern of others. Programs such as Alcoholics Anonymous are specialized on the needs of men, focused on the reasons they drink, occasionally even thick in some of the abusive attitudes that led to the women drinking. Government programs for women are seldom available at all.

Technology can involve the full workplace panoply of computers and chemicals; or it can involve the labor-saving gadgets and chemical innovation of home place. Medical technology, however, is of special importance. The removal of birth from home to hospital and development of intensive care for premature infants has greatly reduced mortality and transformed the birthing experience. The development of infant formulas to substitute for mothers' milk has removed the mortal crisis of inadequate lactation, has freed infant care from the sole proprietorship of a mother, and has transformed the experience of bonding, as well as that of work. Such formulas, aggressively promoted for profit, have also resulted in infant death from diarrhea and malnutrition where the human resources of adequate money, potable water, fuel, and cleanliness did not comport with safe usage.

Thinking about women in the developing world stirred by the changes described in Chapter 4, and more, it is easy to imagine many cultural ecologies of health emerging. Rural-urban migration can mean the shift from contaminated village wells, malarious mosquitoes, inadequate food, no income opportunity, illiteracy, extended families, and life-threatening pregnancy to safe drinking water, few vectors, good food, vaccination and basic health care, dwelling in plastic hovels in a tidal swamp, and work in a garment sweatshop or years of sexual slavery—to suggest just one possibility of contrasting ecologies. What scenarios might be promoted by the empowerment of women to claim education, reproductive health care, small loans, job and other opportunities envisioned in the International Women's Conference in Beijing 1995? Realizing the low fertility ending the demographic transition and living in an economically developed country which recognizes that women have human rights does not, however, mean the disappearance of health differences between men and women.

Heart disease continues to be a greater cause of both mortality and morbidity among men than women, but after menopause it becomes the major cause of death and the most common life-threatening morbidity for women. Differences among the races in stroke, breast cancer, diabetes, and other causes of mortality suggest anything but gender unity (Vignette 7-1, Table 4). Native Hawaiians have the highest mortality rate for breast cancer (37.2/100,000). The first generation of immigrants from Japan had the low rates of Asia, but succeeding generations have gone up. Asian-American women have the highest suicide rates under 24 and over 65. they are particularly at risk for osteoporosis because of relatively low bone density, small frames, and lower early calcium intake (nondairy culture) Diabetes is 60% more frequent among African American women than among white women. Obesity, intrinsic (i.e., not understood) high blood pressure, and stroke are higher. Maternal mortality is more than four times as likely among African American women than among whites, even among college-educated women with health insurance. HIV/AIDS disproportionately affects African Americans and is a leading cause of death for women under 45. Within-gender (group) differences raise the same questions about poverty, status, culture, and biology discussed in Chapter 7 more generally.

As Vignette 7-1, Table 2 illustrates, a wide variety of differences continue between the health status of men and women. What component of the differences

VIGNETTE 7-1, TABLE 4. Leading Causes of Death: United States, 1990–1994

| | Death rate per 100,000 | | | | | |
| | Total population | | Whites 15–64 | | Blacks 15–64 | |
Cause	Female	Male	Female	Male	Female	Male
Heart attack	226.8	259.4	35.6	110.2	61.9	118.2
Stroke	84.2	59.0	13.1	15.6	35.3	46.6
Lung cancer	51.5	^95.4	33.1	56.2	31.9	81.6
Breast cancer	41.9	1.3	33.6	1.2	42.2	1.3
Diabetes mellitus			9.5	11.8	25.5	26.2
Transportation accidents			18.5	49.1	16.8	57.6

Note. Data from Centers for Disease Control and Prevention (*www.nytimes.com/specials/women/data/90-94.htm*).

in arthritis is due to different experience of occupation and what to hormones or diet? Is men's greater hearing impairment due to occupational hazard, or to cultural behavior regarding music, guns, or power motors? What could be the cultural ecology of more feminine hay fever, sinusitis, and bronchitis? Or are these differences all due to women crying to the medical system at the least sniffle while men endure in silent agony?

8

Disease Diffusion in Space

There are only two ways in which anything, whether it be an idea, a type of tree, a sophisticated new plan for financing hospital care, or an infectious agent of disease, can come to be found in a particular location. Either it developed there independently or it somehow moved there from another place. Movement is by far the most usual explanation of the existence of phenomena at a particular location. An understanding of the mechanisms that influence the spread of any phenomenon and its spatial pattern is at the core of the geographic study of diffusion.

The term "diffusion" implies a spread or movement outward from a point or beginning place. Diffusion research by medical geographers can be divided into two basic categories. Some studies focus on the spread of medical innovations within a health care delivery system. Examples of such research are investigations of the diffusion of tomography scanners in the United States (Baker, 1979) or abortion facilities in the northeastern United States (Henry, 1978), wherein the central concern has been the development and spread of new ideas and goods. More common, however, are studies of the diffusion of infectious diseases, especially nonvectored infectious diseases. In these studies many of the conceptual and methodological concerns of epidemiology and geography have been combined. Geographers, however, want to know not only how a disease spreads in a population but how that spread occurs over space; not only how many cases might occur at a future point in time but *where* those cases are likely to occur.

Western civilization has long had a general recognition of the existence and importance of diseases diffusion. Disease quarantine, which could involve an individual, a household, or even an entire community or country, at least tacitly implies the existence of *disease diffusion*. Indeed the term comes from the medieval port city of Raguna when, in 1377, it tried to seclude incoming vessels for 40 days in an effort to prevent importation of plague. In the United States, Noah Webster's *A Brief History of Epidemic and Pestilential*

Diseases traces the spread of several late 1700s epidemics across New England (Webster, 1799). At about that same time William Currie was also describing the geography of a number of epidemics in the United States (Currie, 1792, 1811). The contagionists investigating the distribution of yellow fever in the early 1800s recognized that the disease was carried from place to place, spread by an infected individual. Although we might find their medical explanations of causation amusing, the quality of their geographic descriptions were, given the severe data limitations, excellent.

Most studies of geographic diffusion have emphasized an explanation of events in a space–time context. The extent and form of human intercourse are critical for both innovation and diffusion. Variables such as distance, the locations of settlements, and the distribution of jobs and facilities all influence the level and direction of interaction. Diffusion is patterned by the configuration of the networks that encourage movement and barriers that discourage it. A major prerequisite of disease diffusion, for example, is the existence of a sufficiently large susceptible population. A sufficiently large immune population, or, more precisely, a sufficiently small susceptible population, can serve as an effective barrier to disease transmission. Knowledge of where a disease has been before and how it moved through population settlements, therefore, can help target vaccination campaigns on transmission channels or establish buffer zones of immune people as barriers.

New infectious diseases and newly virulent or antibiotic-resistant strains of old ones have appeared in recent decades. The evolution and emergence of new disease agents largely as a result of changes in land use and transformation of population mobility are discussed in Chapters 3 and 4. That development lies in the cultural ecology of population–behavior–habitat interactions. This chapter focuses on one aspect of behavior, population mobility and moving around elements (i.e., agents and vectors) of a disease system (Chapter 2). Whether they spread only locally, such as Legionnaire's disease, or diffuse as great world pandemics, such as HIV/AIDS, the threat of emerging diseases challenges the development of diffusion prediction that relates not to the mathematical or virtual space of differential equations but to real towns needing real health care personnel for people at specific locations.

TERMINOLOGY

Epidemiological Terminology

Epidemiologists are concerned with disease infections moving through a population (one that seems not to exist distributed in space but as a whole occupying a point). Many of the terms discussed in Chapters 1 and 12 were developed to describe this process. A person can be infected but never develop symptoms (*subclinical*), or can develop a disease but not pass the infection to another person (*viremia, dead end*). How likely is a disease to develop in an infected person (*pathogenicity of the agent; resistance of the host*)? How virulent is the infection that occurs (*case fatality rate*)? How likely is the infection to be passed on (*secondary attack rate*)? How long is it between infection and when a person becomes infectious to others (*incubation period*, which is actually a little different from period and time to symptoms, because people with some infections start to "shed" the disease agent in respiratory droplets, etc., before they actually develop symptoms such as fever)? People who have not yet been infected but can be are *susceptible*. Those who have already had the disease, in reality or through vaccination, and can no longer be infected are *immune*. Those who are actively able to pass the agent on are *infectious*, and for some diseases it is possible for individuals to have passed through the course of the disease and no longer have symptoms themselves yet still shed disease agents and be *carriers*.

Knowledge of these parameters enables researchers to model and predict future developments and possible intervention strategies and outcomes when an epidemic starts. If *this* many people are infected at a point in time, the argument goes, and this is the incubation period, the secondary attack rate, and the proportion of the population susceptible, then at the next point in time *that* many people will be infected. Calculations can be complicated. The proportion of susceptibles may vary with such characteristics as age, vaccination history (sometimes substituted for by income and education levels), prevalent health status, or genetically given resistance, for example. Nevertheless, epidemics in a population are often mathematically reduced to a set of differential equations. With such knowledge the need for hospital beds or the economic impact of work absenteeism and such matters can be predicted for the whole population. Researchers can model the comparative advantage of targeting various population subgroups for a vaccination drive, for example. Far too often in such efforts, however, the question of *where* is left out.

Much has been learned about the movement of a new infection through a population. An epidemic typically follows an "s-shaped curve," or logistic curve (see Vignette 8-1). At first only a small proportion of the population is infected (early innovators, in geographic parlance). The numbers of infected people increase exponentially at first, but then growth slows down as the proportion of susceptibles decreases and susceptible individuals become increasingly difficult for the agent to contact. The epidemic finally wanes, leaving a small proportion of the population uncontacted. If the population is not of a critical size, the disease then becomes extinct. If a population is large enough to produce continually enough new susceptibles (usually children), the disease may become endemic. Eventually it may circulate like such "childhood diseases" as mumps and measles.

Whole populations do not, of course, occupy a point in space. Diseases diffuse over space because population in all its diversity is distributed over space. All such parameters as vaccination coverage, age, income, education, ethnicity, and settlement size vary over space. Day-care centers, schools, and medical facilities are located in space. Contact is made in space and must overcome distance to occur. The remainder of this chapter is about geographic modeling of disease diffusion, surely the purest application of the spatial analysis tradition of geography discussed in Chapter 1.

Types of Diffusion

The geographic process of diffusion goes on constantly and affects many aspects of our lives. Information about someone's death or illness is usually spread mouth to mouth, friend calling friend or telling neighbor. If a new product becomes available, such as a new contraceptive or medical treatment, at first supply will be limited and people will need to travel to a large urban area or specialized medical center because the innovation will not be available locally. Perhaps a foreign student has finished medical study in a U.S. university and is returning home to practice and teach the new techniques he has learned. These examples are medically related, but they could as well be about political rumor or a new sports franchise or the ongoing restoration of the American bald eagle to regions in which it was recently extinct. They are examples, respectively, of expansion, hierarchical, and relocation diffusion.

Relocation diffusion involves the introduction of an innovation to a new location that is not part of the network or system of interactions from which it comes. It often involves leaps over great distances and intervening populations. People with knowledge may migrate to a new place, for example, as when Italian immigrants taught New York Irish Americans to make pizza. We have studied several examples of relocation diffusion in earlier chapters. The movement of plague bacilli from burrowing rodents in central Asia to rodents in European cities to burrowing rodents in American, Argentinian, and South African grasslands constituted a whole series of relocation diffusions. When hunters who had depleted the local raccoon population captured raccoons from a Florida population in which rabies circulated and introduced them into the woods of West Virginia, they set off an epizootic of raccoon rabies that has diffused across a region currently extending from Massachusetts to North Carolina. Relocation diffusions happen. Modeling and prediction efforts usually begin with their arrival.

Expansion, contact, and *contagious diffusion* are often lumped together or used interchangeably. "Adoption of innovations" which takes place through contact between people is strongly affected by distance. Geographers speak of the "friction of distance" and measure "distance decay." This simply means that the farther apart people are, the less likely they are to have contact or interact. The strong affect of distance causes the process of contact diffusion to have a distinctive pattern which is sometimes likened to an ink spot spreading on paper or to ripples moving out from a stone thrown into water. The larger term here is "contact diffusion." The major difference among these types of spatial diffusion is that ideas can travel over telephone and electric lines and such with almost no friction of distance, whereas a contagious microbe must be transmitted from one individual to another within some physical proximity. Ideas are frequently disseminated to millions of people at a time via television or the Internet. The movement of people is required for contagion. (The transmission of germs through fomites, such as infected blankets, is rare.) Although most geographical literature is concerned with expansion diffusion, it is perhaps more technically correct to speak about diseases spreading through contact diffusion.

The final type of diffusion, *hierarchical*, is characterized by disease agents moving among urban areas according to their relative size. Some of the most important theoretical constructions in geography have for decades addressed the regular spatial arrangement of settlements (including cities) of different sizes and how population size relates to economic functions and the distance decay (and hence market regionalization) of such activities as wholesaling and retailing. The settlements of different size and function are referred to as *central places*. These exist in a framework of hierarchical relationships among which goods, ideas, money, and especially people, move up and down (Figure 10-7). The tension between the numbers of people necessary to support sales of a business or service and the friction of distance that people must overcome to reach it forms flows of people which can be regionalized into "market sheds" (analogy from watersheds, in which rain flows downslope into separable riverine systems) with distance decay "cones" of demand (see Figure 10-8). When a disease agent diffuses, it moves through the interaction of people up the urban hierarchy to the largest city and then is said to *cascade down the hierarchy* to other cities (Figure 8-1).

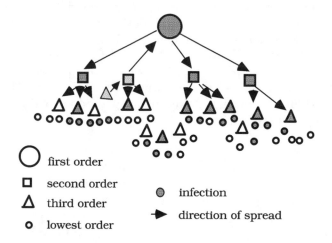

first order

second order

third order

lowest order

infection

direction of spread

FIGURE 8-1. Infection cascading down the urban hierarchy.

Networks and Barriers

Diffusion occurs over a web, or backcloth, of places, people, and the communication links through which information, people, and goods flow. The diffusion of a given phenomenon might be studied at several different time periods in order to gain knowledge about changes in network structure. Alternatively, research on the simultaneous diffusion of the same or similar phenomena in different networks could illuminate the impact of types of network structures. These strategies are pursued by several of the studies discussed later under modeling.

In opposition to networks, which pattern and support diffusion, barriers slow and shape the process. Barriers have three basic effects. *Absorbing barriers* simply stops an innovation. Populations vaccinated against smallpox are an example of an absorbing barrier: Unable to contact susceptible persons, isolated cases had no chance to diffuse, and smallpox disappeared. Sparse populations in arid lands can behave like absorbing barriers to disease diffusion. *Reflecting barriers* channel and intensify the local impact of a diffusion process while blocking its spread to another locale. For example, the presence of lakes or unbridged rivers may cause rabid raccoons to turn back and limit an epizootic to a territory; or the presence of a hostile ethnic group or gang may cause people to shop at a certain place or travel in one direction instead of another. Finally, the barrier may be *permeable,* allowing some diffusion but slowing the process. Most international borders are permeable barriers.

Barriers are often physical—oceans, deserts, mountains, rivers, and so forth. Broad barriers such as oceans or deserts were effective barriers to contact diffusion during the period of slow transportation. The disease might run its life course during the journey and never reach the destination. Aboard a ship, the susceptible population might be too small to maintain the contagion through the course of a trip. Rapid transport today has almost eliminated the effectiveness of such barriers.

Cultural barriers are especially important in the diffusion of styles of health care. The Chinese carried their medical system with them as they migrated to Southeast Asia earlier this century (relocation diffusion). Comparatively few people indigenous to that area have chosen to adopt the Chinese system, however, perhaps indicating the cultural separation of the population groups. It has spread more, for example, among the Thai, who are Therevada Buddhists, than among Malays, who are Moslems. Programs such as child vaccination, family planning efforts, and AIDS prevention programs diffuse in a similar way with varying types of constraints.

DISEASE DIFFUSION

The characterization of infectious disease as either endemic or epidemic is often inadequate, as a disease can be both. A disease heretofore nonexistent in an area may suddenly appear, often virulently and in the absence of cultural buffers (Chapter 2). More commonly, an endemic disease develops in epidemic proportions, perhaps seasonally. How and whether it develops depends on several well-known factors (Burnet & White, 1974, pp. 118–119). The first of these are the qualities of the microorganism that influence its relationship with a human host. These qualities include the number of organisms needed to initiate symptoms and produce clinical disease; for most agents subclinical infections also produce immunity. Second are the number of organisms shed by a carrier of the infection, the period of shedding, the method of shedding into the environment, and the survival time of infectious organisms in the particular environment outside a human host. Third is the probability of contact with a susceptible host during the period of infectiousness, a factor influenced by the agent's virulence as well as the numbers and distribution of susceptible people. A fourth factor is the population's immunity, whether from prior infection, vaccination, or genetic predisposition.

The diffusion of infectious disease moves both through population and over space. Most studies and efforts to model and predict the course of diffusion start with a time series. An epidemic starts when the incidence of cases exceeds expectation, whether that expectation is no disease at all or an endemic clutter of occasional cases. Many diseases follow a cyclical pattern in which a virus or other agent contacts a cohort of susceptible children, born since the last epidemic, and spreads rapidly within the group. After a while, as the proportion of immune members of the group increases, it becomes more difficult for a disease agent to contact a susceptible person and the rate of spread slows down (the logistic curve, again). The periodicity of measles epidemics, for example, especially in less populated areas, was regulated by the fairly consistent number of children born each year and the substantial minimum susceptible population needed to maintain the infection (Cliff, Haggett, & Smallman-Raynor, 1993; Cliff & Haggett, 1983). Artificial immunization has greatly reduced the number of measles cases today, but any relaxation in the completeness of vaccination could reestablish a susceptible population. Such was the case in the early 1980s when numbers of college students began coming down with measles. The relatively new vaccine they had received as small children was found to confer less than permanent immunity. The college epidemics were stopped by requiring all students to get booster shots immediately.

The regularity that results according to these known factors has led to major developments in deterministic modeling. These follow the general approach begun by Bailey (1957, 1975): susceptibles–case incidence–infectives–removals–immunes. Because these models generate epidemics which become extinct, the influential Hamer-Soper model added birthrates at the beginning to generate a continuously susceptible population. The size of population and its subpopulations can then be fed into the differential equations to generate predictions that are mathematically satisfying. The development, mathematics, and applications of these models are thoroughly explained in Thomas (1992). The geographer's frustration at the spatial blindness of these models and modelers is well expressed in Gould (1993), especially his chapters "Time But No Space: The Failure of a Paradigm" and "The Response: How Many Bureaucrats Can Dance on the Head of a Pin?"

The remainder of this chapter discusses ways the diffusion of contagious disease over space can be visualized and modeled. For the most thorough and graphic explanation and presentation on the subject, readers should consult Cliff and Haggett (1988) or, more mathematically, Thomas (1992). Geographic disease diffusion research is often based on models developed to study other types of innovations and applied outside the area of health concerns. These general models have been extended and expanded to fit the special circumstances of disease diffusion. The studies by Brownlea (1972) on hepatitis, Haggett and others on measles (Cliff et al., 1993; Cliff & Haggett, 1982; Cliff & Haggett, 1983, 1988; Cliff, Haggett, & Ord, 1986; Cliff, Haggett, Ord, & Versey, 1981; Haggett, 1976), Stock (1976) and Kwofie (1976) on cholera, Pyle on cholera (1969) and influenza (1984, 1986), and Gould (1993) on AIDS are used in the following section to look at the diffusion of disease as a geographic subject. A final section brings these and other geographic studies to focus on the pandemic of AIDS.

MODELING DISEASE DIFFUSION

Most of the epidemiological research in disease diffusion has involved microscale field investigations which rely on relatively small samples. The range of scales used by geographers in diffusion studies offers a different view. A long-range advantage to broad-scale models of disease diffusion is their possible importance for forecasting, even for place. If we can identify those variables (centers, barriers, population distributions, spatial processes) that consistently influence the diffusion of a particular disease, or if the geographic diffusion pattern of a place is repetitive and thus predictable, health officials could focus vaccination programs and health education on blocking or minimizing outbreaks. We will look at models of hierarchy, distance decay, stochastic diffusion, "gravity models" of population potential and spatial transformation, and spatial autocorrelation. Finally, we examine how these approaches have been employed to better understand measles, influenza, and AIDS. We end the discussion of AIDS with a consideration of context and consequences, and the limitations of this spatial analysis.

Diffusion over Distance and through Hierarchy

The two processes—contact diffusion, which involves traversing distance over time, and hierarchical diffusion, which involves the channeling of contact through the population interactions that create the urban hierarchy—were discussed previously. Figure 8-2 illustrates how they are expressed. Try to identify four types of diffusion in the diagram before reading further.

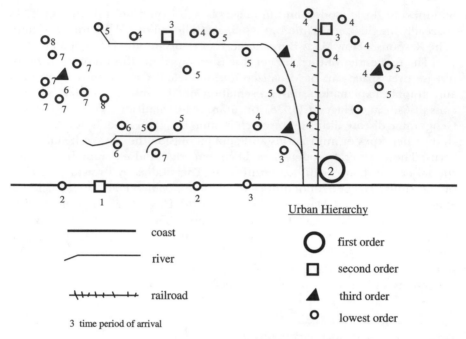

FIGURE 8-2. Distance decay and urban hierarchy.

Contact diffusion is best expressed as taking place when the disease agent arrives later at places farther away from the source. Traversing distance dominates the movement of the disease along the coast and up the lower river in the diagram. The movement along the upper river becomes more complex at the appearance of hierarchical diffusion. The infection moves up the urban hierarchy from the second-order coastal city to the first order quickly. All the large cities of second functional order get the infection immediately after the coastal primate city does (first order). As the disase cascades down the hierarchy, the size of the urban place becomes more important than distance to be traversed. Of course, contact diffusion begins to occur locally from each of the infected urban places, too. Radial diffusion from a settlement to the nearest settlements is obvious, especially among the cluster of villages in the west. They get the disease so much later than the other places, despite the third-order urban place and despite the proximity to the initial settlement infected, that a strong barrier effect is clearly present. It is easy to visualize rugged interfluvial mountains and perhaps a hill tribe ethnic group. Relocation diffusion, of course, occurs when a ship arrives at the coastal port and introduces the first infection to the coastal settlement system. This composite diagram of diffusion types was inspired by the patterns of diffusion of cholera in West Africa actually mapped and analyzed by Stock (1976). The relationships of distance and hierarchy can be represented on a graph, similar to what Stock did. Figure 8-3 portrays distance from the coastal primate

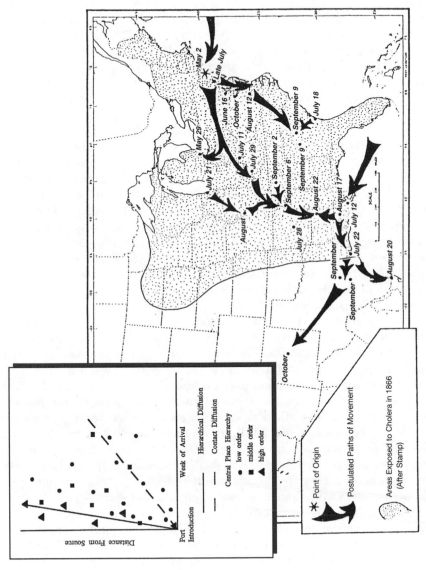

FIGURE 8-3. Diffusion of the 1832 cholera epidemic in the United States. From Pyle (1969, p. 66). Copyright 1969 by Ohio State University Press. Reprinted by permission.

271

city on one axis and the period of the disease's arrival on the other. The symbol used to represent places indicates their status in the urban hierarchy. It is clear from the major vector that hierarchical diffusion has become most important as size of place dominates distance in time. The minor vector, however, suggests the presence of an unintegrated system within the country, perhaps similar to the lower river valley of Figure 8-2, in which distance is still the dominant factor for diffusion. This perspective on disease diffusion was first developed through studies of cholera diffusion by Pyle (1969), whose map of cholera spreading in 1866 appears in Figure 8-2 also. These two conceptually important studies, by Stock and Pyle, are described later.

Cholera is an acute intestinal bacterial disease that is internationally reportable to the World Health Organization. Its symptoms of severe diarrhea and vomiting result in mortality from severe dehydration and consequent shock and cardiovascular collapse. If untreated, case mortality may be more than 50%. The bacterial agent, *Vibrio cholerae*, has two accepted "biotypes" and may be developing a third. The cholera vibrio, biotype *cholerae*, has an ancient endemic focus in the Ganges Valley of India. Indeed, the dreadful black Hindu goddess of death and disease, Kali, has her own temples in Calcutta (people who die of cholera often turn black as their blood congeals). Humans are its only host, although the vibrio can survive in the dense organic matter, algae, and zooplankton of the Ganges delta. Genetically, it includes a set of genes inserted by a plasmid to make it a human pathogen, which suggests that a plasmid crossed from some kind of animal bacteria to the normally harmless, widespread aquatic vibrios of delta ecosystems when the Ganges' sytem was simplified and organically polluted by people (Wills, 1996) Cholera is transmitted through contamination of water or occasionally food by fecal matter or vomitus. The cholera vibrio is sensitive to heat, acidity (stomachs), dry conditions, and ultraviolet light and does not survive for long in most environments. For millenia cholera has broken out epidemically in India when pilgrims returned to their homes from periodic Hindu festivals in the sacred Ganges. By the early 19th century international trade networks and population mobility had developed to spread cholera to southeast and southwest Asia, where the Hajj to Mecca became a center of diffusion. Soon, in six 19th-century pandemics, cholera spread from the Ganges to the great ports of India and then through Suez and on to Europe and North America. Each pandemic was cleared elsewhere and collapsed back to only India. In the 20th century epidemics seemed effectively limited to Asia. Then, a World War II–era epidemic introduced cholera to the eastern islands of the Indonesian archipelago, where it stayed and evolved into the El Tor biotype. El Tor cholera has a lower case mortality (i.e., it is evolving toward commensalism; see Chapter 3, this volume). Infections may involve only diarrhea, or even no symptoms at all. Infective but unknowing carriers of the disease resulted in the World Health Organization dropping the last pretense of control through vaccination, which is no longer required for travel (and was never more than partially effective in the short term). The new cholera has spread since 1961 to the southern states of Europe and the (former) Soviet Union, entered the United States and Japan where sanitation contained it, and apparently for the first time spread to West Africa (where it has stayed). In the 1990s, the agent was brought in ballast water by ships from Southeast Asia to Peru's coastal algae, and it then diffused through South America.

Pyle was the first to realize that the diffusion of a disease such as cholera could be used to analyze the spatial structure of a country. That is, the pattern of the diffusion could illustrate the type of transportation system, the development of national economic integration, and the evolution of a functioning urban hierarchy of commercial and mobility interactions. Even before germ theory and vital statistics, the arrival and presence of cholera in a place were noted in the local newspapers. Pyle studied the diffusion of three major cholera epidemics in the United States by developing the methodology depicted in Figure 8-3. The first epidemic, in 1832, was introduced (relocated) at several points: the riverine ports of Canada, New York City, and New Orleans. Diffusion occurred along the Atlantic coast and the riverine systems, arriving clearly the farther the later in a system dominated by water transport. The second epidemic, in 1849, occurred when the hierarchical structure of the United States urban system was emerging. Railroads were becoming important, although much of the interior was not yet connected to the East by rail. The epidemic was introduced in New York City and New Orleans. From these cities it diffused up the rivers and along the coast in two separated regions, but within each region, hierarchy, size of urban place, had emerged as the major predictor of how soon the epidemic would arrive. By the time of the third epidemic in 1866, the rail system was well established but did not cross the continent. Cholera was again introduced in New York City, but the epidemic now moved through the country as one system with urban hierarchy determining time of infection. Even the exceptions (residuals) served to emphasize the structure: Detroit was infected early for a city of its size, clearly because of its proximity to nearby Canadian cities; San Francisco was infected more than a year late for a city of its size, but of course the transcontinental railroad was not yet built though pioneers still walked or sailed there; and Washington, DC, which then was almost deserted during summer, did not receive the epidemic until Congress convened in the fall.

The arrival of El Tor cholera in West Africa (1970–1975) in a "virgin" or totally susceptible population provided Stock the chance to develop one of the most comprehensive and conceptually clear studies of diffusion. He examined the applicability of existing diffusion models. First he needed extensive fieldwork to identify, locate, and map the local timing of the outbreak of cholera throughout the region. He identified at the village level behavior that buffered or increased risk. This ecology was modeled as a local system. It involved such things as caring for the sick and preparing the dead for burial, washing hands, eating with hands out of common plates, use of latrines, and presence of local medical service. Then, addressing regional scales, he identified and developed four models (which are generically represented in Figure

8-2) to describe the overall diffusion pattern.

There were three models of contact diffusion: coastal, riverine, and radial. Fishermen carried the disease along the coast and it spread from coastal villages to nearby towns. Diffusion along the Niger River also was dominated by the friction of distance. Larger towns received the infection no earlier than smaller towns closer to the origin. The radial pattern of contagious diffusion was identified around Lake Chad. Here the disease intensity was particularly virulent, and as people fled the lake area there were no developoed transportation routes or natural channels to structure the diffusion paths. People from a village fled to the nearest ones around, from which people fled outward to the next ones. Only in Nigeria had a clear example of hierarchical diffusion emerged. Coastal diffusion introduced cholera to the primate city of Lagos, from which river, bus, and rail routes emanated. A settlement's level in the urban hierarchy rather than its distance from Lagos determined when the epidemic arrived. Overland transportation routes channeled diffusion. The least affected areas of the country had low population density, little urbanization, and undeveloped transportation.

Stock's monograph emphasizes the complexity of the geographic structure of diffusion. All the basic models had some applicability. Immune populations, deserts, and sparsely populated areas were permeable barriers, but rivers, coast, and developed overland routes helped channel movement. Stock suggested that the linear pattern along the Niger River loosely resembled the 1832 cholera diffusion along the internal waterways of the Untied States discussed earlier, whereas the hierarchical diffusion in Nigeria more closely resembled the 1866 United States epidemic's structure. The difference between Nigeria and Mali in economic development in the early 1970s thus seems similar in spatial expression to the past structural development of the United States.

Local Diffusion by Chance: Stochastic Simulation

There have been few attempts to apply to disease diffusion the simulation methods formulated by Hagerstand which have otherwise been very useful in modeling innovation diffusion (see Vignette 10-3). This may be because the influences on the multiple waves of an epidemic are very complex. The aging but best example of the application of stochastic diffusion simulation to disease is a study of infectious hepatitis in Wollongong, Australia (Brownlea, 1972).

The infectious hepatitis virus is transmitted through fecal contamination. The virus is robust and tolerant of a wide range of environmental conditions. Water, fish, seafood such as oysters, and pet hair may be vehicles for disease transmission. Brownlea identified cyclical fluctuations in the number of cases reported. During epidemic years, incidence rates of 2 per 1,000 or more affected mainly children and showed an equal sex ratio, strong spring seasonality, and no spatial concentration. During interepidemic years, rates were rather uniformly 0.3 per 1,000, affected all ages, and showed little seasonality and no spatial concentration. Because hepatitis is often poorly reported, Brownlea aggregated cases over 15 years and used a Poisson probability test to determine just where active spread was present. He identified the center of this as a wave that moved spatially through time and labeled it a "clinical front."

Brownlea developed several models for hepatitis behavior at different scales within this industrial–suburban, rapidly growing region. The basic model was based on Hagerstrandian-type stochastic simulation of a random walk (Vignette 8-2, Figure 1). Assuming a closed population, equal chance of diffusion in all directions, and essential community immunity as the epidemic passed, he simulated a random diffusion in which the clinical front would advance as a ring from Wollongong's initial node. Time periods for measurement were determined by incubation period. The bulges and bends in the actual, observed advance of the clinical front—that is, the deviation from the random—he attributed to ecological parameters he had identified which op-

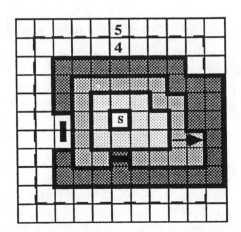

SIMULATED DIFFUSION   **OBSERVED DIFFUSION**

— —   time unit boundary   ▢   time 1

2   time unit   ▨   time 2

▯   grid for mean information   ▨   time 3
        field probability surface

                                         ➤   channeling characteristic

S   source   ▬   barrier characteristic

FIGURE 8-4. Simulation of the diffusion of infectious hepatitis.

erated as barriers or channels (Figure 8-4). Modifying the simulation to fit the actual disease behavior by adjusting the cell probabilities showed that concentration of young families, light sandy soils, concentration of older people, and a polluted lake used for fishing and swimming were important parts of the physical and sociodemographic surfaces that retarded or channeled epidemic diffusion. Recalibration of cell probabilities led to a close match between the simulated and real diffusion patterns.

These findings were applied to the movement of "the clinical front" among the settlement nodes in the study area. Brownlea found that the disease diffused from each population center, exhausting the susceptible population at the core and rippling out to the surrounding nodes. If a peripheral node developed a sufficient concentration of inmigrants and young children, it became a new center of infection and node of diffusion. The first exhausted node was occasionally reinfected from the surrounding, newly active nodes, which caused the in-filling epidemiological pattern of the interepidemic years. The model laid a bais for explaining the disease's rhythmicity and spatial patterning and provides a powerful example of using Hagerstrand's stochastic simulation for analysis of disease diffusion.

Approaches from the Family of Spatial Interaction Models

One of the most robust nomothetic models in geography is the Gravity Model, the prototype for geographic modeling of spatial interaction. It has been widely used to account for, and predict, an amazingly wide variety of flows: job migration, telephone traffic, airline passenger movements, mail delivery, commodity shipping, and the spread of information, among many others. Because it is about interaction, contact, flow, connection, and the spatial patterns that result, it is also about the diffusion of disease.

The basic concept is elegantly simple. The greater the number of people who live in two places, the greater the likelihood of contact between them, but the further apart the two places are, the less the likelihood of contact between them. We would expect more people to move, write, or telephone each other between Chicago and Philadelphia than between Chicago and Houston. We would expect more of such contact between New York City and Washington, DC, than between New York City and Buffalo, New York. In an important way, even the hierarchical diffusion discussed earlier is "gravity model thinking" as the likelihood of interactions between the populations of the largest cities overwhelms the friction of the distance between them. If, furthermore, instead of the attraction between only pairs of places, we consider the influence of all places in a study region upon each other's contacts, we create a surface of potential interaction among people called *population potential*. Vignette 10-1 develops the calculation and mapping of population potential.

The Gravity Model was derived from efforts in the 19th century to analyze society "scientifically" and create a "social physics." The inverse relationship between the attraction of population size (such as mass) and the discouragement of distance seemed obviously analogous to Newton's gravity model. Some of the terminology used today, such as "potential," is derived from this physics. Obviously, however, the surface of the earth and the spatial arrangement of its settlements do not exist in a void; such things as direction, road routes, mountain and sea barriers, really matter. It was easy to account for the different "frictions" of distance encountered by different modes of movement—whether by foot, car, plane, etc.—by varying the exponent on the distance (instead of dividing by distance-squared *à la* Newton) until the formula worked. After this empirically determined "calibration," other more elaborate ways were developed using constants to "constrain" the model so that the total flow predicted out from an origin or into a destination equaled the actual total flow observed. The computation of gravity model predictions of migration, for example, has become very complicated. The model is also so far from the original physics that a new theoretical rationale has been developed in terms of maximum likelihood and maximum entropy (Wilson, 1974) The large literature on the gravity model and other models of spatial interaction can be conceptually approached for general understanding (Abler, Adams, & Gould, 1971; Gould, 1984; Senior, 1979) or more advanced and mathematically sophisticated explanation (Cliff & Haggett, 1988, 1989; Thomas, 1992).

The family of spatial interaction models and their derivatives can provide a way to put real space into diffusion within population. For example, the former Soviet Union used to collect remarkable incidence data, daily reports from more than 100 cities, and had developed detailed mathematical models of the diffusion of influenza within its population. These formulas ignored distance between the cities in that vast country. These models had been adapted by British epidemiologists and others to the kind of data available in the West but remained aspatial. When Pyle used the gravity model to put distance (between cities) into predictions using their approach on U.S. data, he showed that distance as well as size (mass) was important by accounting for 70% to more than 80% of the variance among U.S. cities. He further added to his prediction by using population potential of the elderly population in his regression analysis (Pyle, 1986).

The following two examples—of Gould using the gravity model as a "spatial filter" to transform the diffusion space of Ohio and of Hunter using a surface of population to explain the basic movement of an influenza epidemic through England and Wales—should clarify the gravity model and provide some sense of the power of these techniques in medical geography.

Diffusion through Transformed Space

Cartographers have long transformed space for analytical purposes. Distances on roads, for example, might be represented by travel time instead of actual miles so that areas get foreshortened or extended. Cartograms, such as demographic base maps, represent the content of a region as space. Indeed, it is impossible to represent the surface of our sphere on a flat sheet of paper without transforming space (Chapter 13). Gould used the gravity model as a "spatial filter" to transform the space of Ohio so that accessibility, in this case to the contagion of AIDS, could be illustrated and used predictively.

Gould mapped the diffusion of AIDS across Ohio's 84 counties and three large cities of Cleveland, Columbus, and Cincinnati from 1982 on. As he claimed and Figure 8-5 shows, there is educational value in the dramatic impact of maps showing AIDS diffusing—and arriving. Instead of dismissing AIDS as spreading in some "other kind of people" or being someone else's problem, the reaction of Ohioans viewing the maps in sequence (and of course locating their own place first) often was "it's coming; . . . it's here!"

The three largest cities of course have a lot of interaction among their populations, as well as contact with large cities outside the state. The gravity model was used to calculate all 3,486 potential interactions among the counties, which are then mapped into multidimensional "AIDS space." The rural counties isolated from other contacts, or places connected by proximity and population size, then show the spatial logic of the mapped pattern of diffusion.

Figure 8-6 shows another population potential surface for England and Wales. After examining the uses of absenteeism at school and work and various other estimates of infamously unreported influenza incidence, Hunter and Young used the incidence of acute pneumonia (primary and influenzal, and well reported) to map the Asian flu epidemic of 1961 week by week on areal and demographic base maps. They located the centroid (itself a kind of gravity model calculation) of cases for each week. They calculated the population potential by county and mapped it in the way discussed in Vignette 10-1. As the figure shows, the center of the epidemic advanced week by week along a ridge of population potential until it reached the "potential mountain" of London. Population potential and week of onset were highly correlated, but not total incidence.

Testing Models of Diffusion with Spatial Autocorrelation

The methodology of analyzing changes in relationship (or similarity) over space by correlating the values of geographic units, such as counties, at sequentially increasing distance for sequentially increasing time can provide a powerful and sensitive analysis of disease diffusion. This method, spatial autocorrelation analysis, is described and developed in Chapter 13 and Vignette 13-1. In this section we look at how, in the hands of masters such Andrew Cliff and Peter Haggett, it can illuminate the disease process and its human geography. The illustrations and models that follow are all from their work (Cliff et al., 1993; Cliff & Haggett, 1982, 1983, 1988; Cliff et al., 1986; Cliff et al., 1981; Haggett, 1976)

Measles is endemic throughout most of the world today. The virus is

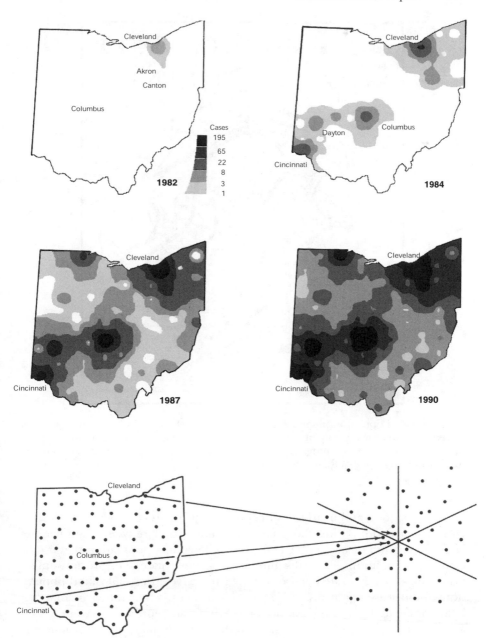

FIGURE 8-5. Diffusion of AIDS in Ohio and in space transformed by the Gravity Model. The Gravity Model can be used as a "spatial filter" to transform the space over which infectious agents spread. From Gould (1993). Copyright 1993 by Blackwell Science. Reprinted by permission.

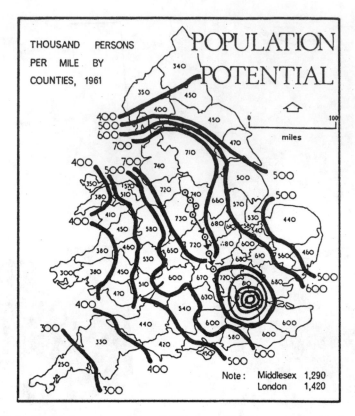

FIGURE 8-6. Population potential and diffusion of influenza in England and Wales in 1957 showing the movement of the epidemic center along the ridge of highest population potential. From Hunter and Young (1971). Copyright 1971 by Association of American Geographers. Reprinted by permission.

highly infectious, and nearly all susceptible individuals contract measles after close contact with an infectious person. Epidemics flare when a sufficiently large population of susceptible children are born in a population that is otherwise more than three-fourths immune as a consequence of previous infection (i.e., at the saturated end of the logistic curve). In small island populations the disease agent disappears, ceases to exist, when the virus that has killed or created immunity can no longer find a susceptible person to infect. There is then no measles in that place until population mobility introduces it again from outside. Numerous mathematical models and island studies have determined that a minimum population size of 250,000 to 500,000 frequently interacting people is needed to generate the new susceptibles and contact rate required to maintain the disease. The difference in these population estimates is undoubtedly related to the relative isolation or intensity of interaction of the people. The need for such a large size of interacting population is strong evidence, as discussed in Chapter 2, that measles could not have existed as a human disease (crossing over from dogs and/or cattle) until the first cities were built in the trading nexus of today's Middle East.

Haggett first studied measles diffusion in the relatively isolated county of Cornwall in southwestern England. He posed seven possible models from what was understood at the time about the process of spread. Which was important: spreading in separate regional systems; from cities to surrounding rural areas; contact diffusion spreading in waves across distance from the largest city; local contagion from one geographic unit to another; contact by people in their "journey to work"; or simply the population size of the places or the population density of the unit areas? He had two waves of measle epidemic to study, a 222-week series from late 1966 to the end of 1970, across 28 political jurisdictions. The genius of this study was to redefine "nearness" to count "joins" in terms of his postulated models, not just spatial contiguity. Each unit could be correlated with its neighbors, but so could commuting origins and destinations, cities of the same class size, units of the same density, and so on. He discovered that different spatial processes of diffusion were more important during different stages in the epidemic, as well as during endemic or epidemic periods. During endemic periods, the population-size model showed the persistent cases of disease in an otherwise weakly structured low level of contagion. Early in the epidemic, population size became less important and waves of contagion effects (shortest distance) and journey to work took over. During the epidemic peak local contagion was most important. As the epidemic waned, it did not shrink in geographic extent but decayed in place, with some tendency for lower-level hierarchical spread to continue. These observations could not be generalized, of course, beyond this one epidemic in this singular place and time. A more ambitious study was needed, on a greater scale.

Cliff and Haggett found in Iceland a large island population system which could be "closed" for analysis as a region and which enjoyed meticulous records kept over more than a century. They followed the introduction, spread, and disappearance of multiple epidemics of both measles and influenza. Over time the population grew large enough to maintain endemic disease, and the infrastructure of transportation, medical care, schooling, and general circulation of information and people was also transformed. They were able to study how intervals, peaking, duration and frequency, age structure, and other dynamics were affected. Spatial autocorrelation methods were the core of the most powerful of these analyses.

As shown in Figure 8-7, they used the method developed in the Cornwall study. They defined "joins" in various ways to test hypotheses of process. The geographic patterns of diffusion of contagious measles and influenza could be expected to reflect population movements for work, schooling, shopping, holidays, and such social activities as visiting relatives. An "index case," or infected person, could theoretically travel to any one of the 50 medical districts (used for epidemiological data). The center of each district could be consid-

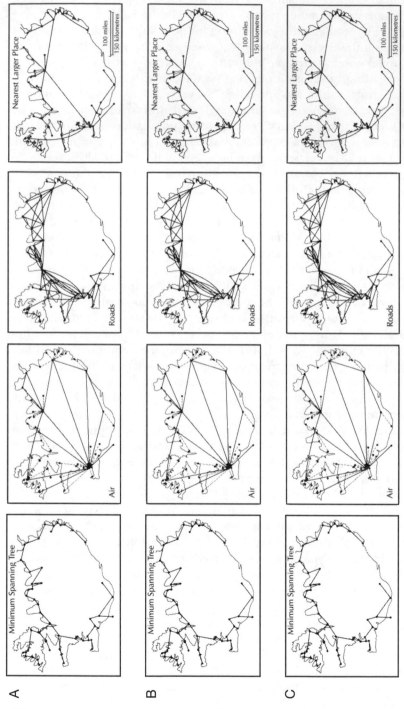

FIGURE 8-7. Join-count statistics for estimating paths followed by influenza and measles epidemics in Iceland, 1945–1970. A, nodes and joins for diffusion models; B, influenza; C, measles. Using spatial autocorrelation to study the links and pathways of diffusion of influenza and measles in Iceland. From Cliff and Haggett (1988, p. 206). Copyright 1988 by Blackwell Science. Reprinted by permission.

ered a "node" linked to each other by links of minimum distance (represented by the "minimum spanning tree," or MST). By defining joins not only in terms of minimum distance but also in terms of airports, road connections, and nearest larger place with or without contiguity (i.e., urban hierarchy) the progression, duration, and concentration in time of successive epidemics of measles and influenza could be examined over decades of change. On each of the histograms in Figure 8-7 the vertical axis plots the number of occasions, in 17 influenza and 8 measles epidemics, on which the black–white statistic (Vignette 13-1) showed that network to be statistically significant at the 95% level in a one-tailed test for positive spatial autocorrelation. Time in months is on the horizontal axis. For "nearest larger place," the bar graph shows nearest larger contiguous place and the line graph shows hierarchical size regardless of contiguity (i.e., pure population). The MST and the road network are said to be "spatially constrained," that is, they represent contagious diffusion in which contiguity and distance are important. The air network and nearest larger place represent hierarchy, nodes, and population connections more important than distance.

The graphs show the importance of contagious spread for both diseases. In the case of influenza (B graphs), for example, the MST was important from 1 month before to 2 to 4 months after and for measles (C graphs) at all stages. The road network was most important during the peak of the epidemic. The influenza epidemics waned in place, not through constriction of territory. So did measles, but it showed some role for urban hierarchical diffusion in filling in the latter stage. Contiguous hierarchy was important for influenza only at the peak and immediately after; pure population-size hierarchical diffusion (the line) was important in the initial spread, during the peak, and until the end. In contrast, for measles unconstrained hierarchical diffusion was never important. For both diseases, the air network was surprisingly insignificant. The researchers speculate that the period of infectivity is too short for both of these diseases for long-term travel to be as important as local contagion. The difference in the importance of population size is likely related to the fact that measles gives permanent immunity to the exposed population, whereas influenza continuously mutates and finds new susceptibles.

As the transport system, school location and residential type, and commercial connections in Iceland changed over decades, so did the frequency, peakedness, duration, intensity, and other characteristics of the epidemics. From studies in spatial analysis such as this a lot can be learned about both the characteristics of the infectious disease and about the connectivity and structure of the human geography. Such knowledge is especially useful for developing strategies for vaccination (such as those used in the eradication of smallpox) and epidemic containment (Cliff et al., 1986).

The Diffusion of Influenza

The "swine flu epidemic" that did not happen in 1976 provides a major example of the need for such knowledge and geographical modeling of diffusion pathways. After the type of influenza isolated in an outbreak at Fort Dix, New Jersey, in January turned out to be the same as that which killed 20 to 50 million people in a world pandemic in 1918–1920, massive efforts were made to vaccinate the entire U.S. population. A particular characteristic of the deadly pandemic was that it killed not only elderly, very young, and other vulnerable people but also healthy young adults. The entire population was at risk. There was no way to target vaccinations, because little was known (or spatially considered, of course) about how such an epidemic would spread. In the end, there was no outbreak. Not only was a large amount of money spent but, because, inevitably, there are some people who have reactions to any vaccination, the serious side effects became more important than the danger of the swine flu epidemic that did not develop. The vaccination campaign created a popular backlash that impugned both science and government. How much better it would have been if the vaccine could have been produced and storehoused while a rational strategy for containment of any outbreak and spatially targeting vaccination coverage was implemented.

The ecology of influenza is intrinsically interesting. Influenza is notorious as an anual winter epidemic. Usually the epidemiological explanation for winter infections is that people gather together inside and so communicate contagion better. Even in places such as prisons, however, places that are crowded all the time, influenza is a winter epidemic. Researchers have inconclusively examined how dryer air, charged ions produced by the static of heating systems (Chapter 5), and such can affect throat mucous or the permeability of cells. It has been suggested that in lower humidity, or perhaps in lower ultraviolet radiation, the virus may survive longer in the air between people, and so be able to infect more of them. Cliff and Haggett have addressed how influenza that is newly epidemic in the Northern Hemisphere in winter becomes epidemic in the Southern Hemisphere in winter, and what happens to it in the tropics all year long (Cliff et al., 1986).

Influenza is one of those few contagious diseases that could have occurred even when human population on earth lacked great cities. There are two reasons for this: Humans share the influenza virus(es) with several animals, especially swine and ducks, and the virus has an extraordinary ability to mutate in gradual (drift) and radical (shift) transformations that baffle the recognition and memory of the human immune system. There are three major strains of influenza known. Influenza C is least known but does not seem to cause epidemic disease. Influenza B causes morbidity in youthful populations and has low case mortality. The pandemics seem to be caused by influenza A strains of virus. Influenza A virus has a coat, or envelope, of glycoprotein in the form of spikes of hemagglutinin (H) and neuraminadase (N) (the strains of the virus are today referenced by patterns identified in these spikes, as H1N1 or H2N3). The hemagglutinin is responsible for binding the virus to host cells. The neuraminadase facilitates release of the virus from infected cells and the spread to others. As "the flu" spreads endemically in a population, continuing all year but spreading especially in winter, the virus changes the angle, bend, and other such properties of its spikes. This gradual "drift" finds enough new susceptibles to continue its presence. Then, with irregular periodicity, the virus rearranges its spikes into different HN ratios and patterns that are not recognized by the immune system ("shift") and the whole population becomes susceptible to a new infection which can spread in a great pandemic wave. This rearrangement seems to occur through genetic exchange as multiple varieties of the influenza virus infect pigs and perhaps ducks, simultaneously. Cultural processes of herding pigs and ducks and agricultural domestication and intensity have played a role in creating pandemics, but the recombination process probably also occurred from time to time in wild birds and mammals in prehistoric time. There has been a tendency for new varieties to emerge from the cultural hearth that domesticated pigs and ducks, southern China, which continues an especially numerous and intense association. This has given Hong Kong special importance as an advance warning surveillance site for the development of appropriate vaccines for the future winter. There was special excitement in 1997 when a kind of chicken flu apparently was transmitted to people for the first time, leading authorities to slaughter all the chickens in Hong Kong. It should be noted, however, that the American Midwest also has an exceptionally intense historic focus of swine and people, and that the great North American flyways (of migrating waterfowl) may be implicated in the early emergence of epidemics. Pyle has noted the xenophobia implicit in naming influenza epidemics for other places. Indeed, the "Spanish flu" (or deadly "swine flu" in today's vernacular) of World War I quite possibly was brought by American farmboys from the Midwest to Europe.

Pyle has tried to discover whether these drifted, endemically epidemic and shifted, rapidly pandemic forms of influenza have different and predictable spatial patterns (Pyle, 1969). Such footprints would be useful in detection but especially important for developing containment and intervention strategies. Using harmonic analysis (Chapter 5) to map the timing of epidemic arrival and peak, he studied centuries of influenza epidemics in Europe and decades in the United States. He reconstructed diffusion pathways to identify patterns of great "frontal" assaults sweeping across continents, patterns of year-to-year continuous advance, and patterns of multiple-node, gradual fill-in. Having seen these footprints of shift and drift, he then combined many of the modeling techniques discussed in this chapter to simulate how the great epidemics of Swine flu, Asian flu, and Hong Kong flu spread in the United States compared with the endemic spread of intervening years. Pyle simulated how influenza would spread randomly if it began in the sites harmonic analysis had designated "repeated events" and if hierarchical diffusion dominated. He added surfaces based on population potential for the elderly instead of city locations. He then used regression to test the prediction of these simulations for the spatial spread of drifting and shifting influenza.

GEOGRAPHIC APPROACHES TO THE PANDEMIC OF AIDS

Among the plethora of emergent and reemergent infections from epidemics of multiple-drug-resistant tuberculosis and malaria to outbreaks of hanta virus, bubonic plague, and ebola, the diffusion of no other agent in recent time has had nearly the profound impact on people and their societies as has human immunodeficiency virus (HIV) and the acquired immunodeficiency syndrome (AIDS) it causes. AIDS is indubitably the plague of the late 20th century. Its spatial diffusion has similarities to other epidemics and can often be modeled and successfully predicted, as we shall see. The basic ecology of the virus is not unique, although the challenge to treatment and development of vaccines is exceptionally difficult. The disease, AIDS, however, has truly been "constructed" in perception, stigmatization, blame, fear, altruism, destitution, new social organization, political invective, and family, economic, and social collapse like no other in our time. The literature, both scientific and humanistic, on AIDS is already vast, while just its geographic contributions continue to accrete by the day. This final section of one chapter cannot do justice to the problem and issues involved. It aspires as a text only to introduce briefly various aspects of the medical geography of AIDS and perhaps inspire further geographical research and insight.

Ecology

The disease agent is different from any other in this book. HIV is a retrovirus in the family of "lentivirus" or slow virus (Gallo, 1986; Huet, Cheynier, Meyerhaus, Roelants, & Wain-Hobson, 1990; Nada, 1989). Slow viruses taking years to produce symptoms have been known to infect many animals but have not previously been associated with disease in people. In animals they are variously known to produce wasting, pneumonia, severe neurological complications, and some types of cancer. HIV consists of a string of RNA (ribonucleic acids) and an enzyme called reverse transcriptase. RNA usually is an intermediary which carries information from a cell's genetic code, DNA, to protein molecules in the cell and causes them to organize in the form of a copy of the DNA. This virus uses its enzyme to "write itself backwards," to copy its own RNA as two chains of DNA, and so is classified as a *retro*virus. The new DNA then works its way into the cell's DNA and waits, apparently until the cell is triggered to start reproducing rapidly by an infection it must fight. The cell then starts to manufacture enormous quantities of the virus's RNA. The HIV is *in* the white blood cells: macrophages, monocytes, and especially "helper" T4-cells which recognize an infection and mobilize the production of the proper antibodies. This is because the envelope of the HIV has two glycoproteins which lock onto molecules (CD4) on the surface of white blood cells and then penetrate the membrane and merge. Thus HIV uniquely accomplishes several things (which took years for researchers to understand): It hides inside the very cells responsible for finding and destroying "nonself"; it destroys those cells, in the process of replicating itself, at the very time they are most needed to fight an infection and so are multiplying and concentrating and optimizing the target for infection by the HIV. Eventually, of course, the white blood cells are so totally destroyed that the everyday infections and cell mutations of all kinds, usually routinely suppressed, run amok.

Many consequences of this disease process are now understood. It is months before antigens to the HIV can be found in the blood and during this time not only will tests be falsely negative but donated blood can be a source of infection. It often is years before an infected person develops symptoms and the vulnerabilities of AIDS, but during this time he or she is infectious to others. Some people, probably because of the frequent challenges to their immune system from sources of multiple infections such as consumption of contaminated water or anal sex, move into HIV replication and develop AIDS years earlier than others. A child, for example, who simultaneously is infected with schistosomiasis, tuberculosis, malaria, and dysentery will not live long. The HIV mutates at an extraordinary rate, several times faster than the influenza virus, which has so far helped confound efforts to develop a vaccine. The "cocktail" of anti-AIDS medicines which has been developed to interfere with the various steps of this process, such as attachment to the cells, fusion, transcriptase, replication, and passage between cells, has been successful in extending life for years and protecting white cells. It is, however, expensive beyond hope for people in developing countries and for some people in the United States. The retroviruses cannot exist in air or water or sunlight and thus cannot be transmitted by casual contact of hands or breath. They have been isolated from fresh blood in the stomach of mosquitoes, but not from the muscle cells or mouthparts (i.e., not replicating or living in the mosquito's tissue, and thus not able to be vectored except, perhaps, mechanically after an interrupted meal is quickly resumed from someone else). The disease agent is contagious between people only through the passage of fluid from one body into another. Because hemophiliacs require transfusions of plasma concentrated from the blood of scores of people to get enough of the clotting factor they need, they are exceptionally at risk. In many places an entire generation of hemophiliacs has died. In many places today intravenous drug users (IDUs) are similarly endangered by the efficiency of infection by injected blood. About a third of babies born to infected mothers are themselves infected, but that rate is going down in developed countries with new treatments for the pregnant women. In most developing countries, an infected child is dead within 1 year and an adult within 2 of developing AIDS.

There are several reasons to be interested in where a disease evolved. Perhaps the most important is that in the place where exposure to a disease agent has been longest, resistance and even immunity to it also is likely to have evolved the most. There must be such a place: Any new virus must result from a mutation of an older one existing somewhere in space. Once understood, any mechanisms of resistance and defense might then be replicated by human technology (as in the production of a DNA vaccine). It is also important to determine whether a new infection is a nidal disease and to identify the reservoir and any vectors or other components of the nidus, if there is one (Chapter 3). Then research needs to determine what the nature of human intrusion or connection with it was. As discussed in earlier chapters, the sheer dimension of land-use change and population mobility in the world today makes new epidemics in the future likely. Any development, even of surveillance and warning systems not to mention intervention or containment, requires more study and deeper understanding of the processes (Morse, 1992).

The HIV evolved in sub-Saharan Africa. Like such disease agents as measles and influenza before it, the retrovirus apparently crossed over to people and mutated into a viable human infection around the middle of the 20th century, although it possibly happened earlier in isolated populations. There are many variants of simian immunodeficiency virus (SIV) which occur widely in various primates (Gould, 1993, summarizing literature in Chapter 2; Grmek, 1990; Huet et al., 1990; Marlink et al., 1994). The first SIV identified, common and without symptoms in African green monkeys although deadly to Asian monkeys, is widespread across the continent but can be genetically separated from human forms. There are two known forms of HIV. HIV-2 occurs among the population of West Africa (with some cases elsewhere in recent years) and is comparatively low in virulence and transmissibility, causing few disease outcomes and less reduction in lymphocytes over a long period. It is extremely closely related to a SIV, which is common in the sooty mangabey monkey population of West Africa. As Gould (1993) put it, there is greater genetic "distance" and variation among SIVs isolated from sooty mangabeys than between them and the HIV-2s isolated from people. HIV-1 was first found in central Africa and has only been recently found in populations in western Africa. It is the virus of the world pandemic. A very closely related virus, probably the source, has been isolated from a subspecies of wild chimpanzees. This may explain why chimpanzees inoculated with HIV-1 in laboratories show symptoms but do not die. It gives researchers an important, although precious, animal model.

There are today at least eight genetic subtypes, or clades, of HIV-1, which have been designated A through H (Osamov, Heyward, & Esparza, 1996). One of the clades, Bl, has become prevalent in North America, Latin America, Europe, Japan, and Australia. This indicates that only one form was introduced and spread rapidly in the 1970s. Clade E is the most transmissible, which partly explains why there are so many cases of HIV in Africa (Levy, 1996). It was introduced in the late 1980s to India, a truly ominous development. It is also not at all certain that a vaccine developed for the North American or European clade, B, would be effective against the others clades. It has proved especially difficult, in any event, to develop a vaccine in large part because of the extremely high mutation rate of the virus because of errors in its process of reverse transcripting.

There are many ways that the virus could have crossed over from our species' nearest relative. The report of an anthropologist who observed monkey blood being injected by one tribe suggests an efficient means that became a rather popular answer (Kashamura, 1973). There are many less exotic means, however. Primates, as one of the largest animals in tropical forests worldwide, are commonly eaten. For example, it is not hard to imagine that butchers and cooks prick themselves as often as surgeons do. As a geographer who has lived among people who keep primates as pets, I (M.S.M.) can attest that monkeys bite each other and children; there is no referee to stop the game because of blood.

The geographical origin of the AIDS pandemic otherwise lies in the mobility change, land development, and urbanization discussed in Chapter 4. Whether or not HIV had infected isolated people previously, this time it took a truck to a city and encountered migrant laborers and tourists and international businessmen. Within tropical Africa there are many ways in which the virus could have been spread. These ways include not only heterosexual sex but also the penetration of skin by unsterilized instruments; knives and needles used for purposes as diverse as circumcision, tattooing, and esthetic scarification; vaccination for smallpox eradication; or currently childhood vaccination for tuberculosis, cholera, whooping cough, and other mass interventions including antibiotic treatments. In developed countries, unsterilized needles have mainly injected heroin. In many developing countries the blood supply remains contaminated. For all the world, however, the overwhelming majority of HIV transmissions has been through sexual intercourse. As a sexually transmitted disease, it is most contagious when people have lesions from other venereal diseases.

Geographic Modeling

When AIDS first came into public view, in 1981 among homosexual white men in the United States, nothing was known of its causes, origins, means of spreading, contagiousness, treatment, or prevalence. Even when the first retrovirus was identified a mere 2 years later and case numbers began to build into the hundreds, knowledge of these things had not advanced much. The first and most enduring reaction of geographers attempting to advance helpful knowledge, was to map it. Mapping proved especially difficult for years because, even when AIDS was reported, legal and scientific concerns for patient confidentiality prevented the release of data. Although two dots put on a county base map at a scale that woud fit a whole state on a single piece of paper would be totally anonymous, conventionally individual data came attached to age/sex/race/income/ethnicity/education and other such variables that, published, could be used to identify someone. (Because an address can identify someone, it is not published in that form.) Behind several years of geographers' frustration, however, lay a more basic problem. Health professionals of all kinds, and most of the public, perceive an epidemic as spreading through a population over time, but they do not envision the process as happening over space or having geographic consequences. We return to this point later.

The first geographic studies attempted to find spatial pattern and so lay the basis for inferring something of process. What was the pattern of prevalence, of recent incidence in various population groups, how extensive, how dynamic, how related to existing spatial models? In the United States, Africa, the world, how was its location related to highway infrastructure and settlement system, to mobility, to international travel for different purposes? How did it relate to demographic structures and fertility levels, prevalence and knowledge of contraception, use of condoms, availability of medical care, and all the other structural and intervention variables? This set of concerns has continued into present involvement in establishing national rural sampling frames that can be used for regionalization and resource allocation (Dutt, Monroe, Dutta, & Prince, 1988; Gardner, Brundage, McNeil, Visintine, & Miller, 1989; Lam, 1996; Lam, Fan, & Liu, 1996; Shannon & Pyle, 1989; Shannon, Pyle, & Bashushur, 1991; Smallman-Raynor & Cliff, 1990; Smallman-Raynor, Cliff, & Haggett, 1992; Stephenson, 1995; Wills, 1996)

The maps show the spread of AIDS to eastern and southern Africa; to New York and San Francisco, then the metropolitan states, then the midwestern and southern and rural areas nationally; early to the great cities of Brazil and Mexico and then to cities across South America; and at the end of the 1980s to Asia. There is clearly a pattern of hierarchical diffusion with local expansion, with suggestions at least of linear diffusion along the interstate highways that have led to studies of drug selling, prostitution, and truck driving. Postulates about these diffusion patterns and population composition led to spatial modeling. Gould's (1993) effort in particular to "predict the next maps" unraveled the spatial processes involved. His use of the gravity model was discussed earlier (Figure 8-5), but that was just a small bit. He established surfaces of AIDS in the United States and cities such as New York that could be useful for prediction and preparation in real places. Gould argued in the international World Health Organization arena for the importance of a spatial perspective when the dominant paradigm was (is) just to subdivide the differential equation of epidemic contagion into smaller and smaller groups, until there are no data at all; that is, not only homosexuals, bisexuals, heterosexuals, prostitutes, IDUs, transfusees, hemophiliacs but also contact rates that might also vary by white, black, Hispanic, Asian, young, old, rich, poor, female, male—tens of thousands of transmission rates reduced to absurdity (p. 161), when the epidemic has moved from here to there.

There are basic differences in approach indicated in these studies that are not simply separations between geographer and epidemiologist. In their space–time models, geographers have been concerned with reconstructing the pathways of HIV diffusion to provide short-term predictions and advanced warning for education, health care provision, community organization and other responses (Gould, 1993; Lam et al., 1996; Loytonen, 1991;

Williams & Rees, 1994). Whether working with the logistic curve to create probability surfaces or using spatial autocorrelation to examine differences among regional structures, the strength of such spatial diffusion studies is the production of realistic local estimates that mobilize, and educate, communities as a whole rather than promoting blame, separation, marginalization, or begrudging of resources on one hand and the endangerment of false security and ignorance among the majority on the other. There are indeed groups of people at greater risk, however. Diluting educational and other efforts by addressing the whole will have less preventive impact than targeting intervention, including any future vaccination, to population groups at greatest risk. Thomas has recognized the theoretical importance of such early warning, pointing out, for example, that "distance from a source may be thought of as a spatial protection which may be enhanced if local behaviours manage to either deflect, or decelerate, the passage of the wave" (Smyth & Thomas, 1996, p. 12). He and others have argued however that long-term policies and targeted interventions require systems models that elicit the underlying epidemic structure (i.e., demographic) and can be used to simulate the impact and effectiveness of alternative public health interventions (Thomas, 1996). Thomas's multiregion models, for example, have demonstrated that population growth rates and risk activity rates are important for simulation and targeting of vaccination and other interventions. Those simulations, however, have not been effective in predicting the observed pandemic pathway and are said to need revision to specify better geographic variations in model values (i.e., back to spatial modeling).

Little effort in all this modeling has been directed at health care delivery and remedial services. Kearns (1996) notes the limited attention to facilities such as AIDS hospice location and indeed to the space of gay men, their experience, evolution of their community-based organizations. There has been some simulation, noted earlier, for targeting public health interventions. The importance of community-based intervention, because of greater effectiveness, is often noted. "Community" is used in the British sense of an interacting subgroup of the population rather than the U.S. meaning of a place in which people interact. One of the most successful intervention programs internationally has involved using peer educators, commercial sex workers, to educate their fellow workers about HIV and AIDS and the importance of using condoms. Because not all bars in any country can be targeted for recruitment into such programs, Welsh (1994) studied the territorial extent of diffusion of information among commercial sex workers and their customers to different bars and to other communities to which they traveled. He used computer mapping and (distance) road buffers determine the locational and other characteristics of the bars most central to the network within a provincial city in the Dominican Republic. Then he successfully used the gravity model to establish the existence of hierarchical diffusion of the information regionally.

HIV has diffused around the world, in space and not just time, but so what? Geographic study of the AIDS pandemic has largely failed to address either the macroparameters of the patterns—global economic restructuring, urbanization, and political domination—or the microlevel constraints on everyday human agency, such as the behavioral choice of women. The best of the studies discussed previously describe or fit the pandemic retrospectively. Useful prediction or interventions for other populations have been lacking, mainly because of insufficient context or resulting insight.

Dimensions, Contexts, and Consequences

More than 40% of HIV infection in the world today occurs in poor females. In at least nine U.S. cities, AIDS is the leading cause of death among all women ages 15 to 45. If such information seems incongruent with the popular image of AIDS as a disease of men, mostly of gays and IDUs, geographic studies have done little to inform or analyze. It is difficult to present much data in this chapter, as everything will be dated and obsolete very soon, but some sense of dimension, proportion, and trend is needed (Farmer, Connors, & Simmons, 1996; Panos Institute, 1986, 1992; Mertens & Low-Beer, 1996; Special Program on AIDS, 1987). The latest data can always be found on the Web page of the World Health Oranization, which links to its country reports and surveillance.

When the first edition of this text was written, in 1987, 40,770 cases of AIDS had been reported to the World Health Organization in 1986 from 91 countries. Although 81% of these were from the Americas (primarily the United States), this was because of more complete reporting. The World Health Organization estimated that there were more than 100,000 cases of AIDS, the majority of which were in Africa. In the United States, 1% of the cases were in children, 2% were blood (i.e., transfusion) related, less than 7% of cases were women, 14.5% were IDUs, 70% gay men, and the remainder both gay and IDUs. HIV had recently been discovered, but little serology had yet been done. It was estimated that there were 5 to 10 million people infected worldwide, including up to 15% of adults in some localities.

The perceptions created by the composition of these early reports of the new disease did a lot of harm. American media and even some medical literature referred to AIDS as "The Gay Plague" and some thought it punishment from God on bad people, although the children and hemophiliacs were troublesome because they were not "to blame." Therefore "normal" people did not have to worry; education in high schools about "safe sex" was objectionable. Funding for research or vaccine development or education explicitly targeted to people at greatest risk was not much of a priority. The disease came out of "deepest, darkest Africa" and probably involved weird or immoral sexual practices. It was easy to deny risk by further marginalizing people with infection. Perhaps, then, it is not surprising that African governments were not very cooperative. African leaders protested that Africans were not homosexuals, did not use drugs, and were being unfairly blamed. The

Americans, probably the CIA, must have created the disease to fight the Soviets. Alternatively, maybe the virus was deliberately tested on Africans to keep them poor and powerless. It did not matter that not even the Americans knew at that time what a retrovirus was or that even in warfare no chemical or biological agent could be used without knowledge of an antidote to protect one's own. Denial was such that several national leaders had to suffer the loss of their sons and whole devastated villages of orphans had to be created before international research, medical care, health education, or other interventions were accepted. Because health researchers think about epidemics in time rather than as spatial processes, this mere snapshot of the early stage of the pandemic was widely perceived as an infection that occurred in populations at risk. Perhaps there was genetic susceptibility involved. In Asia, the epidemic potential was therefore dismissed because it was not occurring (there) in any Asian population. AIDS was obviously a *farang* disease, Thais said; perhaps it was genetic, or resistance to it was. As the epidemic started in Thailand at the end of the 1980s, denial and concern to protect the tourist industry let the storm gather.

Worldwide reporting of AIDS to the World Health Organization continues to be unreliable. AIDS has become the fourth leading cause of death worldwide (third in sub-Saharan Africa). In 1998, 2.2 million AIDS deaths were reported. As this edition is written, about a million and a half AIDS cases have been reported in the last year, for a cumulative total of more than 7 million cases. Serology has become much more common worldwide. The World Health Organization estimates that more than 25 million adults (42% female) and 1.5 million children are living with HIV/AIDS (as compared, for example, with almost 500 million infected with malaria). This is predicted to exceed 40 million by the year 2000. It is difficult to assess death from AIDS because it also underlies the millions of deaths worldwide from epidemic tuberculosis and malaria. Of 1.191 million AIDS deaths reported from sub-Saharan Africa in 1994, 40% were female and 23% children (who usually live only a year and so are more important in mortality rates than prevalence rates). More than 13 million people are infected. This is more than 5% of all adults ages 15 to 49 in the region, with a sex ratio of 1:1. In southern and southeastern Asia (i.e., mainly India and Thailand) about 5 million people are infected. The highest prevalence rates, approaching 2%, are in Thailand, Burma (Myanmar), and devastated Cambodia. In Latin America about 1.5 million adults are infected, for an overall prevalence of 0.5% but more than 70% of infections occur in the largest countries, Brazil and Mexico. Most early infections were among homosexual and bisexual men. The now 18% female proportion is increasing. The Caribbean region, with prevalence rates of 1.5%, has only 250,000 infections. Northern Africa and the Middle East are early in the epidemic and have only a 250,000 infections and low prevalence rates; and in East Asia the infection was introduced so recently that prevalence barely registers yet. The epidemic is recent, small, but rapid in Eastern Europe and Russia. Western Europe has around 800,000 infected, more than 80% male. In the United States and Canada, almost 1 million people are infected, about 20% female. The still lowest incidence but most rapid rate of growth of infection is among women. Heterosexual sex now accounts for about 13% of transmission in the United States, as compared with more than 70% globally. The proportion of infections associated with male-with-male sex has fallen to 40%. AZT therapy has greatly reduced perinatal transmission. Blood-related transmission is now very rare.

Such numbers are numbing but it is hard to absorb meaning from them. One way is to search for patterns. "Type 1" and "type 2" patterns have been discriminated, in geographical parlance often called the "north" and "south" model and their hybridization (Wood, 1988). Type 1 is north (just think United States) and HIV transmission is concentrated among promiscuous homosexuals, IDUs, victims of blood contamination, women infected by bisexual or IDU partners, and babies born to them. These are groups that can be marginalized, some say, and there is not a general epidemic threat: this denies, of course, that the most rapidly growing "group" is women with no known risk exposure, even through their partner's behavior. Type 2, or the South pattern, is characterized mainly by heterosexual transmission, especially through prostitution, with serious impact also from a contaminated blood supply, medical needles, and practices such as scarification or circumcision that also may involve contaminated blood. Drugs in most places are not involved. Most places with those characteristics, such as the Caribbean, got HIV, however, by hierarchical diffusion through tourism and business from IDUs and homosexual tourists from the North.

In the early years, the Centers for Disease Control declared that being ethnically "Haitian" was by itself a risk factor. Perfectly healthy people lost their jobs as a result. HIV was probably introduced to Haiti from the United States. Its broader pattern in the Caribbean is a reflection of the slave trade, of neocolonial plantation and trade structures, and of more recent economic reallocations, displacement from land, and power realignment with the end of the Soviet threat. As Farmer (1992) puts it, after following the struggle for health and livelihood of Haitian villagers and describing the political and economic structures and anthropological meanings of their lives:

> One way to avoid losing sight of the humanity of those with AIDS [that is, not just to accumulate information on genes and mores and myths] is to focus on experience and insights of those who are afflicted. . . . Link the large-scale events and structures of the world AIDS pandemic to the lived experience and commentary of people. . . . For Aids in Haiti is about proximity rather than distance. AIDS in Haiti is a tale of ties to the United States, rather than to Africa; it is a story of unemployment rates greater than 70 percent. AIDS in Haiti has far more to do with the pursuit of trade and tourism in a dirt-poor country than with [exotic sexual or religious rituals]. (pp. 262, 264)

Similarly, in East Africa AIDS is not simply a matter of diffusion along highways with truck stops and prostitutes and the majority of men away from their families laboring in mines or plantations or urban factories. It is the history of the mobile labor force which was created by colonial economic policy, of apartheid, of currently unstable governments, of war and environmental refugee movements; and more broadly of urbanization, rapid population growth, land-use change, and the developmental impacts discussed in Chapter 4. Writing about public health study of the global pandemic in general, Farmer, Connors, and Simmons (1996, p. 242) discusses studies that note the association of HIV with cigarette smoking but ignore the also present association with dirt floor in Haitian slum, or those studies that examine biological forces in such detail as "mucosal and squamous epithelial discontinuity and integrity in the susceptibility to AIDS of Nairobi sex workers" but ignore the social causes found in the same studies and results that "prostitutes from the lower socioeconomic group were more than twice as likely as their counterparts in the higher socioeconomic group to be infected with HIV." Socioeconomic factors that drive the spread of HIV usually are effectively ignored. In this last section, two examples are briefly considered for some diffusion context.

Thailand

Thailand has the highest prevalence of HIV in Asia. India will soon overwhelm world statistics in numbers of victims, but the northern region of Thailand is already being overwhelmed with dead and orphans. In 1986, six cases of AIDS were reported to the World Health Organization. They involved homosexual men back from study and work abroad and a pair of IDUs from the port. The Thai perception that AIDS was a foreign disease was confirmed by this and the exposure elicited little concern when no positive serology was found in clinics. Within 6 years 500,000 people were infected. The AIDS-specific mortality rate in the year 2000 is expected to exceed the current mortality from all other causes combined for the young and middle-age population. In 1989, a "sentinel system" was established which monitored blood sampled from IDUs, female commercial sex workers, blood donors, sexually transmitted disease (STD) clinics, antenatal clinics, and army conscripts. Maps of antenatal clinic prevalence from December 1991 to 1994 show the rapid spread from Bangkok to the northern provinces and southern beach resorts and over a couple of years to the northeastern provinces (Brown & Sittitrai, 1995, pp.16–17). Prevalence in northern antenatal clinics in Chiengmai and Chiengrai had then reached more than 10%. At first AIDS reached peak age incidence in the late 20s, but over a decade the peak of incidence has shifted older by 5 years. Infection with the HIV most often occurs from ages 20 to 30. In mid-1994, sexual transmission accounted for 75.5% of AIDS cases: 1% of this was transmitted by homosexual or bisexual men; 66% by heterosexual men. Intravenous drug use accounted for 8%, and blood for only 0.3%. Mother-to-child transmission, however, caused 8% of cases (Brown & Sittitrai, 1995, from which the statistics are taken; Institute, 1992; Shaeffer, 1994).

In 1995, about 45,000 Thais died from AIDS, more than 10% of them children; that year 65,686 new cases were diagnosed, 7% of them children. Because children die more quickly, usually in a year, they do not accumulate in the prevalence rates. There were more than 140,000 people living with HIV/AIDS, and more than 177,000 who had already died. In 10 years those numbers are expected to be 832,000 dead, 10% children, and more than 1 million people then infected. These numbers occur in a population of 60 million growing to 65 million (2% prevalence).

There are ways that the epidemic is similar to the pattern in the South. It is mostly transmitted by heterosexual sex. Because men infect their wives, transmission to children through pregnancy and nursing constitutes a large component of the epidemic. In rural hospitals in northern Thailand more than 30% of women in a few antenatal clinics have tested positive for HIV. In 1993, military conscripts were 3.7% positive. The economic consequences in loss of labor, numbers of orphans, and medical care are devastating. The Thai government has made good general health care available to most of the people, but by 2000 the cost of hospitalization for AIDS alone will be more than 1 billion baht ($50 million). In Chiengmai, already more than a third of hospital beds are occupied by AIDS patients. As in Africa, there are great microgeographic variations in parental death rates. These reflect the spatial diffusion expressed in the local times of arrival of the virus. The impact has been greatest on northern Thailand, but despite dangerous complacency it is coming in other regions which are just spatially lagged. As in Africa, the father usually dies before the mother, because he was infected first. The widows have a priority need for counseling and support. Family and community-based care are critically important and in need of strengthening.

There are also important differences, however. Thailand has a vigorous economy and rapidly rising average standard of living. Although it is still a predominantly rural and agricultural country, the Thai people have lowered their fertility to replacement. In some ways this increases the economic and demographic impact of AIDS morbidity and mortality. Studies in Africa have shown that most extended families can absorb one or two deaths before economic circumstances decline drastically, but in small, more nuclear Thai families, the mortality of working adults has immediate dire consequences. Most care is given by wives who often have to stop work themselves, putting the family standard of living into a downward spiral. Thailand has increased mandatory education to 9 years, but orphans cannot afford uniforms and books or fees. The costs of the children to grandparents who are usually very poor forces their withdrawal from school and intensifies the problem of child labor abuse, including child prostitution. On the positive side, there is a vigorous family planning effort that has not only lowered fertility but also made condom usage available and familiar to all. After a few years of initial government denial and concern for its tourist economy, the Thai people elected a new government which put the leadership responsible for the famously successful family planning efforts in charge of AIDS prevention. New HIV infections have stabilized at around 89,000 a year, and the infection rate for new conscripts has begun to fall. Because of the cumulative effect of HIV infection, however, the most dreadful onslaught of AIDS is yet to come.

The calamitous and extremely rapid spread of HIV in Thailand has concentrated attention on its sex trade (Brown & Sittitrai, 1995; Fairclough, 1995; Gould, 1993). To these studies, surveys, and commentaries I (M. S. M.) add interpretation from 30 years' experience with the country. Visits to brothels were indeed pervasive, common, and casual in traditional Thai culture. Most women accepted the view that it was the nature of men to seek variety and stimulation and that their casual pleasure did not necessarily diminish their devotion as husbands and fathers. Nevertheless, most use of prostitutes fell into two categories: Single young men were introduced to sex and taught by experienced older women; and the brothels entertained on special occasions or provided hospitality to visitors such as government officials. Police reassignments and commemorative parties, military recreation, and business conventions provided routine occasions. Some ethnic Chinese merchants also sometimes had "minor wives" or concubines of indeterminate permanence. Most Thai men once married, however, stayed with their families in their villages and had little opportunity or desire to hurt their wives. The brothels that existed throughout the countryside were of a different nature than those today, too. One brothel in a northeastern district town of 6,000, for example, had, in 1966, three prostitutes. Two were widows whose children slept together in a back room; the third was a mentally retarded woman in her 20s whom the widows took care of and called "little sister." Their biggest source of income was the district police, several of whom (as civil servants of the central government) had been stationed there away from their families.

The texture and dimension of commercial sex in Thailand was transformed by the Vietnam war. Before the war only about 40,000 Americans were based in Thailand, an American ally, at any given time, but during the war hundreds of thousands came from Vietnam for "rest and recreation." The demand for prostitutes and the flood of money in base towns and Bangkok sent "merchants" to villages far and wide searching for girls. At first deception was important. Village girls were solicited to be hotel maids and restaurant waitresses or dishwashers. Soon more money than a farmer would see in years, enough money to pay off the usurious loan and save his land or to send the other children to college, was offered for a future debt bond on a daughter. Most daughters were proud and happy to be able to help their impoverished parents and siblings. Northern Thailand was especially targeted because women in the northern mountains had long been considered the most beautiful in the country because of their lighter skin. The main railroad trunk line ran between Chiengmai and Bangkok. The north had become a tourist destination for Thai silk and teak and temples. People in the poorest region, the northeast, mostly ethnic Lao or Khmer, usually resisted the solicitations, although they suffered more from unreliable rainfall and crop failure. When drought destroyed their livelihood, 1 million desperate people could flood into Bangkok looking for work. In normal years tens of thousands of men went during the dry season, when they could not work on their farms, to work in construction or transportation. Their biggest squatter slums grew up around the port. Youth of all kinds migrated to the primate city for educational, training, and entertainment opportunities.

There was a crisis in several sectors of the Thai economy when the U.S. military was asked to leave after the war ended. As trade relations grew with booming Japan, Taiwan, Singapore, and Germany, however, a diversified tourism became a more important source of foreign exchange and employment. Thailand offered a beautiful and unique culture. The religious sculpture and temples were beautiful, the people smiling and friendly (having never been a colony, people in Thailand had developed little resentment or inferiority complex), delicious new food awaited on beautiful beaches. In a few years the brothels and recruitment network found more commercial opportunities than before as more than 5 million tourists a year visited the kingdom. After "visit Thailand year," 1987, advertising "the land of sex" was taken over by foreign tour operators. A German firm began to import Thai women and rent them out by the month (with returnable deposits) for business. Jumbo jet loads of Japanese businessmen are said to find it cheaper to fly to Bangkok for a weekend, stay in a luxury hotel, play golf all day, and fulfill their fantasies all night than to pay golf fees in Japan.

Thai society has changed in important ways. The country is rapidly industrializing, especially through textile and micro-lectronics, and urbanizing. Both of those processes mean mass movement to Bangkok, the primate city that dominates the urban hierarchy, and mass slums with destitute children. Values of consumerism seem to have swept aside Buddhism. In a 1990 survey, 50% of single men went to brothels. A new generation has grown up, especially in the north, who think it normal to treat women as a commodity. A few women become wealthy and many view commercial sex work as an easier job—often with air conditioning—than working in a rice field in the sun. The main alternative, when available, is working 60-hour weeks in a sweat shop. Middlemen now make "green loans"—like advances for rice crops at planting time—and build dream houses for fathers understanding that when their daughters in primary school finish their mandatory education, they will be indebted. At the same time, the opium growing of the Golden Triangle, which once was almost entirely for export, together with the civil war against the central Burmese government hegemony, has fostered the addiction of increasing numbers of hill tribesman and has corrupted law enforcement at all levels.

Therefore, within a couple of years of the relocation diffusion to Bangkok, HIV had moved from IDUs to commercial sex workers, and within another year the third phase had exploded in the male clients. As the businessmen, soldiers, college students, and laborers went home, the fourth wave burst in their current and future wives and girlfriends. By 1994, just 7 years after first detection, 7.6% of AIDS cases were infants. Northern Thailand was the first region to face the tragedy. As commercial sex workers became more infected, the industry extended to solicit, sometimes by force as actual slaves, new and younger women. Hill tribe girls in Burma are sold by addicted fathers or driven by the Burmese military onslaught across the border as refugees. The utterly destitute women of Cambodia were induced to fill the brothels that Thai businessmen set up for the United Nations troops that brought elections to the killing fields. The Khmer Rouge killed and starved 2 million people there 20 years ago, but the children who survived now struggle in a current population of 11 million that is already 2% positive for HIV.

New York City

In the United States nationally, the epidemic in the 1990s seems to have "stabilized" or at least slowed. This is usually ascribed to behavioral changes involving safer sex and public health interventions. Over time the virus may also be lowering its virulence or people their infectiousness (viremia). Cultural buffers have improved to protect the blood supply and change sexual behavior. New therapies have decreased the death rate in 1996 among all groups, and there has been an overall slowing of the epidemic (<5% case increase annually, compared with 18% increase a decade ago). That still means, however, that the number of people with AIDS increases 10% a year. The HIV prevalence rates have become more disproportionate and are now as follows: blacks, 177 per 100,000; Hispanics, 90 per 100,000; and whites, 30 per 100,000 (Council, 1997).

Once introduced, the virus went quickly to the top of the urban hierarchy, New York City (regionally known, simply, as "the city"). The costs of the epidemic, from the loss of talent to the expense of care, took a heavy toll and received a lot of attention. The virus progressed from an infection of gay men to IDUs to the girlfriends of users and then to those who prostitute themselves to support a cocaine habit, and thence to the heterosexual clients from the suburbs. What has been less noticed, however, is regionalization and expansion of the epidemic within the city and what it shows of spatial expression of social processes in the human geography of this country in general. The ideas and analysis which follow are based primarily on the work of Rodrick Wallace (Gould & Wallace, 1994; Wallace, 1990, 1991, 1993; Wallace & Fullilone, 1991; Wallace, Huang, Gould, & Wallace, 1997; Wallace & Wallace, 1995)

The AIDS epidemic in New York City is well described by Wallace as a "synergism of plagues." The prevalence of HIV is spatially associated, or regionalized, with drug abuse, violent death from homicide and suicide, low birthweights, high unemployment, crowded housing, arson, population mobility, and displacement. Wallace analyzes how the process began in the bourough of the Bronx in the late 1970s in what had been viable and famously vibrant ethnic communities. Rental housing became overcrowded even as employment and tax base moved out and education in public schools deteriorated. During the 1980s, national policies of "benign neglect" of the cities became local policies of "planned shrinkage" within New York. As incidence of arson, drug pushing, street crime, drug and alcohol abuse, and suicide, as well as low birthweight and infant mortality, increased in the southern Bronx; fire and police and medical services were withdrawn. A "meltdown of the sociogeographic structure" and social networks followed, hollowing out a burned-out section and displacing people to surrounding areas in an expansion–diffusion of social pathology. Medical service became gridlocked. Schools further deteriorated, as did employment opportunities. After discussing the improper policy role of government in triggering the syndrome, Wallace examines the critical thresholds of investment that would be required for "community recrystalization" which are, of course, much higher than would have been required to prevent meltdown. As the citywide population shifts (as in school pupils) diffused, an "interrelated nexus of behaviors adversely affecting both public health and public order" also transferred HIV to new marginalized communities. The poverty rates of communities surrounding the city became highly predictive of diffusion. The commuter network of the city is extensive. People from Long Island commonly commute more than 2 hours each way. First with commuting homosexuals and IDUs but, as the pathologies spread, increasingly through the heterosexual sex trade, the HIV expanded to the suburbs. In other cities, too, the spead of AIDS from the "hollowed-out center" of "physically and socially devasted, politically and economically abandoned high density minority neighborhoods to the suburbs as a single, spatially extended disease ecosystem" was confirmed. "Our empirical results contradict the conclusions of a recent National Research Council report that AIDS will be largely confined within marginalized urban populations. In reality U.S. urban apartheid, particularly its continuing disruption of minority social structures, has markedly accelerated the diffusion of AIDS into suburban communities" (Wallace & Wallace, 1995, p. 333.)

    One of the most important insights from this research is the foreshadowing of how future epidemics may spread. Regarding the current greatly increased housing and service problems in the city and emergence of multiple drug resistant tuberculosis, Wallace et al. (1997) observed:

> The devastation from that first burnout contributed materially to the return of TB, having an impact like a war. The social disintegration and forced migration of population resulting from another wave of burnout will overwhelm existing TB control programs—including the recently implemented program of Directly Observed Therapy—resulting in markedly increased numbers of patients who fail to complete their arduous six-to-nine month program of antibiotic therapy. This is the prescription for generating multiple-drug-resistant TB, as patients repeatedly enter the hospitals, are partially treated, and then are lost in the maelstrom of burning neighborhoods.
>
>   New York City's resistant TB strains can be expected to hopscotch betwen urban ghettoes along the national travel net—most cities did something equiva-

lently stupid to New York's ghetto fire service cuts—and then to ooze out along the commuting field into the suburbs: New York City greatly dominates the nation's urban hierarchy.

AIDS and TB are relatively slow diseases. . . . Both have had a similar incubation within marginalized populations concentrated in U.S. urban travel centers—the action of social vectors. We now await something from the increasingly global economic exploitation of the world's outback. . . . Ecological disruption and agricultural expansion . . . are increasingly likely to bring dangerous pathogens. . .

These may not be so slow. (p. 946)

OTHER EPIDEMICS

Maybe nothing is more inherently "geographical" than the study of the diffusion of disease at a variety of appropriate scales. This chapter has looked at the "social physics" of how disease agents diffuse through settlement systems with social contexts. Many epidemic infections which need study were not considered. Intervention in the recurrent epidemics of viral meningitis in West Africa come to mind. Perhaps the epidemic of rabies, which continues to spread in the eastern United States and Canada, especially among raccoons, is a more accessible target. Contagious diseases have an ecology, but their characteristics, impact, and prediction are especially appropriate for spatial analysis.

REFERENCES

Abler, R., Adams, J., & Gould, P. (1971). *Spatial organization: The geographer's view of the world.* Englewood Cliffs, NJ: Prentice Hall.

Bailey, N. J. T. (1957). *The mathematical theory of epidemics.* High Wycombe, England: Charles Griffin.

Bailey, N. J. T. (1975). *The mathematical theory of infectious diseases and its applications.* High Wycombe, England: Charles Griffin.

Baker, S. R. (1979). The diffusion of high technology medical innovation: The computed temography scanner example. *Social Science and Medicine, 13D,* 155–162.

Brown, T., & Sittitrai, W. (1995). *The impact of HIV on children in Thailand.* East West Center Program on Population, University of Hawaii and Thai Red Cross Society Program on AIDS, Honolulu, HI.

Brownlea, A. A. (1972). Modelling the geographic epidemiology of infectious hepatitis. In N. D. McGlashan (Eds.), *Medical geography: Techniques and field studies* (pp. 279–300). London: Methuen.

Burnet, M., & White, D. O. (1974). *Natural history of infectious diseases* (4th ed.). Cambridge, UK: Cambridge University Press.

Cliff, A. D., & Haggett, P. (1982). Methods for the measurement of epidemic velocity. *International Journal of Epidemiology, 11,* 82–89.

Cliff, A. D., & Haggett, P. (1983). Changing urban–rural contrasts in the velocity of measles epidemics in an island community. In N. D. McGlashan & J. R. Blunden (Eds.), *Geographical aspects of health* (pp. 335–348). London: Academic Press.

Cliff, A. D., & Haggett, P. (1988). *Atlas of disease distributions: Analytic approaches to epidemiological data.* Oxford, UK: Blackwell.

Cliff, A. D., & Haggett, P. (1989). Spatial aspects of epidemic control. *Progress in Human Geography, 13,* 315–437.

Cliff, A. D., Haggett, P., & Ord, J. K. (1986). *Spatial aspects of influenza epidemics.* London: Pion.

Cliff, A. D., Haggett, P., Ord, J. K., & Versey, C. R. (1981). *Spatial diffusion: An historical geography of epidemics in an island community.* Cambridge, UK: Cambridge University Press.

Cliff, A., Haggett, P., & Smallman-Raynor, M. (1993). *Measles: An historical geography of a major human viral disease from global expansion to local retreat, 1840–1990.* Cambridge, UK: Blackwell.

Council, A. A. (1997). *AIDS forum.* Washington, DC: C-SPAN.

Currie, W. (1792). *Historical account of the climates and diseases of the United States of America.* Philadelphia: Dobson.

Currie, W. (1811). *A view of the diseases most prevalent in the United States of America.* Philadelphia: J. & A. Y. Humphreys.

Dutt, A. K., Monroe, C. B., Dutta, H. M., & Prince, B. (1988). Geographical patterns of AIDS in the United States. *Geographical Review, 77,* 456–471.

Fairclough, G. (1995). A gathering storm. *Far Eastern Economic Review, 158,* 26–30.

Farmer, P. (1992). *AIDS and accusation: Haiti and the geography of blame.* Berkeley: University of California Press.

Farmer, P., Connors, M., & Simmons, J. (Eds.). (1996). *Women, poverty and AIDS.* Monroe, ME: Common Courage Press.

Gallo, R. (1986). The first human retrovirus. *Scientific American, 224,* 88–98.

Gardner, L. I., Jr., Brundage, J. F., McNeil, J. G., Visintine, R., & Miller, R. N. (1989). Spatial diffusion of the human immunodeficiency virus infection epidemic in the United States, 1985–87. *Annals of the Association of American Geographers, 79,* 25–43.

Gould, R. R. (1969). *Spatial diffusion* (Resource Paper No. 4). Washington, DC: Association of American Geographers Commission on College Geography.

Gould, P. (1984). *The geographer at work.* New York: Routledge.

Gould, P. (1993). *The slow plague: A geography of the AIDS pandemic.* Cambridge, MA: Blackwell.

Gould, P., & Wallace, R. (1994). Spatial structures and scientific paradoxes in the AIDS pandemic. *Geografiska Annaler, 76B,* 105–116.

Grmek, M. (1990). *History of AIDS: Emergence and origin of a modern pandemic.* Princeton, NJ: Princeton University Press.

Hagerstrand, T. (1952). *The propagation of innovation waves.* Lund, Sweden: Gleerup.

Haggett, P. (1976). Hybridizing alternative models of an epidemic diffusion process. *Economic Geography, 52,* 136–146.

Henry, N. F. (1978). The diffusion of abortion facilities in the northeastern United States, 1970–1976. *Social Science and Medicine, 12D,* 7–15.

Huet, T., Cheynier, R., Meyerhaus, A., Roelants, G., & Wain-Hobson, S. (1990). Genetic organization of a chimpanzee lentivirus related to HIV-1. *Nature, 345,* 356–359.

Kashamura, A. (1973). *Famille, sexualité, et culture: Essai sur les moeurs sexuelles et les cultures des peuples des Grands Lacs Africans.* Paris: Payot.

Kearns, R. (1996). AIDS and medical geography: embracing the Other? *Progress in Human Geography, 20,* 123–131.

Kwofie, K. M. (1976). A spatio-temporal analysis of cholera diffusion in western Africa. *Economic Geography, 52,* 127–135.

Lam, N. S.-N. (1996). Use of space-filling curves in generating a National Rural Sampling Frame for HIV/AIDS research. *Professional Geographer, 48,* 321–332.

Lam, N. S.-N., Fan, M., & Liu, K.-B. (1996). Spatial-temporal spread of the AIDS epidemic, 1982–1990: A correlogram analysis of four regions of the United States. *Geographical Analysis, 28,* 93–107.

Levy, J.A. (1996). HIV heterogeneity in transmission pathogenesis. In J. M. Mann & D. J. M. Tarantola (Eds.), *AIDS in the World II: Global dimensions, social roots, and responses.* (pp. 177–186). New York: Oxford University Press.

Loytonen, M. (1991). The spatial diffusion of human immunodeficiency virus type 1 in Finland, 1982–1997. *Annals of the Association of American Geographers, 81,* 127–151.

Marlink, R., Kanki, P., Thior, I., Travers, K., Eisen, G., Siby, T., Traore, I., Hsieh, C.-C., Dia, M. C., Gueye, E.-H., Hellinger, J., Gueye-Ndiaye, A., Sankalé, J. L., Ndoye, I., Mboup, S., & Essex, M. (1994, September 9). Reduced rate of disease development after HIV-2 infection as compared to HIV-1. *Science, 265,* 1587–1590.

Mertens, T. E., & Low-Beer, D. (1996). HIV and AIDS: Where is the epidemic going? *Bulletin of the World Health Organization, 74,* 121–129.

Morse, S.S. (1992). AIDS and beyond: Defining the rules for viral traffic. In E. Fee & D. M. Fox (Eds.), *AIDS: The making of a chronic disease.* Berkeley: University of California Presss.

Nada, P. (1989). AIDS viruses of animals and man. *Los Alamos Science, 18,* 54–89.

Osmanov, S., Heyward, W.L., & Esparza, J. (1996). HIV-1 Genetic variability: Implications for the development of HIV vaccines. *Antibiotics and Chemotherapy, 48,* 30–38.

Panos Institute. (1986). *AIDS and the Third World.* London: The Panos Institute and Norwegian Red Cross.

Panos Institute. (1992). *The hidden cost of AIDS: The challenge of HIV to development.* London: Panos Publications.

Pyle, G. F. (1969). The diffusion of cholera in the United States in the nineteenth century. *Geographic Analysis, 1,* 59–75.

Pyle, G. F. (1984). Spatial perspectives on influenza inoculation, acceptance, and policy. *Economic Geography, 60,* 273–293.

Pyle, G. F. (1986). *The diffusion of influenza.* Totowa, NJ: Rowman & Littlefield.

Senior, M. L. (1979). From gravity modeling to entropy maximising: a pedagogic guide. *Progress in Human Geography, 3,* 179–211.

Shannon, G., & Pyle, G. (1989). The origin and diffusion of AIDS: A view from medical geography. *Annals of the Association of American Geographers, 79,* 1–24.

Shannon, G. W., Pyle, G., & Bashushur, R. L. (1991). *The geography of AIDS.* New York: Guilford Press.

Smallman-Raynor, M. R., & Cliff, A. D. (1990). Acquired immunodeficiency syndrome (AIDS): literature, geographical origins and global patterns. *Progress in Human Geography, 14,* 157–213.

Smallman-Raynor, M. R., Cliff, A. D., & Haggett, P. (1992). *London international atlas of AIDS.* Oxford: Blackwell.

Smyth, F., & Thomas, R. (1996). Preventative action and the diffusion of HIV/AIDS. *Progress in Human Geography, 20,* 1–22.

Special Program on AIDS. (1987). *Strategies and structures: Projected needs.* Geneva: World Health Organization.

Stephenson, J. (1995). AIDS data animation maps evolving US epidemic. *Journal of the American Medical Association, 274,* 784.

Stock, R. F. (1976). *Cholera in Africa.* Plymouth, England: International Africa Institute.

Thomas, R. (1992). *Geomedical Systems: Intervention and control.* London: Routledge.

Thomas, R. (1996). Modelling space–time HIV/AIDS dynamics: Applications to disease control. *Social Science and Medicine, 43,* 353–366.

Wallace, R. (1990). Urban desertification, public health and public order: 'planned shrinkage,' violent death, substance abuse, and AIDS in the Bronx. *Social Science and Medicine, 31,* 801–813.

Wallace, R. (1991). Traveling waves of HIV infection on a low dimensional, sociogeographic network. *Social Science and Medicine, 32,* 847–852.

Wallace, R. (1993). Social disintegration and the spread of AIDS—II: Meltdown of sociogeographic structure in urban minority neighborhoods. *Social Science and Medicine, 37,* 887–896.

Wallace, R., & Fullilone, M. T. (1991). AIDS deaths in the Bronx 1987–1988: Spatiotemporal analysis from a sociogeographic perspective. *Environment and Planning A, 23,* 1701–1724.

Wallace, R., Huang, Y.-S., Gould, P., & Wallace, D. (1997). The hierarchical diffusion of AIDS and violent crime among U.S. Metropolitan Regions: Inner-city decay, stochastic resonance and reversal of the mortality transition. *Social Science and Medicine, 44,* 935–947.

Wallace, R., & Wallace, D. (1995). U.S. apartheid and the spread of AIDS to the suburbs: A multi-city analysis of the political economy and spatial epidemic threshold. *Social Science and Medicine, 41,* 333–345.

Webster, N. (1799). *A brief history of epidemic and pestilential diseases.* Hartford, CT: Hudson & Goodwin.

Welsh, M. J. (1994). *Peer educators' geographic range of effect: An analysis of an AIDS intervention in the dominican republic.* Doctoral dissertation, University of North Carolina at Chapel Hill.

Williams, J. S., & Rees, P. H. (1994). A simulation of the transmission of HIV and AIDS in regional populations within the United Kingdom. *Transactions of the Institute of British Geographers, 19,* 311–330.

Wills, C. (1996). *Yellow fever, black goddess: The coevolution of people and plagues.* New York: Addison-Wesley, Helix Books.

Wilson, A. G. (1974). *Urban and regional models in geography and planning.* New York: Wiley.

Wood, W. (1988). AIDS north and south. *Professional Geographer, 40,* 266–279.

FURTHER READING

Adesina, H. O. (1984a). The diffusion of cholera outside Ibadan City, Nigeria, 1971. *Social Science and Medicine, 18,* 421–428.

Adesina, H. O. (1984b). Identification of the cholera diffusion process in Ibadan, 1971. *Social Science and Medicine, 18,* 429–440.

Angulo, J. J., Haggett, P., Meghale, P., & Perderneiras, C. A. (1979). Variola minor in Braganca Paulista County, 1956: A trend–surface analysis. *American Journal of Epidemiology, 105*, 272–280.

Argulo, J. J. (1987). Interdisciplinary approaches in epidemic studies—II: Four geographic models of the flow of contagious disease. *Social Science and Medicine, 24*, 57–69.

Becker, C. M. (1990). The demo-economic impact of the AIDS pandemic in SubSaharan Africa. *World Development, 18*, 1599–1619.

Cohn, S.E., Klein, J.D., Mohr, J.E., van der Horst, C.M., & Weber, D.J. (1994). The geography of AIDS: Patterns of urban and rural migration. *Southern Medical Journal, 87*, 599–606.

Henry, N. F. (1978). The diffusion of abortion facilities in the northeastern United States, 1970–76. *Social Science and Medicine, 12D*, 7–15.

Nijkamp, P., & Reggiani, A. (1996). Space–time synergetics in innovation diffusion: A nested network simulation approach. *Geographic Analysis, 28*, 18–37.

Okeyo, T. M., Baltazar, G. M., & Johnston, A. (1996). *AIDS in Kenya: Background, projections, impact and interventions.* Kenya, Africa: National AIDS and STDs Control Programme, Ministry of Health, and National Council for Population and Development.

PAHO. (1996). New emerging and re-emerging infectious diseases. *Bulletin of the Pan American Health Organization, 30*, 176–181.

Pollitzer, R. (1959). *Cholera.* Geneva: World Health Organization.

Pyle, G. F., & Furuseth, O. J. (1992). The diffusion of AIDS and social deprivation in North Carolina. *The North Carolina Geographer, 1*, 1–10.

Shaeffer, S. F. (1994). *The Impact of HIV/AIDS on education: A review of literature and experience.* Paris: IIEP/UNESCO.

Smyth, F. M., & Thomas, R. W. (1996). Controlling HIV/AIDS in Ireland: The implications for health policy of some epidemic forecasts. *Environment and Planning A, 28*.

Thomas, R. W. (1993). Source region effects in epidemic disease modeling: Comparisons between influenza and HIV. *Papers in Regional Science, 72*, 257–282.

Thomas, R. W. (1996). Alternative population dynamics in selected HIV/AIDS modeling systems: Some cross-national comparisons. *Geographical Analysis, 27*, 108–125.

VIGNETTE 8-1.   Diffusion Waves and the Logistic Curve

It is often convenient to think of diffusion as waves of innovation and acceptance spreading geographically (Hagerstrand, 1952). These innovation impulses tend to lose their energy with distance from the source of the innovation. If we plot the acceptance of a new idea, or the onset of a disease contagion, for a series of time periods against the distance from the source, we can see how the innovation gradually fades with increased distance (Vignette 8-1, Figure 1). During each successive time period the locus of greatest initial acceptance of contagion is further from the source. During the first several periods the total volume of acceptance increases; after that, the number of new acceptances decreases with each successive period. The summation of all these time curves across space and through time results in a pair of bell-shaped curves. The geographic bell is centered over the original innovation point and identifies a declining share of the total population ever accepting the innovation with increasing distance. The second bell graphs the overall pattern of volume of acceptance (or contagion) from a small number of innovators through the great bulk of acceptors to a final few laggards.

The course of a diffusion process may be described with a logistic curve (Vignette 8-1, Figure 2). The curve is described by the formula

$$P = U/1 + e^{(a-bT)}$$

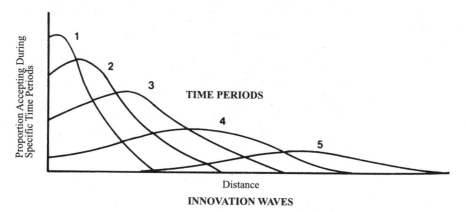

VIGNETTE 8-1, FIGURE 1. Innovation waves. Adapted from Gould (1969, p. 11). Copyright 1969 by Association of American Geographers. Adapted by permission.

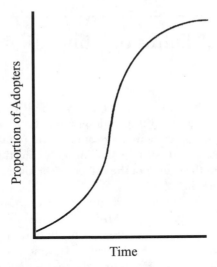

Time

VIGNETTE 8-1, FIGURE 2. Logistic curve. Many diffusion studies have identified the characteristic s-shaped curve of volume of adoption through time. Adapted from Gould (1969, p. 20). Copyright 1969 by Association of American Geographers. Adapted by permission.

where *P* is the proportion of adopters, *T* the time at some point in the diffusion process, *U* the upper limit of the adoption (10 if everyone accepts the innovation), *e* the base of natural logs (2.7183), and *a* and *b* particular values that describe the location and shape of the curve (*a* identifies the height above the time axis where the S-shaped curve starts, and *b* how quickly it rises). Because *a* and *b* define a particular curve so that it is like no other, they are parameters (constants in a relational expression that determine how two or more variables change together). The logistic curve can be thought of as a cumulative frequency curve derived from the bell-shaped curve of innovation acceptors.

VIGNETTE 8-2.   Diffusion Simulation

The geography of disease diffusion can be very complex. Within a small group, the probabilities of contact (and thus of infection) can be nearly random. However, the probability of contact between groups is often related to distance. How can this idea of a contact field, with the likelihood of infection decreasing with increasing distance from the source of the infection, be turned into an operational model to predict future diffusion?

Hagerstrand (1952) used the bell-shaped curve of probabilities of contact to determine a mean information field (MIF), or an area in which contacts might occur (Vignette 8-2. Figure 1). The greatest likelihood of contact is within the central cell fitted directly over the innovator. Distance decay in the chance of contact is equal in all directions. Hagerstrand used the MIF to initiate a stochastic simulation of the diffusion process. To prime the MIF, the range of numbers from 0 to 9,999 was assigned to each of its 25 cells on the basis of the cell's probability. Thus, each corner cell would receive 96 of the 10,000 digits, while the central grid gets 4,432.

The printed MIF can be used as the basis for the simulation process. The driving force that powers the model is a table of random numbers from 0 to 9,999. In a simple form of the model, one innovator exists. The MIF, which can be thought of as a grid floating over the underlying population, is centered over that innovator. He or she has the opportunity to pass the innovation to two other individuals. Those acceptors will be somewhere under the MIF grid. A random number is drawn to determine the grid location of the first acceptor. There is a nearly 45% chance that the acceptor will be in the same cell as the innovator and a less than 1% chance that the acceptor will be in one of the corner cells. Let us assume that the first acceptor is located under the cell immediately to the left of the innovator and the second acceptor is within the central cell. Thus, after the

.0096	.0140	.0168	.0140	.0096
.0140	.0301	.0547	.0301	.0140
.0168	.0547	.4432	.0547	.0168
.0140	.0301	.0547	.0301	.0140
.0096	.0140	.0168	.0140	.0096

VIGNETTE 8-2, FIGURE 1. Mean information field.

first generation (the first set of transfers), two individuals in two cells of the map now have the innovation. In each subsequent generation each individual with the innovation becomes an innovator and can pass it to two other persons. In generation 2, then, the floating MIF centers over each of the new acceptors, each time with a random number drawn to identify the locations of the next acceptors. In generation 3 these four will join the early acceptors, four individuals passing the innovation to eight others.

The ultimate pattern of diffusion may vary greatly from simulation to simulation. For example, if the first acceptor was to the left of the innovator, that might pull the pattern in that direction, which is known as direction bias. If the patterns resulting from many simulation exercises are combined, however, their overall pattern would approximate the bell-shaped curve with its high point centered over the innovator.

This Monte Carlo simulation model can be modified in many ways to better approximate reality. Is the innovator an especially powerful transmitter of the innovation? Then allow that individual several new contacts each generation while the other generations of innovators have only one. Is the disease very infectious? We can allow every innovator and acceptor to infect several new individuals each generation. Suppose the underlying population is unevenly distributed. This population can be used to create a set of normalized probabilities, with each cell's probability based not only distance from the innovator but also on its share of the total population. Barriers can be incorporated into the model as well. A permeable barrier (such as immunity levels) might mean that only every fourth attempted passage of the innovation into a cell beyond the barrier is successful. Other types of barriers can be similarly incorporated.

The opportunities for modification of the basic model to more precisely simulate reality are nearly limitless. However, the goal should be to model the essence of the diffusion process and to reduce to a minimum the number of modifications to the MIF model. The critical essence of the model is that it enables identification of these primary influences and suggests some approximation of their relative importance. Even a simple model, however, is difficult to run by hand. High-speed computers make feasible the great volume of arithmetic manipulations in a simulation modeling.

9

Health Care Delivery Systems Worldwide

This chapter presents an overview of health care issues that is broader than the usual geographic perspective. A process as complex as trying to prevent or cure illness cannot successfully rely on any one approach. Geographers will apply their own techniques to solving problems of disease and health, but they should be aware of other approaches.

The chapter begins with a definition of a medical or health care delivery system, along with an introduction to the concept of medical pluralism and a multidisciplinary approach to studying health. Following that is a summary of the beginnings, development, and diffusion of the world's major medical systems and how those systems are implemented in the health care delivery systems of several individual countries.

HEALTH CARE DELIVERY SYSTEMS

Combatting the insults that bring about illness requires appropriate physiological and immunological responses. All vertebrate life has evolved biological defense mechanisms: What makes humans unique is the addition of cultural responses to disease. Medical systems are part of the cultural response to disease.

What is a medical (or health care) delivery system? It consists of ill people and of practitioners who diagnose and treat illness. A good medical system also tries to enhance health before illness. Prevention, a healthy care environment, and good relationships between patients and medical personnel are important. Furthermore, patients and practitioners exist within a wide context of social institutions and beliefs involving health education, dietary taboos, government policies concerning the distribution of health re-

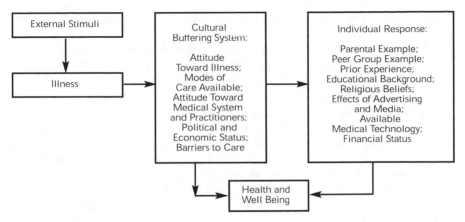

FIGURE 9-1. Interaction of the basic elements of a health care delivery system.

sources, the social and financial status of population groups, and ideas people have about what causes disease. The study of medical systems should not be too narrowly focused: Many studies have treated health problems, health personnel and facilities, the location of services, and the use of services as four separate entities when they are interrelated in health care delivery systems.

A *system* consists of a variety of distinct elements and interactions among them. A medical system consists of elements such as disease agents; hosts; vectors; cultural, economic, and environmental conditions; caregivers; government regulation; human behavior; and intervention, including the interactions among all of these (Figure 9-1). In any system, positive and negative feedback mechanisms are at work. As examples, consider that patients' experiences with a caregiver could lead to more or fewer referrals to that caregiver; an improvement in the urban environment could reduce visits to a care provider; and health education for a particular population group could result in improved diet, which in turn results in a more disease resistant physical state.

THE MULTIDISCIPLINARY APPROACH

Because health care delivery involves or intersects with a large part of human culture and the environment, its study must involve contributions from many areas of inquiry. The scientific study of medicine is essential. The natural sciences are emphasized: basic fields such as biology and chemistry and newly developed specialties such as genetic engineering and molecular biology. The branches of public health—epidemiology, health administration and education, environmental health, and biostatistics—are involved in the study of health care. In the last few decades, social science has become very much involved.

Cultural norms are as important as the biological characteristics of a disease in defining health and ill health. Eyles and Woods (1983), and Jones and Moon (1987) discuss the inextricable relationships between disease, health, and society. They point out that disease may be defined as abnormal biological deviation, but the question is, Who decides what is normal? "Normality is what prevalent social values hold to be acceptable or desirable, and in contrast to the biomedical notion of universal generic diseases, the social view accepts that what constitutes disease can vary temporally, culturally, and indeed, geographically" (Jones & Moon, 1987, p. 5).

Each of the social sciences has made a contribution to the study of health care delivery systems (Table 9-1). There are at least two reasons to be aware of these contributions. First, a knowledge of other approaches aids in understanding the spatial aspects of health care delivery. For example, the distance people are willing to travel to a hospital may be influenced by their social class. Second, the factors that each social science discipline emphasizes in studying medical systems can be seen as constraints on how a system can actually function. There are many social, economic, and political factors in society that help determine how disease is perceived and how treatment will be provided and accepted (Gesler, 1991).

TABLE 9-1. Social Science Contributions to Health Care Delivery Study

Discipline	Contribution
Anthropology/sociology	Comparative health care systems
	Beliefs about illness causes and effective treatments
	Characteristics of patients and practitioners
	Patient–practitioner relationships
Economics	Medical costs, cost-benefit analysis, and regulation
	Private and public payment plans
	Health care and economic development
Geography	Analysis of location of health care facilities
	Direction and distance of movement to facilities by patients
	Allocation of patients to facilities under various social conditions
	Effects of place (culture and environment) on quality of health care
History	Evolution of the major medical systems
	Changes in illness prevalence and treatment modes
	Awareness of historical inertia
Political science	Impact of type of medical system
	Role of public and private power-wielding groups
Psychology	Societal influences on mental and physical illness
	Doctor–patient relationships and effects on health
	Physiological factors in substance abuse

MEDICAL PLURALISM

The existence and use of multiple sources of medical care, traditional and modern, defines *medical pluralism*. This may mean pluralism in the sense that several systems of medicine coexist, giving multiple choices to individuals, or it may mean pluralism within a particular system, allowing patients access to various levels and types of care. There is cultural pluralism in every country. The varieties of religions and languages in India, of tribal backgrounds in Nigeria, of social status in Brazil, and of ethnicity in the United States, are all examples of cultural pluralism.

It should not be surprising that medical pluralism exists throughout the world as well. Still, we tend to be ethnocentric; that is, we feel that our cultural group and our traits are superior to others. Certainly this is true of the attitude of most Westerners toward health care. The biomedical, or modern or Western, system, with its firmly entrenched elements of physicians, nurses, technicians, hospitals, clinics, high-technology equipment, drug industry, and research laboratories, is *the* medical system for most people in the industrialized world and also for elite groups in the Third World. Alternative medical systems, however, exist and flourish. In North America, for example, one may find holistic health care, chiropractic, lay midwives, *espiritismos* and *curanderos* among Hispanics, and root doctors among blacks. All systems have strengths and weaknesses and work in different ways, according to the beliefs and expectations of the people served, but they all "work" or they would not be tolerated.

Many of the first Western doctors who visited non-Western countries in the past assumed that health care did not exist in those countries and that biomedicine would be filling a vacuum. Non-Western medicine, however, continues to serve most of the world's health needs. Despite attempts to extend biomedicine to all parts of the globe, it is too expensive for most people, and not culturally relevant for many. The significance of pluralism for the poorest Third World countries is that although virtually all nations want access to modern health care for their citizens, the means and resources for this often do not exist. Thus, after self-treatment, traditional medicine is the main provider of health care to local, especially rural, populations.

HISTORY OF THE WORLD'S MAJOR MEDICAL SYSTEMS

Medicine in Prehistoric and Ancient Times

Evidence from paleopathology (the scientific study of disease in former times) shows that the precursors of human disease are far older than humans. The bones of dinosaurs, for example, show evidence of damage from arthritis. When humans evolved over 2 million years ago, many potentially harmful pathogens already existed. We can surmise that before the neolithic revolution (around 8000 B.C.) humans suffered mostly from pathogens that could survive in small, nomadic populations or that were transmitted by animals. As humans settled into agricultural communities, they were exposed to a variety of new diseases to which they had immunological responses. These diseases, which included measles, smallpox, whooping cough, diphtheria, and tuberculosis, depended for steady transmission on the presence of relatively large groups of people living in close proximity.

It is assumed that humans have always made attempts to combat disease. Concrete records of specific treatments are scanty. There is evidence that trepanning (trephining) was practiced by neolithic humans. This technique, often the work of a skilled surgeon, was primarily used to bore holes into the skull. The main purpose for trepanning is not clear; it may have been performed to relieve headaches, to remove bone fragments following an injury, or to let evil spirits out of people afflicted with epilepsy.

The first solid evidence of medical practice has been found in the primary culture hearths that produced the earliest written records. The medicine of these ancient civilizations had roots in the supernatural, and practitioners were essentially priests. There is evidence, however, of empiricism, practical organization, and the beginnings of public health. Egypt was famous in ancient times for its medical techniques. Physicians and dentists practiced there as early as 2700 B.C. The earliest known legal code, the code of King Hammurabi of Babylon (2250? B.C.), contains laws on malpractice and setting medical fees. The Indus Valley and North China were the birthplaces of the *ayurvedic* and Chinese medical systems. The Yellow Emperor's medical treatise codified the thoughts of Chinese medical practitioners on disease causation and treatment. Written between 2600 and 1000 B.C., this is the world's oldest medical text. Public health and medical practice in the New World, reported by the European explorers of the 15th and 16th centuries A.D., was on a par with the rest of the world. In particular, the Spaniards highly praised the sewerage systems of the Incas.

Origins of Professional Systems

As societies developed in complexity, a variety of systems of treating illness developed. Four traditional systems, Chinese, ayurvedic, galenic, and unani, have developed and persisted for centuries (Figure 9-2). A fifth, biomedicine, has its roots in 2nd- or 3rd-century Greek culture. Biomedicine is sometimes also called Western medicine or modern medicine. All these systems are professional; they are highly organized and have an established array of techniques and codes of conduct. All have a highly developed pharmacopoeia and long and progressive histories, and they serve very large populations today.

Chinese medicine developed during the Chou dynasty (1121–225 B.C.) and the Han dynasty (206 B.C.–A.D. 221). Disease was considered to be the re-

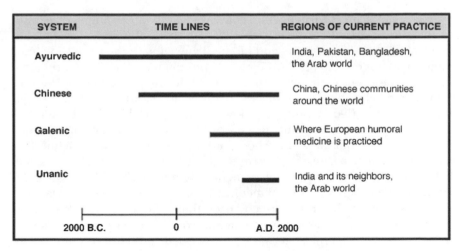

SYSTEM	TIME LINES	REGIONS OF CURRENT PRACTICE
Ayurvedic		India, Pakistan, Bangladesh, the Arab world
Chinese		China, Chinese communities around the world
Galenic		Where European humoral medicine is practiced
Unanic		India and its neighbors, the Arab world

2000 B.C.   0   A.D. 2000

FIGURE 9-2. Time line of professional medical systems.

sult of disharmonies in the body, between humans and the environment, and even throughout the universe. The treatment of disease arose from philosophical concepts such as that of *yin* and *yang*, which are the negative and positive principles of universal life. Yin stands for things such as earth, moon, darkness, and femaleness, and yang symbolizes heaven, sun, light, and maleness. The life energy *ch'i* flows through the "meridians" of the body. The meridians touch the skin at special points that can be stimulated by heat, pressure, or needles in the healing technique of acupuncture. China remains the core area of the practice of Chinese medicine, but it is practiced wherever Chinese people have migrated. Its influence has been greatest in Korea and Japan, part of China's cultural sphere.

The origins of *ayurvedic* medicine, which means "the science of living to a ripe age," can be traced to the migration of Aryans into the Indus Valley and the development of Harappa culture around 2000 B.C. By the 6th and 5th centuries B.C. the Indian medical system had approached its present form (Basham, 1976). In this system, disease represents a disequilibrium of the humors (wind, bile, mucous, and blood), and cures attempt to reestablish a proper balance. Health is related to *karma*, or the effect of good and evil deeds, in both former lives and one's present life. Practitioners of ayurvedic medicine must have a comprehensive knowledge of pharmacopoeia and understand well the influences on health of climate and morality.

Ayurvedic medicine is important for both rural and urban Indians. Its core area is North India; South India has many ayurvedic practitioners but also established the *siddha* system, which employed substances that purportedly could transform base metals into gold as well as aid in rejuvenating the human body. Although siddha has its origins in the Dravidian culture of South India, in diagnosis and treatment it generally corresponds with ayurvedic medicine. Indian migrants have carried their ancient medical practices to other parts of the globe, particularly to the Arab world.

Galenic medicine, unani, and biomedicine all have their roots in Greek medicine. Hippocrates (460?–377? B.C.), from the island of Cos, represented the culmination of early Greek medicine. By his time, the idea of the four fundamental elements in nature (hot, dry, wet, and cold) and the four bodily fluids, or *humors* (blood, phlegm, yellow bile, and black bile) had been developed. A healthy person maintained a proper balance of these humors, which originated from four parts of the body and were associated with the four fundamental elements. Disease and treatment depended on proper or improper balances among the humors and elements. Hippocrates' *On Airs, Waters, and Places* was the first great classic of medical geography: It associated certain diseases with certain climates and recognized that cultural practices and social institutions can change or temper climatic conditions. Hippocrates denied that disease had supernatural causes and stressed careful observation of patients. One of the many statements ascribed to Hippocrates is, "Persons who are naturally very fat are apt to die earlier than those who are slender" (Hippocrates, 1939, p. 305).

After the time of Hippocrates, many humoral and nonhumoral schools of medicine arose in Greece. Only with the coming of Galen of Pergamon (A.D. 130–201) did humoral medicine gain the upper hand. Galen, the "father of experimental physiology," was a Greek residing in Rome. He was physician to the emperor Marcus Aurelius. His experimental insights became important texts, first for the Islamic Arab civilization and in the early Renaissance for Western Europe. He modified the Hippocratic idea, that an equilibrium of humors could be achieved, by teaching that physical, cultural, and demographic factors could cause one of the four humors to dominate and produce a unique "temperament": sanguine, phlegmatic, choleric, or melancholic.

The *galenic* body of medical thought held sway in Europe for 1,500 years. Galenic practice began to lose its importance only over the last 300 years. When Europeans began exploring and colonizing the world after A.D. 1500, galenic medicine diffused along with many other cultural traits.

The Arabs took over the system of Greek medicine in the 7th and 8th centuries A.D. and called it *unani* ("Greek" in Arabic). In common with other early medical systems unani had a strong ethical element and stressed the importance of the doctor–patient relationship in healing and the influence of beliefs on disease and health.

Western incursions into the Arab world in the 19th century led to the decline and eventual stagnation of unani. Biomedicine supplanted unani to a large extent. Unani is still important in South Asia, where it was introduced by Moslem conquerors. Unani exists alongside systems like ayurvedic, siddha, and biomedicine in India, Pakistan, Sri Lanka, and other South Asian countries. Some of these countries have established state and private pharmaceutical companies that produce unani drugs. Unani is also important in other areas of strong Moslem influence, Southeast Asia in particular.

Biomedicine arose out of the galenic medical tradition. Practitioners of galenic medicine in post-Renaissance times were sympathetic toward experimental physiology, which led to many important medical discoveries (such as the circulation of blood). Biomedicine advanced during the development of scientific method and inquiry: The 19th-century discoveries in bacteriology gave scientific medicine its present high status. These discoveries, collectively *germ theory*, focused on the idea that infectious diseases are caused by microorganisms. Two outstanding bacteriologists were Louis Pasteur (1822–1895) of France and Robert Koch (1842–1910) of Germany. Pasteur identified the organisms that produce anthrax and fowl cholera and worked on vaccines for these diseases; he also developed an antirabies vaccine, although rabies is caused by a virus and viruses could not yet be identified. Koch identified the bacteria that caused wound infections, developed better techniques to identify bacteria, and discovered the germ that causes tuberculosis. Several other scientists entered the new field of bacteriology, and between 1875 and 1905 about two dozen disease agents were found. During this period there were also discoveries in serology and immunology; disease vectors such as the tsetse fly and *Anopheles* mosquito were identified, surgery and gynecology advanced, and anesthetics and antiseptic conditions became part of operating procedures.

Public health improvements were of great significance in the 19th century. In fact, modern sanitation movements preceded bacteriology. Increased life expectancy in the Western world between 1850 and 1950 was due more to preventive than to curative medicine. Germ theory merely confirmed the validity of the ancient idea that cleanliness was important to health.

In terms of biomedicine's organization, two movements are most important. Specialization was spurred by the rapid accumulation of vast amounts of new information in diverse areas of medicine. Professionalization tightened ethical and educational standards within established medicine, partly in response to proliferation of nonscientific, nonestablishment health practitioners. For example midwifery clashed with professional obstetric and gynecological groups in the 19th century. Such organizations as the British Medical Association (1832) and American Medical Association (1847) were formed.

Of all the world's major professional medical systems, biomedicine has clearly been the most widely diffused. This medical system has become synonymous with the culture of illness and health in many Western countries, and the Third World has adopted it to varying degrees. Each European power introduced biomedical practices to its colonies. The first European physicians to work in most colonial nations were too few in number to care for any but colonial and military personnel, other Europeans, and a limited number of native persons in the upper social strata (Phillips, 1990). When it was recognized that many diseases are contagious, programs were initiated to treat larger populations that were in contact with Europeans. Despite this, health for colonial people remained as poor as it had been in precolonial days.

Biomedicine had little real impact in the Third World until after World

War II, when the colonial governments began to train native assistants in Western medicine while others went abroad to study medicine. When the colonized countries gained their independence, a native elite had acculturated to Western medicine. This elite perpetuated the Western medical hegemony. Since then biomedicine has played a major role in the mortality transition, one of the primary reasons for today's population growth in developing areas (see Chapter 4).

The relationships among biomedicine and other health systems in the United States have shifted over the last century. Medical pluralism in the United States is represented by the primary, or establishment, biomedical system, plus alternatives such as holistic health care, lay midwifery, chiropractic, Christian Science, homeopathy, root doctors, *espiritismos*, and *curanderos*. These alternatives are based on paradigms that differ from those of the dominant medical system within a society. Some of these alternatives cross ethnic and socioeconomic boundaries; others are confined to certain groups and localities.

The relative importance of the biomedical and alternative subsystems in the United States has shifted over space and time in response to cultural change. The temporal shift can be partially understood in terms of the changes in biomedicine since 1850. The system has gone through three stages, or phases of a dialectical process: thesis, antithesis, and synthesis. At the beginning of stage I, humoral ideas dominated the practice of medicine. Following discoveries in germ theory toward the end of the 19th century, modern biomedical practice began to emerge and gain ground. At the same time, some traditional practices, such as lay midwifery, declined in importance. In stage 2 some successful innovations (e.g., certain surgical procedures such as anesthesia, skin grafting, and artery clamps) proliferated, biomedicine expanded rapidly, and doctors began to enjoy a high status socially and financially. However, around 1950 the establishment system began to be criticized for neglecting the whole person; for its overemphasis on reductionist, biomedical thinking; for a slavish devotion to high-technology cures; and for accelerating costs. Some people began to turn to other systems of health care. During this stage, for example, holistic health care (HHC) started to be adopted by significant numbers of people. Stage 2 witnessed clashes among medical subsystems for control of resources and consumers. Attacks by the American Medical Association (AMA) on chiropractors and midwives is one example of this struggle. In stage 3, treatment innovations began to gain ground and old ideas were revived; each of the new subsystems began its own evolutionary cycle. The possibility for new syntheses arose at this stage. Thus, nurse midwives have emerged as a synthesis of lay midwifery and biomedical nursing, and many doctors have begun to practice in holistic settings (Gesler, 1991).

Geographer Isabel Dyck and others are critical of biomedicine on the grounds that it is less holistic, with heavy reliance on technological and pharmaceutical interventions in the illnesses of individuals (Dyck, 1992). Dyck points out that a particular environment may be labeled "unhealthy," but treatment of the individual is biomedicine's main concern and is practiced in isolation of the context of the "sick" individual's life. Dyck argues that the practice of medicine is but one factor in the health of individuals (Figure 9-3), with the organization of work, social networks, and government institutions and practices either contributing to health or being detrimental to it. Thus, the geography of health and by extension health care, is inextricably linked to the geography of cultural belief and practice. This theme is echoed in Chapters 10 and 11 as well.

Alternative Medicine

The cultures of preindustrial, traditional societies usually are complex and deal with the environment in sophisticated ways. Traditional medicine exists in various forms and under a range of names, including nonprofessional, indigenous, or traditional, although the more inclusive term "alternative medicine" is widely used today. Practitioners of traditional medicine are called healers, native doctors, shamans, or medicine men. The study of traditional medical systems has emerged in the discipline of *ethnomedicine*, which involves the study of beliefs and practices stemming from indigenous cultural development (Good, 1987).

Four general types of traditional practitioners may be identified: spiritual or magicoreligious healers, herbalists, technical specialists such as bone setters, and traditional birth attendants. The first category, *spiritual healers*, is the most common and includes respected healers and charlatans alike. Religion and magic have always been closely tied to healing in traditional soci-

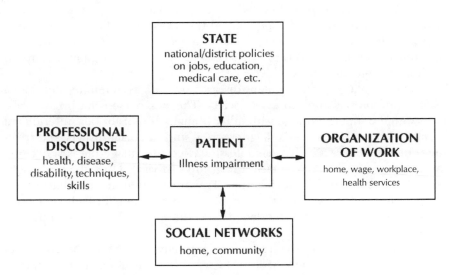

FIGURE 9-3. Factors in the health of individuals.

eties. Supernatural beings are believed to affect, among other things, illness and health. The healer mediates between the supernatural, the patient, and the community (Good, 1987). *Herbalists* focus on the use of medicinal plants to cure illness. Knowledge of herbal formulations is sometimes codified, sometimes simply passed down from healers to apprentices. Recently, research efforts into the nature and potency of herbally derived medicines have been expanding in Western nations. *Bone setters,* as the term implies, have a somewhat narrow focus, but in some places, their practice resembles that of chiropractic. *Traditional birth attendants* assist mothers at childbirth. The necessary skills may be acquired by helping experienced attendants deliver babies, or through modern training efforts sponsored within clinics and hospitals in many communities throughout the world. In Mexico, primarily poor illiterate women, living in remote areas with difficult access, rely on midwives. Because of this, the Mexican government implemented rural health programs in the late 1970s to train indigenous midwives (Parra, 1993).

Most traditional medical systems are confined to limited areas and specific populations, scattered throughout every continent (Gesler, 1984). Various Native Americans of both North and South America, numerous African tribes, and a variety of groups in Asia practice traditional medicine. It is estimated that traditional healers are the basic providers of health care in various guises for up to 90% of the rural population in South Asia and Africa. Various prescientific medical systems may involve directly or indirectly 80% of the world's population (Phillips, 1990).

Although it is difficult to generalize about the medical practices of all these people, some ideas and techniques are widespread. For example, diagnosis and treatment can be carried out by immediate family, kin, and/or group leaders as well as by healers. The various treatments held in common include the use of medicinal herbs, prayers, the sacrificing of animals, exorcisms, the wearing of sacred objects, and the transferral of disease from one person to another. Such treatments often depend on an intimate knowledge of intracommunity relations to be successful. They are especially effective in dealing with mental illness.

A healer may be a judge; many diseases are seen as stemming from violations of the morals and mores of society. The sick person has broken relations with the supernatural or with other humans and his or her suffering is a social sanction. The healer's diagnosis is a kind of social justice, and treatment often involves a cathartic confession. Because village life is very close-knit, tensions must be resolved for the group's survival. Thus, the healer also plays a role of creating "psychic unity." Treatment often includes having sick people, their relatives, and other people bring out their ill feelings toward each other. The healer's knowledge of community conflicts is important here.

Another function of the healer is to entertain, to perform before an audience (Good, 1987). Many Africans expect ritual treatment to be included along with medication. Music, drama, storytelling, myth making, dance, and fantastic costumes become part of the healing ritual. The healer may even go into a trance. These efforts can inspire intense emotion in the audience and have a positive effect on the group's everyday behavior.

In many African societies, much less distinction is made between material and spiritual worlds than in Western nations. Illness may be viewed as having a social or spiritual origin, in addition to physiological causes. A psychosocial approach to medicine is therefore applied in African medicine where a person's body, mind, and soul are conceived as an indivisible whole. A medicine may be both a substance administered to treat and prevent illness or anything used to control the spiritual cause of illness. Although biomedicine appears to be eclipsing traditional treatment in sub-Saharan Africa, indigenous remedies can be just as effective and much cheaper, more accessible and easily understood by local populations than their biomedical counterparts. Madge (1998) maintains that proven indigenous remedies ought to be incorporated into formal medical curricula and outreach programs for students and professionals before such knowledge is lost.

Stepan (1983) describes four categories of local or national legal regulation of traditional medicine: exclusive, tolerant, inclusive, and integrated. *Exclusive* systems of regulation allow only the practice of modern biomedicine. The justification for a ban on other forms of practice is that it protects the public from unqualified practitioners, but it has the effect of sustaining a monopoly on the part of the scientific medical hierarchy. Exclusivity has little effect in countries or regions where expensive biomedicine is inadequate and unable to satisfy even the most basic health needs, and where the people have always depended on traditional forms of healing. Exclusivity was introduced into many European territories during the colonial period, and traditional healers have since had little if any legal standing or official recognition. Western medicine was introduced to Korea by American missionary and Japanese (Western trained) doctors at the end of the 19th century. The Korean governments have since established policies of promoting Western medicine while suppressing and ignoring traditional practices (Son, 1999).

In *tolerant* legal systems, such as those of Germany, the United Kingdom, former British colonies, and some Latin American countries, the practice of various forms of alternative medicine is legally tolerated, though biomedicine is the dominant form and the practice of medicine is strictly regulated. Uganda, Sierra Leone, and Ghana allow any system of therapeutics, provided its practitioners are trained and recognized by their community. Some former French African colonies have been slow to extend legal status to traditional medicine, and countries such as Lesotho and Swaziland attempt to limit the practice of traditional medicine in one way or another (Phillips, 1990).

Inclusive systems consider both biomedicine and traditional medicine legal. This usually occurs where popular traditional systems predate modern medicine. In South Asia, indigenous medicine is part of the state-regulated structure of health care. In India, there is a Central Council of Medicine that is responsible for the regulation and teaching of ayurveda, siddha, and unani (Stepan, 1983). Pakistan and Sri Lanka also recognize traditional medicine within their official medical establishments. Since it achieved independence, India has allocated considerable funds to the development and teaching of traditional medicine.

China has a medical system that is regarded as *integrated*; that is, there is official government promotion of a single medical system in which the training of health practitioners in both biomedical and traditional systems takes place. The policy of the World Health Organization is to encourage some form of integration to optimize health care coverage. In fact, as the misunderstanding, skepticism, and fear once expressed about alternative medicine by Westerners fade gradually, alternative forms are being increasingly accepted in modern societies.

NATIONAL/REGIONAL EXAMPLES

The following descriptions of health care systems provide examples from places with a wide range of disease patterns, levels of industrialization, and government systems.

Tropical Africa

All African nations south of the Sahara (with the exception of South Africa) are, by most economic and demographic indicators, considered part of the developing world. It has been estimated that some 218 million persons in tropical Africa were without access to health services in 1990; the average population-to-physician ratio was well over 5,000 to 1 in these nations (Instituto del Tercer Mundo, 1994). This is in stark contrast to 13 nations in Western Europe and North America, which have an average ratio of 484 to 1 (Organization for Economic Cooperation and Development, 1990).

Long before European contact, traditional medicine, with its rituals of magic and religion, was an important influence in African society. Europeans who arrived in Africa in the 19th and early 20th centuries brought with them modern medical systems that emphasized curative practices but did not exclude ideas about disease prevention. Consonant with their mission of natural resource exploitation, colonial governments quickly turned coastal towns into shipping centers. In so doing, they developed industries that attracted many foreigners and rural migrants. These entrepots, called *primate cities*, grew to many times the population size of the next smallest settlement. The government also imported modern health facilities, primarily for the use of colonists and their military forces. Meanwhile, the vast majority of the population remained in rural villages, and their health care was in the hands of traditional nonprofessional healers or missionaries.

Today, the situation remains much the same. Especially outside cities, traditional medical practitioners remain the principal providers of health care for most Africans. In Zambia, for example, some 80% of the population resides in villages but only have access to a small proportion of the formal health care available (Akhtar & Izhar, 1986b). In Swaziland, the vast majority of the population uses the services of traditional healers. In Malawi, in the late 1980s, some 5,000 traditional practitioners served a population of almost 8 million (Phillips, 1990). In Mauritius, despite a rapid pace of modernization, this multicultural society continues to rely on both biomedicine and alternative sources of care, including ayurveda, homeopathy, Chinese medicine, and others. According to Kalla (1995), alternative medicine predominates over biomedicine.

It is common in Africa to find a complex web of modern, traditional, military, governmental, and voluntary organizations providing a wide ranges of health services. Phillips (1990) points out that when a choice of therapies is available, the decision to select one over the others is often not a function of user characteristics or attitudes but is strongly conditioned by political and economic factors, or simply by the relative accessibility of the service. In Ghana, unregulated itinerant drug vendors have emerged as a new breed of health providers in the absence of other sources (Oppong, 1998). In Zimbabwe, a strong effort was made in the 1980s to improve government primary health care in rural areas. Medical school enrollments increased at the national university, but the effort was undermined when many of the graduates abandoned government health service for private practice where the remuneration is considerably higher (Woelk, 1994).

In some African nations, such as Gambia, Somalia, Rwanda, Angola, and Ethiopia, poverty, drought, and political strife have combined to create a nightmare of illness and injury for rural and urban residents alike. In these countries, defense spending consumes a greater proportion of gross national product (GNP) than does education, and military facilities account for a large proportion of hospital beds and doctors (Akin, Guilkey, Griffin, & Poplin, 1985). In areas where daily life is disrupted by combat, virtually all available health facilities and medical supplies might be in military hands.

Often charitable or religious organizations or international aid agencies establish health facilities in Third World countries. Such facilities generally provide health care free, or nearly free, to residents in the vicinity. This service can provide substantial amounts of care and medical supplies. In Malawi, the organization Médecins Sans Frontières provided care for refugees in formal camps; in Zambia, missionary societies at one time contributed almost all rural health care; in Zaire, in the mid-1970s, missionaries provided considerable amounts of the country's rural modern health services; and mission hospitals in Ghana are estimated to maintain nearly a third of all hospital beds. Charitable organizations have a tendency to focus on primary health care, particularly in villages and rural areas. In some nations, volunteer organizations are more or less formally integrated into the national health care system.

China

When China opened its frontiers to trade with Europe in the middle of the 19th century, visiting missionary doctors introduced biomedicine. It was embraced to the extent that it was effective on illnesses for which traditional medicine had no cures. Prior to the Communist revolution of 1949, China was a poor nation, rife with disease (widespread malaria, schistosomiasis, typhoid, and tuberculosis), high infant mortality, and severely limited medical resources (one doctor served more than 7,000 people).

Following the establishment of the People's Republic, a massive health campaign was launched that succeeded in eliminating venereal disease and subduing schistosomiasis and infectious diseases. Integrating traditional and Western medicine, simple paramedical training was given to peasants and soldiers. Instead of sending out teams of public health experts to halt disease and destroy pests, the entire populations of many areas were educated in such basic ideas as composting human waste to destroy pathogens or elimination of snails that transmit schistosomiasis.

During the Cultural Revolution (1966–1969), the Chinese embarked on a rural cooperative medical care system with a three-tier structure of health care delivery. Primary health care was provided by the *Barefoot Doctor* program based at village clinics. Each clinic was staffed by one or a few doctors, midwifes, and health aides and served between 1,000 and 3,000 people. At the township level, a health center supervised the village clinics and provided a greater range of preventive and curative services. Township centers had an average of 16 health care personnel and served a population of 15,000 to 50,000 persons. These centers were general health institutions that provided both preventive and curative services. At the top of the hierarchy was the county hospital, which provided care to between 400,000 and 1.3 million persons. The county organization also supervised township clinics and provided the greatest range of primary and specialty services. Ninety percent of villages were covered by such schemes in the mid- and late 1970s (Xingyuan et al., 1993). This system resulted in substantial improvements in China's health and is widely regarded as a model of community-based primary health care. Life expectancy has risen to 71 years and the infant mortality rate has fallen to about 30 per 1,000 live births (Population Reference Bureau, 1999). However, regional improvements have been uneven. The health of a region is mainly a function of the prosperity of that region. Some of the more remote regions rely predominantly on traditional medicines; the more cosmopolitan areas rely more on a Western-style approach (Rosenthal & Frenkel, 1992).

The Chinese health care system is highly centralized and multisectoral. It consists of the national health sector administered by the villages, townships, and counties; the military health sector; the industrial health sector, which includes the health organizations of factories, mining, railway, and postal industries; and others, including public security, education, and civil administration.

In his writings about the Chinese medical care system, geographer Christopher Smith provides evidence that, because of the continuing changeover in the collective economy, many of the cooperative medical care schemes have been compromised. During the 1980s agricultural reforms made it possible for many of China's peasants to increase their incomes significantly. A new era of consumption accompanied this rise in wealth, which fed a growing demand for more individualized and higher-quality health care. As a result, many doctors resigned from public hospitals to establish their own private practice. In the mid-1980s, more than 30% of all rural health care facilities were privately owned (Smith, 1993). The number of Barefoot Doctors currently practicing is down. Villages are no longer able to finance their clinics and many have closed or have been transformed into private practice centers. In 1989, fee-for-service clinics accounted for almost 60% of all village health care centers, and only 5% of rural residents were covered by the old cooperative system. In the absence of state support and control, physicians and other care providers have gradually increased their fees. "Although this seems quite natural to Western observers, the danger in the Chinese countryside is that without the guarantee of collectively provided health care, the market mechanisms may leave the poorest areas and the poorest households relatively underserved" (Smith, 1993, p. 765).

China has attempted to fit its health care into its social fabric. How successful has it been in providing health care for all its people? For the most part, national reforms have been judged successful, both from within and without. Against great odds, an innovative approach to health care and maintenance has emerged, driven by political ideology and determination and making creative use of available resources. Still, there is inequality in access to health care, some of which has materialized in the reform era (Smith & Fan, 1995). Rural areas are still disadvantaged in comparison to urban places, and preventive efforts for chronic disease and efforts to institute individual lifestyle changes remain weak (Smith, 1998). Living in the city (as opposed to the countryside) carries with it an urban "passport" which legitimizes one's status and provides access to whatever services are available in that city. Transitions in the economy have created a rural-to-urban migration stream as people relocate in an attempt to improve their quality of life. This "floating population" has discovered that health care and other services are not necessarily universal rights or entitlements in their urban destination. Few of these "floaters" are provided with health care benefits by their employers. A sociological attribute—where one is employed—also has an impact on the individual's access to health care. Employees in the prestigious state sector have always enjoyed access to the best of the available services. The world continues to watch as China's economy encourages a private medical sector and experiments with private health insurance.

India and Sri Lanka

As Europeans began to arrive on the Indian subcontinent in the 15th to 16th centuries, three of the traditional professional systems discussed previously already existed there. Ayurvedic medicine was found in most areas, siddha was concentrated in southern India, and unani, a Moslem import, was also practiced. The British and others introduced biomedicine, and immunization campaigns and treatment centers slowly began to reach the mass of people. As in many other parts of the Third World, Christian missions also supplied health care, often in remote areas.

Today, reflecting India's mixed economy, health care delivery is supported from both the public and private sectors. India and Sri Lanka both have highly diversified and pluralistic health care systems, and both have taken serious steps to promote traditional medicine nationally on a large scale. Both traditional professional and Western-trained doctors have private practices and charge fees for service on a profit-making basis. Traditional medicine in India parallels biomedicine in terms of professional organizations, practitioners' enjoyment of high social status, and training institutions. The preparation of some traditionally based medicines occurs at an industrial scale. Factories manufacture and package a wide variety of commonly prescribed products.

India has significant regional and rural–urban differences in wealth, language, religion, social status, and other culture traits. Its heterogeneity results in spatial and social imbalance in the quantity and quality of available health care. Whereas over three-quarters of India's population is village based, the vast majority of hospitals and medical specialists are in the cities. In the mid-1980s, Mumbai (Bombay), Calcutta, and New Delhi had population-to-physician ratios of about 500 to 1, while elsewhere the ratio is over 7,000 to 1 (Akhtar & Izhar, 1986a). These inequities can be traced back to colonial days, when economic activities focused on port towns and strategic sites. The hinterlands with their indigenous populations were virtually ignored in every way.

Health care in India is typically dispensed in conventional settings, such as clinics and hospitals, but many rural communities do not have such facilities. In the southern state of Tamil Nadu, the government has sponsored traditional health care delivery through mobile clinics in an effort to reach these communities. Hyma, Phillips, and Ramesh (1994) report that although this innovation is a reasonably cost-effective approach to reaching low-income rural people with traditional health care, the effectiveness of these early efforts has been limited by inadequate advance advertising and infrequent and inconsistent scheduling. Patients report general satisfaction with the mobile facilities, although it has been suggested that more and better-trained staff would improve the service.

Several medical systems may exist side by side in India and Sri Lanka, often in competition with one another. The traditional professional systems generally have government approval and thus official status. The health care system of Sri Lanka is a highly diversified pluralistic one. Cosmopolitan medicine is available either free of charge from government-run hospitals and dispensaries or from private practice physicians for a fee. Several forms of traditional medicine are available. The government recognizes only those indigenous practitioners who have gained their education through a rigorous apprenticeship to a professional ayurvedic physician. Sinhala medicine provides the majority of traditional medicine on the island, usually dispensing only herbal remedies (Nordstrom, 1988).

The importance of traditional medicine is evident in Sri Lanka's official circles; there has been a Ministry of Indigenous Medicine in the government since 1980. Unfortunately, most doctors coming out of medical school prefer to specialize. Few have a desire to be involved in primary health care or teach. Furthermore, because most medical students come from cities, they know little of rural problems and are reluctant to practice in rural settings. Thus, like China, a substantial rural, poor population in India and Sri Lanka remains underserved.

The Commonwealth of Independent States

Like presocialist China, prerevolutionary Russia's health care system was inadequate to the needs of its population. Under Communism, access to health care was a major priority because it would enable establishing and maintaining a productive work force. The Soviet ideal of a health care model was one that was typified by a high level of public ownership and public funding and, like any other industry, by a high degree of central planning. The spatial organization of health care facilities followed rather closely the structure of central and local governments, which were based on population size.

The spatial–functional organization had seven hierarchical levels. The lower three levels, where basic care was provided, consisted of clinics that served rural farm areas (dispersed population, under 500 people), rural villages (500–2,500 people), and neighborhoods in towns and cities (3,000–65,000 people). In districts (40,000–150,000 people), treatment was usually given in polyclinics, the point of entry for most people. Further up the hierarchy were regional health departments (which serve 1–5 million people), ministries of health in the 15 republics (5–50 million people), and at the top the central Ministry of Health (responsible for about 250 million people).

Serious attempts were made to provide comprehensive service to the entire population. Treatment was free for half the population, and the rest made nominal payments only for drugs and other healing aids. The system boasted plentiful facilities and personnel. Much of the service was provided in the workplace. There were, however, inequalities and imbalances in access and quality. The system was rigid and unresponsive to individual needs. Job status was instrumental to the quality of service received. Some patients of relative wealth or privilege were able to circumvent the usual approach and gain access to an informal, more responsive system of care.

Primary health care was inadequate because almost all doctors were specialists. It focused on intermediate services rather than health outcomes. The Soviet system featured a higher physician–population ratio than could be found in other European nations; however, medical professionals were simply state employees and had weak status and influence, which led to low morale. The same level of service was not provided in all the 15 republics, and as elsewhere in the world, rural areas were at a disadvantage. The Soviets found it relatively easy to provide remote facilities, but despite incentives to doctors and other medical personnel to go to these places, members of the medical profession were able to resist such assignments. In an effort to supply care to rural areas, paramedics called *feldshers* were successfully employed.

Following the collapse of the Communist regime, the Commonwealth of Independent States (CIS) became responsible for their own health care delivery. These systems are smaller than the old central planning model and have problems that are more complex and difficult to solve with limited resources and constant political upheaval (The same may be said of other former Communist Eastern European states. (See Millard, 1995, for a discussion of post-Communist Poland.) There is some enthusiasm for a Western-style, free-market approach, with both health insurance and private payment choices. There is even talk of redirecting the emphasis away from curative services to illness prevention and health promotion. Enabling legislation was passed in 1991 to phase in programmatic changes over several years, but inflation and persistent poverty have a tendency to dampen citizen eagerness to pursue healthy lifestyles.

Variations in the quantity and quality of health care offered within and between the states will gradually evolve as relative differences in wealth and security and the viability of local political support become apparent. The states have no experience with the provision and administration of health services through insurance schemes. For those republics that have the resources, health care financing will be based on compulsory employer-supported insurance or will be funded from local taxes. It is possible that cartels will develop among providers, leading to price fixing and cost sharing. Insurance is not expected to provide comprehensive coverage, which will result in a demand for private supplementary insurance. A two-tier care system is likely to evolve—one for those who can afford no more than the basic insurance and another for those who have the means to purchase private supplementary insurance (Curtis, Petukhova, & Taket, 1995).

Sweden

The Swedes for many centuries have remained a close-knit group with focused national goals and a common cultural heritage. It is a fundamental principle in Sweden that all citizens are entitled to equal health care regardless of where they live and their economic status. Health care delivery in Sweden is often cited as the premier example of a welfare state system.

The first fully organized health care delivery system was established in 1960. It was notable for its attempt to create a functional–spatial organization. A geographer, Sven Godlund, was asked to conduct a study to determine which cities should become regional centers in the new system. The functional aspect is based on the minimum or threshold populations required to support different levels of facilities, such as large and small hospitals, clinics, and health centers. At each level of service is a geographic space in which accessibility to facilities is optimal. At the highest, regional level are large hospitals that provide many specialist services. Smaller hospitals with fewer beds and specialists provide service at the county level. District hospitals comprise the third level; these are often too small or poorly located to be effective. The most basic care is provided at the commune or township health centers. There are some regional imbalances in physician distribution, as some counties are more attractive to doctors than other, usually rural, counties.

Responsibility for comprehensive health services and for medical care is the duty of 26 county councils. A national health insurance system, financed by state and employer contributions, providing comprehensive medical and dental benefits, has existed since 1955. Physicians in the system receive a salary. Private health care exists on a limited but growing scale. About 5% of the nation's physicians, mainly in large cities, are in full-time private practice. A similar proportion of doctors are employed in private-sector industrial health outside the county council system.

In 1970, following an agreement between the central government, the county councils, and the Swedish Medical Association, physicians were made employees of hospitals, given fixed working hours and salaries, and were forbidden to accept fees for private care of patients in hospitals or outpatient facilities. Even private practice outside the hospital system has been restricted. In the 1980s, this policy was challenged by opposition conservative parties, who favored increased private practice. In the 1990s, Sweden, like other advanced Western nations, saw an increase in demand for technically sophisticated and expensive procedures and for long-term care for the aged.

In a country that already spends over 30% of its GNP on the public sector, there is resistance to additional taxation; changes will have to be made through redistribution of medical care personnel and resources from curative specialties to primary health care, especially in underserved areas. Already there is some experimentation in counties to allow municipalities to take over responsibility for primary health care. One county council has even decided to allocate financial resources to primary health care clinics, which can then purchase medical services from hospitals both within and outside the county (Wennstrom, 1992). There also have been attempts to provide more long-term care for the elderly and outpatient as opposed to hospital surgery. What is happening in Sweden is symptomatic of what occurs in all advanced developed nations, where critics claim that the "system" has been unresponsive to and has not planned adequately for structural changes in the population and its health needs.

It is generally acknowledged that Sweden, as well as other northern and western European nations, provides a high standard of technically excellent health care to its citizens. However, it is also recognized that medical care alone is inadequate to manage the problem of ill health. There is a growing demand for preventive health programs, involving the reduction of smoking and alcohol consumption and cleaning up the environment.

United Kingdom

Britain's National Health Service (NHS), which was established by law in 1946 and began to function in 1948, was seen as part of the new social order in Europe following World War II. The idea of equality of access that had been gathering force for some time in the United Kingdom was set out in four propositions: (1) The NHS should meet all acute and chronic medical needs, (2) health care should be universal and free to all citizens and bona fide foreign visitors, (3) funding would come from collective taxation rather than from payments by patients, and (4) the medical groups within the system would have professional independence.

The NHS struggled with organizational problems from its inception, which is typical for such a large undertaking. For years, the system was a model of inefficiency and duplication of service. Responsibility for health care was divided among hospital authorities, local governments, and 134 executive councils. The sizes of administrative regions and populations served were extremely varied. In 1974, an integrated, three-tiered structure was imposed to establish centralized control and decentralized execution. At the top was the Department of Health and Social Security. At the next level were 14 regional health authorities. The local level was governed by approximately 100 area health authorities. In 1982, the lowest level was abolished in favor of 192 smaller units called district health authorities. This move was intended to allow for more local decision making.

The NHS emphasizes the role of the general practitioner (GP) as the primary caregiver. The GP is the first health care contact for 97% of all residents in the United Kingdom. Patients with problems beyond the scope of general medicine are referred to specialists or hospitals. Though NHS care is free, the number of paying patients that GPs take is growing. In fact, some GPs are reluctant to take many NHS patients. This trend threatens to undermine the whole idea of the NHS and to produce two levels of care.

In 1990, parliament passed the National Health Service Reorganization and Community Care Act, which introduces elements of free enterprise into the NHS (Jefferys, 1992). Under this legislation, hospitals are given greater freedom to cut costs and manage their financial resources. The object is to introduce competition among hospitals such that the most efficiently managed ones will attract more patients and the best physicians. This has raised the concern that some hospitals will be able to avoid admitting cases that require heavy expenditure and extended stays, and that the remaining hospitals will be obliged to admit more costly cases with diminishing resources.

The legislation also provides for greater management of physicians. Family practitioner committees (FPCs) were formed to, among other things, initiate consumer surveys of satisfaction with provider services and to provide GPs with advice on professional procedures. GPs provide their FPCs with an annual report on their activities and practice development proposals, as well as information on their preventive medicine activities. Targets are set, and physicians who reach them are remunerated accordingly, whereas those who do not receive only minimum payment. A mandatory retirement age of 70 has also been established for some physicians.

The government's objective is to establish an element of competition which it considers has been missing since the NHS was founded. Physicians who oppose these changes argue that improvements in the quality of care are likely to come from peer cooperation rather than competition. They feel that GPs should have fewer rather than more patients on their lists if they are to provide them with sufficient time and attention. GPs who practice in affluent middle-class communities will have an advantage over GPs who practice in poor communities in terms of meeting preventive medicine targets. Since enactment of this legislation, a new government has taken power in the United Kingdom. It remains to be seen whether modifications will be made to the reform measures of the 1990 Act.

Geographers John Eyles and John Mohan have written extensively and critically about restructuring and other health care policies in Britain and elsewhere. Those interested are referred to the further readings at the end of the chapter.

Australia

Australia is the only developed country that, in the space of 20 years, moved from a system based on voluntary health insurance to a comprehensive tax-funded system—and repeated the process. In the 1930s, when the establishment of a national health system was first discussed, the medical profession established a firm and lasting position on health services: voluntary insurance with freedom of choice of doctor for patient and patient for doctor, opposition to the supply of medical services by the government, and insistence that patients partially reimburse care providers for their services.

In the early 1940s, the Labour Party took power. Labour established its own health care agenda with the simple position that health services should be treated the same as educational services, that is, it should be free and available to everyone and financed from tax-generated revenue. In a historic judgment, the Supreme Court declared Labour's first major health care plan unconstitutional in its regulation of the activities of physicians. Labour respond-ed by attempting to alter the constitution, and in the ensuing legislative struggle, a compromise was reached. A comprehensive health care scheme would be allowed, but at the instigation of the Australian Medical Associa-tion, wording was inserted into the referendum that disallowed "any form of civil conscription." This was a crucial amendment, as it limited government intervention in the staffing of health and welfare programs. It also ensured protection for the medical establishment and power to set fees for services.

It was the Conservative government, in the early 1950s, that actually in-troduced the first comprehensive health care scheme, and since then there have been several quite different systems in operation as the national govern-ment changed from Conservative to Labour to Conservative and back. When-ever Conservative coalitions governed, the voluntary insurance provision was in effect, allowing caregivers to charge partial fees for services. Whenever Labour was in power, some form of universal coverage was available, fi-nanced from taxes. In the mid-1970s, when Labour was voted into office, the party introduced a compulsory insurance scheme called *Medibank*. Funded from tax revenue, everyone was entitled to basic medical and hospital care without a financial means test. In December 1975, only 6 months after the es-tablishment of Medibank, the Liberal party was elected to power and Med-ibank was dismantled. In the confusion that followed, government withdrew its funding of community health centers. Commercial insurance companies entered the health field, offering, to those with good health histories, low-priced catastrophe insurance. Free of regulation, providers had a tendency to maximize the use of expensive technology and to order exhaustive tests while escalating fees. There were accusations of widespread fraudulence of claims for medical services among providers. With health system inequity as a major campaign issue, the Labour party was reelected in 1983, and there was an im-mediate return to comprehensive health coverage under the new term "Medicare." This is the scheme that has formed the basis of Australia's health care system since, although changes continued to be enacted, some to re-strain costs, others to reconcile political pressures brought by the medical profession.

Basically, the Australian system offers universal access to needed health care, regardless of ability to pay. The primary care physician, or GP, is the point of entry into the system for virtually all patients. Primary medical care is fee-for-service private practice with free choice of medical practitioners. No government benefit is payable for specialist services without a GP referral. There is a national list of prescription pharmaceuticals, funded by the com-monwealth government. Motivated by budgetary considerations, it has be-come necessary to impose patient copayments that vary according to the pa-tient's ability to pay. Prescription drugs are one of the most expensive elements of any comprehensive health program.

Hospital services are available to all citizens at no charge. Nonhospital medical care is also provided through subsidized voluntary insurance. The medical association has retained the right for physicians to bill patients directly for partial payment of services. Free medical care is available to retired persons and their dependents. In this case, doctors are paid directly by the government at a discounted rate. It has become necessary to establish a separate program for long-term care for the elderly. As a result, nursing homes have proliferated and become a major system element in their own right.

In conclusion, Australia's health care system is institutionally modeled largely on the British system, but it operates more like the Canadian system (discussed next). Influences for change, especially social and ideological, come from the United States. The system is a mixture of public and private components that is complicated by the autonomy of the various states in their health policies. As is the case in all developed countries, there are problems of escalating costs and medically underserved areas both within cities and in the rural hinterland. Labour's preferred policies are continually frustrated by the intransigence of the medical profession. Opposition parties have learned that health is one of the most important social issues to the electorate, and they no longer seriously attempt to bring back the free-market provisions of earlier times (Burrows, 1992). Hall (1999) reports that insurance premiums between 1989 and 1996 rose, on average, 9.8% annually, outstripping the consumer price index of 2.9% per year. Support for private health insurance was a component of the commonwealth reform agenda in 1998. The Commonwealth/State Health Care Agreements included a clause "to recognize and support the significant role that the private sector plays in the provision of health services in Australia and the right of Australians to choose private health care."

Canada

Like the United Kingdom and Australia, Canada's philosophy of health care follows the principle that all citizens should have equal access to medical care regardless of ability to pay. In Canada, jurisdiction over health, education, and welfare is the responsibility of the 10 provinces, which creates the possibility of 10 separate provincial approaches to health care planning and delivery.

Despite their historical ties to Britain, Canadians have never, strictly speaking, had a national health care system like that of the United Kingdom. In the first half of the 20th century, medical practice in Canada was laissez-faire; that is, each province defined its own medical care system. Canada lagged behind the United States in developing social legislation in general and health services legislation in particular. After World War II, Canada's federal government enacted important social programs such as social security, but the government was initially unsuccessful in establishing a national medical insurance plan.

The cornerstone for a national system in Canada was laid in the mid-1950s, with national legislation for coverage of hospital care and related diagnostic services. By 1961, all 10 provinces were operating hospital insurance programs, with the federal government contributing half the funds. Medical insurance was added in 1968. By 1971 all the provinces and northern territories were participating fully in the combined medical and hospital services program that came to be known as *Medicare*. Today, coverage is comprehensive (i.e., pays for all medically needed services rendered by physicians or hospitals, without limit), universal (i.e., available to all eligible residents on uniform terms and conditions), portable (i.e., benefits "follow" the citizen moving across provincial boundaries), and offered by nonprofit public organizations and agencies accountable to the government. The federal government intervened one more time in 1984, passing the Canada Health Act. This legislation consolidated previous health insurance legislation and reduced federal transfers to provinces that allowed hospitals to levy user fees or doctors to charge patients more than negotiated charges.

Canada has demonstrated a capacity to deliver universal, high-quality medical care for considerably less per patient than is the case in the United States (Inglehart, 1986). Yet, the cumulative effects of provincial and federal legislation have contributed to the creation of more hospital beds and greater overall economic access to medical care among the Canadian population (Gesler, Hartwell, Ricketts, & Rosenberg, 1992). As a result, health care costs have risen to the point where Rosenberg and James (1994) refer to the Canadian system as the "second most expensive health care system in the world" behind the United States. Federal support for health, postsecondary education, and social services has been steadily reduced as successive governments have struggled with massive national indebtedness. Meanwhile, it is evident that low-income individuals and families are underserved, as are rural compared to urban individuals and families (Anderson & Rosenberg, 1990).

Fundamental conflicts exist because government cannot fund universal health care, balance its budget, and allow physicians to retain their professional autonomy while giving consumers free choice of providers. Provinces continue to expand the scope of covered benefits while trying to control costs. Physicians and hospital management are caught in the middle (Inglehart, 1990). Countless hospitals have been consolidated under regional governance mechanisms. Health professionals' tolerance for change has been sorely stretched by the pace, scope, and scale of institutional downsizing. The wave of hospital closures and cutbacks has been disturbing to the public. Hospitals are not only symbols of health care availability; they also contribute to local economies, particularly in sparsely settled places. Each institution faces pressures from local citizens and its medical staff to be "all things to all people" (Naylor, 1999).

United States

Health care delivery in the United States is unique among large industrialized nations in that it provides health care through an entrepreneurial system. The main source of health care for most citizens is in a private market of thousands of independent medical practitioners, pharmacies, clinics, and so on, subject to significantly less government regulation than in other developed countries. As noted regarding the national systems discussed previously, policies developed to provide efficient and equitable health care entailed either direct government provision of health services or significant government involvement in various schemes of national health insurance, planning, and regulation. In the United States, however, there has always been a reliance on private markets as the favored instrument of allocation of health care for all but a few categorical programs.

The result of this political and economic philosophy has been fragmentation, a collection of systems and subsystems that are based on local and institutional initiatives. There have been attempts at national, state, and local planning, but for the most part each segment (e.g., hospital services, community health services, emergency medical services, and pharmaceutical supplies) has gone its own way. As in other sectors of life, in the United States a wide range of special-interest groups has had an impact on health care policy. These groups include major industrial interests; organized labor; federal, state, and local health planning agencies; hospital organizations; professional physician groups; and the insurance industry. Attempts to bring order out of this chaos have met with limited success.

A brief history of the U.S. system will help explain the current situation. Health care in early colonial days followed European traditions of private treatment for those who could pay and church-run charity hospitals for those who could not. William Penn established the first almshouse in 1713 in Philadelphia. Benjamin Franklin is credited with setting up the first hospital in 1751 in the same city. Other cities followed suit. During the 18th and 19th centuries, hospital growth was slow, but by the end of the period many hospitals had established medical schools. Germ theory and new medical knowledge gave impetus to construction of many health facilities in the first half of this century. Voluntary (community organization, church, fraternal, etc.), short-term hospitals predominated during this free-wheeling era, when there was no overall planning. Meanwhile the Public Health Service was increasing its size and scope, and some local governments were assuming responsibility for the indigent.

Several federal legislative acts have attempted to organize the U.S. health care delivery system. The Hill–Burton Act of 1946 was the first of these. The main emphasis of Hill–Burton was to provide government support for hospital construction in "needy" areas. Need was defined simply as a bed-to-population ratio, without regard for population differences. Population and hospital demand data were obtained at the county level and within metropolitan areas at the census tract level. The states had responsibility for needs assessment and planning. Hill–Burton also led to the establishment of many state health planning agencies, mostly voluntary. There was much variation in the amount of planning and regulation among states.

In the 1960s, the major emphasis of national health policy was on redistribution: increased government expenditures for the poor and aged. With a Democratic administration in power, *Medicaid* was established to provide medical care to the poor who received government payments and to others unable to pay medical costs. *Medicare* made similar provision for the elderly. Both programs are administered by the states, with financial support from the federal government. Both pay for outpatient treatment, physician fees, hospitalization, surgery, and equipment such as walkers and pacemakers. Hospitals were paid their costs—without restriction—plus 2%, and lower-cost substitutes to hospitals were not covered. Over the years, health care costs rose dramatically. Many thought that insufficient controls on these programs were to blame.

Comprehensive health planning (CHP) and regional medical programs (RMPs) were also begun in the mid-1960s. The former program replaced Hill–Burton and provided funding for both state and metropolitan area planning agencies, as well as to health programs within institutions of higher education. RMPs were established to focus on degenerative diseases, mainly heart disease, stroke, and cancer. The geographic boundaries of RMPs were not clearly defined, so territorial conflicts resulted. Both programs were opposed by the major medical organizations, which saw them as government interference within their bailiwicks, and they were eventually abandoned as more conservative political forces prevailed at the national level.

Another landmark in U.S. health care legislation came in 1974, with passage of the National Health Planning and Resources Development Act. This act was an attempt to update and revise existing programs and to foster cooperation among the national, state, and local health care planning agencies. The new program called for each state to create clearly defined health systems agencies (HSAs). HSA populations were to be between 500,000 and 3 million. HSA boundaries were to coincide with other administrative units as much as possible. The HSA became the basic unit for determining health care needs, administering federal funds for approved programs, and reviewing and evaluating programs. Each state formed a board of consumers and providers, all appointed by the governor of the state for the purpose of health services planning. The 1974 act by no means overcame the problems presented by earlier programs. Although consumers were supposed to be a majority on state planning boards, many felt that providers had the dominant voice in planning decisions. Providers continued to resent government interference and complain about the bureaucratization of health care delivery, the costs of maintaining HSAs, and the long review process.

Health care costs have escalated dramatically in the United States over the last several decades. From 1950 to 1990 the amount spent on health care rose from $12.7 billion to almost $700 billion, or from about 4% of the gross domestic product (GDP) to 12.3% of the GDP (Getzen, 1992a). Why such a massive increase? The increase in demand for medical services, fueled by government redistribution programs and by tax incentives associated with employer-purchased health insurance, caused rapid increases in medical prices and expenditures. Cost-based payment for hospitals and separation of the payment to hospitals and physicians provided little incentive for physicians to be concerned with their use of the hospital or for hospitals to be concerned with efficiency. Furthermore, state laws inhibited price competition among health providers and the development of changes in the way care was delivered. The over-65 population is increasing, and this has increased the demand for expensive life-extending services; many inner-city poor obtain free medical care in hospital emergency rooms, but so far these are not significant causes of higher expenditures. *Inflation and rising GNP far outweigh all other causes* as explanations of rising health expenditure (Getzen, 1992b). Still, some 15% of the population (over 30 million persons) are without adequate economic protection for health care costs.

The current health care delivery system in the United States shows very little spatial rationalization, despite the intention of the 1974 act to establish a kind of spatial–functional system of HSAs. There are spatial imbalances in resources, accessibility, and utilization, however these may be measured. Planning has had varied success in different regions of the country, partly because power groups with conflicting interests combat each other.

Several recent developments in the U.S. health care system should be mentioned. The concept of a health maintenance organization (HMO), although it has been in existence since World War II, has gained more acceptance as a health care alternative in recent years. The basic idea is that health care is prepaid. Subscribers to the HMO pay a set fee in advance for certain types of services and then receive whatever treatments they require. HMOs operate on the principle of economies of scale; for HMOs to function they must cover a minimum of approximately 20,000 families (Feldstein, 1992). In 1997, HMOs enrolled nearly 67 million people (up from just over 9 million in 1980). Like Britain's NHS, access to specialty physicians in an HMO is through a "primary" physician. Advantages of the HMO system include physician group practice, which gives doctors flexibility and a chance to consult with colleagues; quicker patient access to physicians; and an emphasis on prevention. Disadvantages are that patients are often preselected, which means that groups such as the unemployed or seriously ill may not be able to participate, and that the traditional right to choose a physician is surrendered. Another type of prepaid plan that has gained acceptance is the preferred provider organization (PPO). PPOs share most of the advantages of HMOs but offer patients a wider range of choices in participating hospitals and physicians.

A second development is an alteration in the way Medicare payments are made to hospitals (40% of all hospital revenues). Payments were based on hospital reports of what treatments cost; since the early 1980s uniform payments to all hospitals have been based on predetermined rates for each of 468 diagnosis-related groups (DRGs). This change was a response to findings that there were wide differences among hospitals in treatment charges, types of treatment, length of stay for similar problems, and use of ancillary resources.

A third development occurred in 1975 when the Federal Trade Commission (FTC) brought suit against the American Medical Association (AMA), charging that the AMA and its constituent societies restricted advertising among physicians. The case was won by the FTC and appealed by the AMA all the way to the Supreme Court, but to no avail. Thus, the courts and U. S. Congress have decided that health care is a business and that, like any other industry, it should be subject to antitrust laws. Such laws assume that a competitive system is more beneficial to society than a regulated one. With the application of antitrust laws to health care, competitive forces began to reshape the delivery system. Advertising has increased, with providers now explaining to the public not only what they do but why they are preferable to competing forms of delivery.

A fourth relatively new service in the health field in the United States is the freestanding ambulatory surgery center (FASC). Improvements in medical technology have made it possible for many tests and procedures to be performed outside the hospital. Studies have shown that 20–40% of all surgery can be performed on an outpatient basis, that is, the patient can be sent home the same day as the surgery. The first FASC in the United States was opened in 1970. By 1987, there were 674 FASCs, and by 1992, there were 1,246 of these facilities, with the greatest proportion found in the southern and western states. This service is one of several modern medical care innovations that have been challenging conventional medical care since the 1970s. American physicians, hospitals, and other organizations have become involved in alternative practice modes mainly because of their cost savings.

Perhaps the most dramatic development in the medical care field in the United States since 1990 is the emergence of *managed care*. Basically, managed care refers to the practice of organizations such as insurance companies and large HMOs to attempt to hold down medical spending by "managing" the financial aspects of the practice of medicine. This translates into companies and organizations specifying how much and what form of health care will actually be allowed to be dispensed by providers. In the United States, the majority of people depend on third party payers to cover most of their medical care costs. Supporters of managed care claim that "unnecessary" drugs, tests, procedures, and welfare programs are what drive up costs. Opponents claim that the managers are interfering with the proper practice of medicine and endangering the lives and health of patients. To be fair, the practice of managing health care is still relatively new and heavily influenced by politics and companies that have a great economic stake in the outcome of the system. Under these conditions, it is inevitable that inequities will arise (Anderson & Poullier, 1999).

Health policy in the United States and in other industrial nations will continue to be driven by attempts to place limits on medical expenditures while providing some level of care to all their citizens through some form of national health service. To adequately care for the poor, more taxes will almost surely be levied and the wealthy will probably retain the ability to purchase more health care outside the system. One relevant research arena for geographers will be to analyze the variations in health outcomes and policies in conjunction with poverty, discrimination, and unemployment inequities between places and regions over time.

CONCLUSION

This small sample of health care profiles suggests the tremendous variety in the ways that nations attempt to deal with illness and health. Cultural attitudes and beliefs, types and severity of illness, government policies, economic resources, the history of traditional and biomedical health services, and the roles of various groups within different societies all play a part. What constitutes the "best" system? Regardless of the mix of governmental or private-sector activity and traditional or modern practice, any society that desires the best of health and longevity of life for its citizens must develop policies to allocate resources equitably and systematically with due respect to its multiplicity of cultures. The present situation in most nations, of allowing inequity to exist in the sense that persons in the same degree of "need" are treated differently depending on their income, ethnicity, or political leanings, can only continue to foster conflict.

However, underlying the problems of inequitable or inadequate health service provision in modern industrial society is what David Mechanic (1994) calls the "failure of the current medical paradigm" (p. 11). Mechanic reminds us of the interconnectedness of health and society. The basic determinants of health have far more to do with social class, family and peer values, education, risk taking, and environmental hazards than with access to practitioners and their technology. Health status is governed by ubiquitous forces we may not be prepared to change: food production and eating patterns; social uses of alcohol, tobacco, and other substances; dependence on automobiles; sedentary lifestyle; and so on. Thus, modern biomedical care may be virtually irrelevant to how we should deliver adequate and equitable care and control costs for those with vulnerabilities and extreme needs.

REFERENCES

Akhtar, R., & Izhar, N. (1986a). Inequalities in the distribution of health care in India. In. R. Akhtar & A. Learmonth (Eds.), *Geographical aspects of health and disease in India*. New Delhi: Concept.

Akhtar, R., & Izhar, N. (1986b). The spatial distribution of health resources within countries and communities: examples from India and Zambia. *Social Science and Medicine, 22,* 1115–1129.

Akin, J. S., Guilkey, D. K., Griffin, C. C., & Poplin, B. M. (1985). *The demand for primary health services in the Third World.* Totowa, NJ: Rowman & Allenheld.

Anderson, G. F., & Poullier, J-P. (1999). Health spending, access, and outcomes: Trends in industrialized countries. *Health Affairs, 18,* 178–192.

Anderson, M., & Rosenberg, M. (1990). Ontario's underserviced area program revisited: an indirect analysis. *Social Science and Medicine, 30,* 35–44.

Basham, A. L. (1976). The practice of medicine in ancient and medieval India. In C. Leslie (Ed.), *Asian medical systems: A comparative study* (pp. 18–43). Berkeley: University of California Press.

Burrows, C. (1992). The ever-changing Australian health care system: A problem of structure. In M. M. Rosenthal & M. Frenkel (Eds.), *Health care systems and their patients.* Oxford: Westview Press.

Curtis, S., Petukhova, N., & Taket, A. (1994). Health care reforms in Russia: The example of St. Petersburg. *Social Science and Medicine, 40,* 755–766.

Dyck, I. (1992). Health and health care experiences of the immigrant woman. In M. Hayes, L. Foster, & H. Foster (Eds.), *Community, environment and health: Geographic perspectives.* Victoria (Canada): University of Victoria.

Eyles, J., & Woods, K. J. (1983). *The social geography of medicine and health.* London: Croom Helm.

Feldstein, P. J. (1992). The changing structure of the health care delivery system in the United States. In M. M. Rosenthal & M. Frenkel (Eds.), *Health care systems and their patients* (pp. 21–36). Oxford, UK: Westview Press.

Gesler, W. M. (1984). *Health care in developing countries.* Washington, DC: Association of American Geographers.

Gesler, W. M. (1991). *The cultural geography of health care.* Pittsburgh, PA: University of Pittsburgh Press.

Gesler, W. M., Hartwell, S., Ricketts, T. C., & Rosenberg, M. W. (1992). Introduction. In W. M. Gesler & T. C. Ricketts (Eds.), *Health in rural North America.* New Brunswick, NJ: Rutgers University Press.

Getzen, T. E. (1992a). U. S. national health expenditures forecast. *Health expenditure analysis letters, 1,* 11.

Getzen, T. E. (1992b). Population aging and the growth of health expenditures. *Journal of Gerontology, 47,* S98–S104.

Good, C. M. (1987). *Ethnomedical systems in Africa: Patterns of traditional medicine in rural and urban Kenya.* New York: Guilford Press.

Hall, J. (1999). Incremental change in the Australian health care system. *Health Affairs, 18,* 95–110.

Hippocrates. (1939). Aphorisms. In F. Adams (Trans.), *The genuine works of Hippocrates.* Baltimore: Williams & Wilkins.

Hyma, B., Phillips, D. R., & Ramesh, A. (1995). *Traditional health care delivery through mobile camps: The unani system of medicine in Tamil Nadu, India.* Unpublished manuscript.

Inglehart, J. K. (1986). Canada's health care system. *New England Journal of Medicine, 315,* 202–208.

Inglehart, J. K. (1990). Canada's health care system faces its problems. *New England Journal of Medicine, 322,* 562–568.

Instituto del Tercer Munco. (1994). *Third World guide 93/94.* Bogota: Garamond Press.

Jefferys, M. (1992). Britain's national health service under pressure. In M. M. Rosenthal & M. Frenkel (Eds.), *Health care systems and their patients.* Oxford, UK: Westview Press.

Jones, K., & Moon, G. (1987). *Health, disease and society: An introduction to medical geography.* London: Routledge.

Kalla, A. C. (1995). Health transition in Mauritius: Characteristics and trends. *Health and Place, 1,* 227–234.

Madge, C. (1998). Therapeutic landscapes of the Jola, the Gambia, West Africa. *Health and Place, 4,* 293–312.

Mechanic, D. (1994). *Inescapable decisions: The imperatives of health reform.* New Brunswick, NJ: Transaction.

Millard, F. (1995). Changes in the health care system in post-Communist Poland. *Health and Place, 1,* 179–188.

Naylor, C. D. (1999). Health care in Canada: Incrementalism under fiscal duress. *Health Affairs, 18,* 9–26.

Nordstrom, C. R. (1988). Exploring pluralism—the many faces of Ayurveda. *Social Science and Medicine, 27,* 479–489.

Organization for Economic Cooperation and Development. (OECD Social Policy Studies No. 7). (1990). *Health care systems in transition* Paris: Author.

Oppong, J. R. (1998, July 13–17). Changing economies and health providers in Ghana: Itinerant drug vendors as a health resource. *Proceedings of the Eighth International Symposium in Medical Geography,* Baltimore.

Parra, P. A. (1993). Midwives in the Mexican health system. *Social Science and Medicine, 37,* 1321–1329.

Phillips, D. R. (1990). *Health and health care in the Third World.* New York: Longman Scientific & Technical.

Population Reference Bureau. (1999). *World population data sheet.* Washington, DC: Author.

Rosenthal, M. M., & Frenkel, M. (Eds.). (1992). *Health care systems and their patients: An international perspective.* Oxford, UK: Westview Press.

Rosenberg, M., & James A. (1994). The end of the second most expensive health care system in the world. *Social Science and Medicine, 39,* 967–981.

Smith, C. J. (1993). (Over)eating success: The health consequences of the restoration of capitalism in rural China. *Social Science and Medicine, 37,* 761–770.

Smith, C. J. (1998). Modernization and health care in contemporary China. *Health and Place, 4,* 125–139.

Smith, C. J., & Fan, D. (1995). Health, wealth, and inequality in the Chinese city. *Health and Place, 1,* 167–177.

Son, A. H. K. (1999). Modernization of medical care in Korea (1876–1990). *Social Science and Medicine, 49,* 543–550.

Stepan, S. (1983). Patterns of legislation concerning traditional medicine. In R. H. Bannerman, J. Burton, & W. C. Ch'en (Eds.), *Traditional medicine and health care coverage.* Geneva: World Health Organization.

Wennstrom, G. (1992). New ideological winds are blowing in the Swedish health care system. In M. M. Rosenthal & M. Frenkel (Eds.), *Health care systems and their patients.* Oxford, UK: Westview Press.

Woelk, G. B. (1994). Primary health care in Zimbabwe: Can it survive? *Social Science and Medicine, 39,* 1027–1035.

World Resources Institute. (1998). *World resources, 1998–99* New York: Oxford University Press.

Xingyuan, G., Bloom, G., Shenglan, T., Yingya, Z., Shouqu, Z., & Xingbao, C. (1993). Financing health care in rural China: Preliminary report of a nationwide study. *Social Science and Medicine, 36,* 385–391.

FURTHER READING

Eyles, J., & Woods, K. (1983). *The social geography of health and health care.* London: Croom Helm.

Gallagher, E. B., & Subedi, J. (Eds.). (1995). *Global perspectives on health care.* Englewood Cliffs, NJ: Prentice Hall.

Health Affairs. An informative policy journal established in 1981. Though most articles refer to the U.S. health system, the publication reports developments in other nations. See, for example, Vol. 18 (3), a theme issue on international health reform.

Kearns, R. A., & Gesler, W. M. (Eds.). (1998). *Putting health into place: Landscape, identity, & well-being.* Syracuse, NY: Syracuse University Press.

Mohan, J. (1990). Health care policy and the state in 'austerity capitalism': Britain and the USA compared. In J. Simmie & R. King (Eds.), *The state in action: Public policy and politics* (pp. 74–94). London: Pinter.

Mohan, J. (1995). *A national health service?* London: Macmillan.

Thomas, R. (1992). *Geomedical systems: Intervention and control.* London: Routledge.

10

Distribution of
Health Care Resources

T he geography of health care embraces two broad areas of study: the spatial properties of health care resources (i.e., *where* the *providers* are and why they are there) and the accessibility, utilization, and planning of health care services (i.e., *where* do *consumers* seek and/or receive care, and why there). This chapter examines the former whereas Chapter 11 addresses the latter. We should point out, however, that the difference between provision of and access to services is sometimes blurred. Thus, some topics in both chapters may appear at first glance to be misplaced.

The classic geographic approach is to describe and explain spatial patterns of health care resources in terms of prevailing political, economic, and cultural processes. Table 10-1 lists, for selected nations, two common measures of resources, public health expenditure as a percentage of gross domestic product, and population per doctor. It is immediately apparent from this table that many nations in Africa, Latin America, and Asia are relatively deprived of trained physicians, and that the nations of Europe and North America expend far higher proportions of their national income than do others. A quick comparison of these statistics with the income of these nations would reveal the resource gap between the wealthier and poorer nations.

Often, explanations consist of statistical relationships that determine the patient's use of medical services (Meade, 1986; Joseph & Phillips, 1984, Chap. 6). However, equally important explanations might consist of government policies or market decisions that define the character and use of health care facilities. This is evident in the recent work by Dyck (1995), Dyck and Kearns (1995), Kearns and Joseph (1993), and Mohan (1998), among others.

Medical and social systems can actually induce particular disorders and adverse conditions in the population. This is termed "iatrogenesis," and it takes several forms. *Clinical* iatrogenesis results when improper medical care produce pain, sickness, and death. For example, antibiotics can be danger-

TABLE 10-1. Public Health Expenditure as a Percent of GDP, Selected World Nations, 1900–1995, and Population per Doctor, 1900–1993

Country	% GDP	Pop. per doctor	Country	% GDP	Pop. per doctor
Africa			**North America**		
Algeria	3.3	1,062	Canada	7.0	464
Angola	4.0	23,725	United States	6.3	419
Burundi	0.9	17,153			
Chad	1.8	30,030	**Latin America**		
Congo	3.6	15,150	Cuba	7.9	275
Egypt	1.0[a]	1,316	Dominican Republic	2.0	949
Kenya	1.9	21,970	Haiti	1.3	10,855
Lesotho	3.5	24,095	Jamaica	3.0	6,420
Libya	3.0[a]	957	Bolivia	2.7	2,348
Mauritania	1.5	15,772	Chile	2.5	942
Namibia	3.9	4,328	Ecuador	2.0	652
Niger	2.2	53,986	Paraguay	1.0	1,231
Senegal	1.1[a]	18,192	Peru	2.6	939
Togo	1.7	11,385	Venezuela	2.3	633
Zambia	2.6	10,917			
Zimbabwe	2.1	7,384	**Asia**		
			Cambodia	0.7	9,347
Europe			China	1.8	1,063
Albania	2.7	735	India	0.7	4,850
Belgium	7.2	274	Iraq	0.8[a]	1,659
Bulgaria	4.0	306	Japan	5.5	920
Czech Republic	7.8	273	Malaysia	1.4	2,441
Finland	6.2	406	Mongolia	4.4	371
Hungary	6.8	306	Pakistan	0.8	1,923
Lithuania	4.8	235	Phillipines	1.3	8,273
Netherlands	6.9	399	Singapore	1.1	714
Poland	4.6	451	Thailand	1.4	4,416
Romania	3.3	538	Vietnam	3.5	2,279
Spain	5.8	261			
Sweden	6.4	394	**Oceania**		
United Kingdom	5.8	780	Austalia	5.8	447
			New Zealand	5.7	518
			Papua New Guinea	2.8	12,754

Note. Except where noted, data are for the most recent year available, within the range 1990–1995.
[a]Public expenditures on health as percent of GNP, 1993.
Data from World Resources Institute (1998, pp. 250–251, 262–263) and Instituto del Tercer Mundo (1994).

ous for those who are allergic to them. *Social* iatrogenesis occurs when health policies reinforce an industrial organization which generates dependency and ill health. The drug industry, for instance, is constantly charged by the media with fostering public dependence on medicine. *Structural* iatrogenesis is defined by medically sponsored behavior and opinions that restrict the vital autonomy of people by undermining their competence to take care of themselves (Illich, 1976; Eyles, 1987). Hospitals, for example, may produce infections that spread rapidly, especially in crowded conditions.

One hypothesis that can be tested is that there is *inequity* in the distribution of these resources; that is, providers locate their offices and facilities in such a way that some segments of the population become (or remain) *underserved.* Underserved may mean different things to different people in different places, and attempts to define and operationalize this term will raise difficulties. Definitions used in Canada and the United States are discussed next.

Inequity implies that there is unmet need somewhere in society. Defining need is not simple, and many possible indices exist. At least three may be identified. First are *direct indicators,* such as overcrowding. Second are *indirect indicators,* which do not necessarily constitute deprivations in themselves but provide evidence for the existence or degree of deprivation. Conditions that aggravate poverty, such as racial or class discrimination are examples of indirect indicators. Third are *interpretative indicators,* which are not direct measures of deprivation but aid the geographical analysis of the distribution of deprivation. An example is the estimated number of immigrants into the United States from places that suffer from extreme poverty or armed insurrection in a given year. These migrants succumb to diseases brought on by malnutrition, stress, and abuse—both physical and mental. Upon arrival in the United States, they are in need of various kinds of health and social services.

There is also the question of how to measure equity. In some contexts, it is used to mean that different people have equal health care resources *available* to them. If every citizen of a nation had a primary care physician available whenever a client felt the need for one, it could be argued that there was equity in the distribution of that particular resource. But, suppose some people are simply able to *use* more primary care providers than others. In that sense, there is some inequity in society. From another perspective, we could argue that equity referred to equal health *outcomes*; that is, virtually every citizen is satisfied with the service he/she receives from the physician. When, say, all poor citizens are provided with the same quantity and quality of medical care with approximately the same expenditures in time and distance, we say that there is *horizontal equity.* When both affluent and poor citizens are provided with the same quantity and quality of medical care, there is *vertical equity* in the delivery system. Most geographic research on equity is horizontal in its approach, but often, both viewpoints are complementary. For example, the supply of medical care available in inner cities or rural areas may be less geographically accessible to some people than to others, and those same providers may discriminate against potential clients on the basis of race or income. There is a substantial literature that addresses service inequity in rural places and inner-city neighborhoods (Gesler & Ricketts, 1992; Ginzberg, Berliner, & Ostow, 1993).

Researchers have attempted to optimize equitable provision and/or economic efficiency. Often these two goals are at odds. Note, for example, the concentration of social and health service agencies in U.S. inner cities—which is efficient for the agencies because overhead costs are lower, clients live nearby, and political opposition to such agencies is minimal. But, what is "optimal" for the clients might include better housing and employment, which is found elsewhere in the city. More about this situation is discussed in the following chapter on access to services. Mathematical models of the location of facilities and their human resources have been and continue to be used to optimize service locations. We first address the definition of resources and acquisition of data necessary for analysis of health care systems and then discuss the methodology of spatial distribution analysis.

For planning purposes, quantitative measures of resource availability are essential, as are measures of the quality of the personnel, facilities, and other resources in an area. However, quantity alone is inadequate to judge equality of resource distribution. For example, the United States has one of the world's highest ratios of health care resources to population, yet there are countries with lower infant mortality rates that possess fewer medical resources.

RESOURCE INVENTORIES

Health care resources include practitioners such as physicians, nurses, and native doctors; facilities such as hospitals, clinics, mental health care centers, nursing homes, health maintenance organizations (HMOs), investor-owned group practices, halfway houses, and the homes of indigenous healers; materials such as antibiotics and medicinal herbs; equipment that ranges from body scanners to tongue depressors; and financial support from private, government, and charitable organizations. Resources are controlled by institutions such as the various national medical, hospital, and herbalist associations and, more recently, insurance and health service management companies. Most geographic studies emphasize the first two resources, personnel and facilities, because data have been more accessible. The other types of resources should not be overlooked, however, because they influence the quality, costs, and administration of care.

In Western countries, information about health care resources is available to the public through a variety of publications, including advertising media and directories. To mention only a few, national data may be obtained through the National Center for Health Statistics, the Health Resources and Services Administration, or the National Institute for Mental Health (United States); Statistics Canada; and the Office of Population Censuses and Surveys or Her Majesty's Stationery Office (United Kingdom). One can find lists of physicians and their specialties in government and medical association publications and telephone directories. Hospitals and other facilities publish financial statements and can supply information on the equipment and medicines they use. Access to patient records is restricted because of the necessity for confidentiality. Investigators may have to rely on interviews to collect information on patient needs, perceptions, and attitudes or the role of community groups in making decisions about health care financing. Government planning agencies often maintain accurate inventories of personnel and facilities as part of their mission to contain rising costs or for purposes of complying with a myriad of regulations. In recent years, it has been possible to obtain some data not only in printed form but on computer-readable disks. This has been particularly useful to researchers who wish to manipulate large quantities of data and perform statistical or mathematical analyses.

In most developing countries, researchers have to rely more on field surveys to obtain the same kinds of information. It is harder to define who is a health care practitioner; traditional healers may play other roles in society and practice medicine only part time. Even information on biomedical systems is not as reliable as in developed countries. Also, it is hard to categorize native doctors because they often have several specialties. Various sources estimate that traditional medicine is the principal source of care for over half of the world's population, yet it remains a resource that is largely invisible to national health accounts. In many developing areas the distribution of pharmaceutical drugs is not controlled, and much open marketing and street selling of drugs goes on that would be difficult to trace.

THE SPATIAL DISTRIBUTION OF RESOURCES

Why do some areas have fewer or more resources than other areas? Spatial analysis is the geographical approach to understanding inequalities in such things as income distribution, food supplies, or health care service. An important issue of equitable service distribution is the contrast between *need* for services and *demand* for them. The economic efficiency criterion emphasizes demand, which is based on use of resources. Some forms of medical care, such as a qualified doctor when someone becomes acutely ill, are considered *necessities.* Other forms, such as corrective plastic surgery, are *luxuries.* In a system in which a fee is charged for care, the quantity of care demanded is inversely related to price. Furthermore, the demand for health services is price inelastic, that is, if the price of the service increases by a certain percentage, the demand for that service may also fall, but by a lesser percentage (Sorkin, 1992). A system that is based on fee for service, such as that of the United States, is biased toward those who have social and financial access to care (vertical inequity). A health system, however, must meet needs. Unfortunately, needs assessment involves costly and time-consuming procedures such as administering health status questionnaires; demographic, epidemiological, and social indicator surveys; and interviews with key personnel within communities.

It should be obvious to the reader that there are complex political and empirical problems in measuring both need and provision (Jones & Moon,

1991; Eyles, 1987, Chap. 2). Furthermore, ecological fallacies are a problem; deprivation at the regional scale is not necessarily congruent with need or resource provision at the local level, because regional averages may mask the diversity between small areas within. This complexity challenges our ability to demonstrate inequality. Equality of distribution generally means that need is equated with expenditure. To fit within geography, we may simply add that needs are met within predefined geographic spaces (horizontal equity). This concept has been termed "territorial justice" (Davies, 1968; Harvey, 1972; Powell, 1990; Smith, 1994). Jones and Moon (1987) illustrate how territorial justice may be represented on a graph (Figure 10-1A). The case where need is met equally at any expenditure level may be described as a line that lies at a 45° angle from either axis and passes through the origin. When measures of need and expenditure in spatial units are standardized or ranked, a place's status may be represented by a the intersection of respective levels of need and expenditure. Observation p in Figure 10-1A demonstrates inequality, that is, an excess of need over expenditure.

The opposite to territorial justice is *inverse care* (Figure 10-1B). Here, the availability of adequate health care tends to vary inversely with the need of the population. Kearns and Joseph (1993) describe the Hokianga district of New Zealand in the 1940s as an isolated and predominantly Maori rural area devoid of adequate medical care. The subsequent establishment by the national government of several "special medical areas" in places such as the Hokianga district was an attempt to correct what was described as an inverse care situation. Sociologist Gabriel Fosu's (1986) description of the mismatch between health care expenditures and population distribution in Ghana in

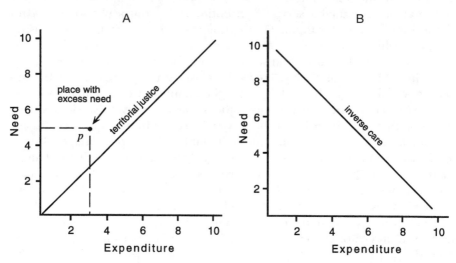

FIGURE 10-1. (A) Territorial justice, and (B) inverse care. From Jones and Moon (1987, pp. 222–223). Copyright 1987 by Routledge. Reprinted by permission.

the mid-1970s is typical of the inverse care hypothesis. At that time, expenditures on specialized hospital care, benefiting only 1% of the population, amounted to about 40% of the nation's health budget. Expenditure on primary health care, serving some 90% of the population, constituted a mere 15% of total health spending.

In developed countries, physicians and hospitals tend to fare relatively better than do their counterparts in the developing world in terms of income, cultural amenities, and availability of supplies and equipment. But even with these benefits, the distribution of practitioners is uneven. For example, Figure 10-2 shows the number of primary care physicians per 100,000 population for 1990 for counties of the United States that are one standard deviation or more above (solid symbols) or below (open symbol) the national average. It is immediately apparent that midwestern and southern counties are more likely to be relatively "underserved," whereas northern and eastern counties have "surpluses" of general practitioners. Although this map shows statistically significant differences, these differences mask many other issues of health care delivery. For example, counties with below-average numbers of physicians are not necessarily "deprived," nor are above-average counties necessarily excessively well off, because medical need varies in both degree and kind from one county to another and from one region to another. Some places may have an excess in specialists and a deficit in primary care doctors (general practitioners).

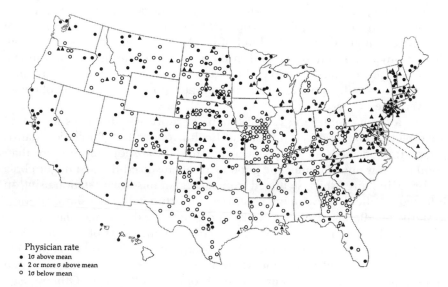

Physician rate
• 1σ above mean
▲ 2 or more σ above mean
○ 1σ below mean

FIGURE 10-2. U.S. counties that exceed or fall below the national average of primary care physicians (general practitioners, pediatricians, and internists) per 100,000 population by more than one standard deviation. Data from Area Resource File System, Health Resources and Services Administration, Rockville, MD.

What constitutes an equitable distribution of resources is ill-defined and controvertible. The demonstration of resource-to-population ratios, like that of Figure 10-2, is a common and oversimplified geographic approach to this issue. Other, more analytical techniques, such as the location quotient, are often used. The location quotient shows the extent to which each of a set of areas departs from some norm, such as regional or national averages. If we are concerned, for instance, with the location quotients of medical resources (doctors, nurses, emergency personnel, etc.) in a set of districts or counties, we could substitute into the equation

$$Q = \frac{X_j}{k}$$

where X_j is district j's proportion of medical resource employment (to total employment), and k is the percentage of medical resource employment in all the nation's districts (a national average). A location quotient of 1.0 would indicate that the medical resource employment in a district was exactly the same proportion of total employment as in the nation's districts. A quotient of less than 1.0 for a district would reveal that employment level to be below average compared with all districts, while over 1.0 would indicate the district had more than its "fair share" of medical resource personnel.

Another tool used by social scientists to measure the level of inequality in the distribution of a resource within a given population is the Gini index. Figure 10-3 describes the generalized application of the Gini index and the Lorenz curve, the geometric interpretation of most calculations in inequality. Ricketts, Savitz, Gesler, and Osborne, (1994) demonstrate how health service researchers might describe the level of inequality in the geographic distibution of physicians nationwide and in individual states using the Gini index. Each diagram of the type shown in Figure 10-3 may represent a particular place, time, or subpopulation, enabling a ready graphic comparison of equality over time or space

In a poor country the establishment of more health clinics in a rural area might look good in a ministry of health report, but if a clinic's staff is poorly trained, beds are dirty, and drug supplies are low, more harm than good may have been done. One good example involved the first major ebola outbreak in Zaire, which stemmed from a Belgian missionary station using an infected needle. In developing countries, unfortunately, such simple devices as sterile needles, latex gloves, masks, and gowns are often unavailable.

Not all planners or social scientists consider measures of spatial maldistribution to be of primary importance. Many economists would argue that market forces should determine where resources are located and that open competition is the best assurance of economic efficiency. Others (e.g., Hemenway, 1982) might say that when the cost of providing care is escalating beyond the financial means of those in need, only the most cost-effective treatment should be provided. In the early 1990s, the state of Oregon, in the

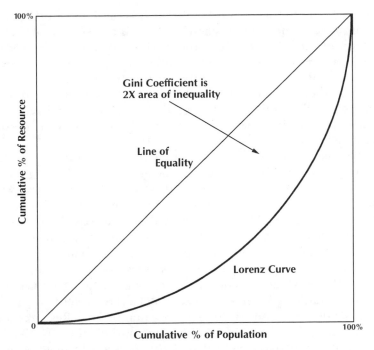

FIGURE 10-3. A generalized Gini Index.

United States, sought to provide medical care through the Medicaid program to its entire uninsured, medically indigent (poor) population. Because the budget for treatment of the indigent population is not unlimited, there had to be a trade-off: fund unlimited services to a defined population or fund a defined set of services to all medically indigent. Choosing the latter, Oregon ranked 709 medical conditions and their treatments on the basis of effectiveness and cost. They then determined that only the top 587 procedures could be funded under existing funding levels. The federal agency that governs Medicaid withheld approval of the plan, arguing that no patient could be denied treatment simply because that treatment would be expensive or because somebody else decided for the patient that his/her life was expendable (Shapiro, 1992). Unless government treats medical care as an entitlement and is committed to fund it unconditionally, some form of rationing, planned or unplanned, is inevitable.

GEOGRAPHIC STUDY OF RESOURCE DISTRIBUTION

Health care resource distribution has been studied at scales ranging from the nation to the neighborhood. The purpose of such analyses is usually to highlight some inequity in spatial distribution, such as rural versus urban, or afflu-ent versus poor. In the United Kingdom there is a strong emphasis on the spatial form of the organization of the National Health Service (NHS; see Chapter 9). When new regional health authorities were created in the Unit-ed Kingdom in the 1970s, the government appointed what is known as the Resource Allocation Working Party (RAWP). RAWP invented a formula for the purpose of distributing funds objectively, equitably, and efficiently to health authorities nationwide. This is an example of a *macroscale* approach to health care management.

Determining physician-to-population ratios by county in the United States (Figure 10-3) is a macroscale graphic method for assessing the equity of personnel distribution. A map of medical specialists by county within a state or a region is an example of a *mesoscale* portrayal. In a further example, Gould and Moon (2000) recently questioned a district-based weighting mod-el used by the NHS which has the effect of restricting provision of health ser-vices to island communities, where populations are small and geographically confined. An analysis of the equity of hospital distribution within a city, illus-trated by McLafferty's analysis of hospital closings in New York City (Figure 10-4), demonstrates a *microscale* schematic (McLafferty, 1989).

National studies may mask differences within regions. Resource inequal-ity is consistently found within administrative jurisdictions. In the United States, ill health related to poverty that threatens inner-city neighborhoods is invisible when viewing national, state, or even county statistics. In most coun-tries rural dwellers have been at a disadvantage in obtaining basic primary health care, much less specialty services, because medical care resources tend to concentrate in urban or suburban places.

A vexing problem in North America is how to provide an adequate level of health care services to its rural population. This problem dates back to the 1960s, when medical school students began to shift away from general prac-tice and into specialty medicine. There was a concomitant drop in the num-ber of physicians establishing practice in rural and nonmetropolitan areas. By 1988, 111 counties across the United States were without a single physi-cian. As a result, studies of medical manpower have been initiated within the United States (Ricketts & Cromartie, 1992). Federal programs, such as the community health centers initiative, have identified underserved communi-ties. Geographers in the United States have been active in the work of rural health services research centers in North Carolina and in the Pacific North-west (Hart, Pirani, & Rosenblatt, 1991). These studies have become increas-ingly sophisticated as mathematical models for specific practitioner need and supply were developed.

In Canada, an underserved area is based on a variety of measures, in-cluding number and type of physicians, population structure and seasonal fluctuation, socioeconomic status of the area, local demand for medical care, availability of housing and facilities for physicians, and the area's health needs and resources (Anderson & Rosenberg, 1990). An underserved county

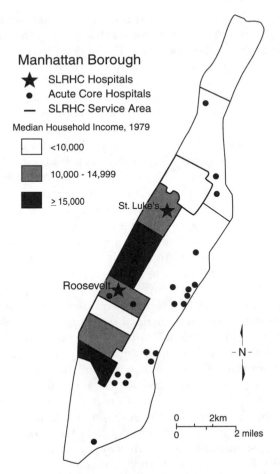

FIGURE 10-4. Median household income and the location of selected hospitals in New York City, 1982. Adapted from McLafferty (1989, p. 146). Copyright 1989 by the Rutgers University Press. Adapted by permission.

in the United States is defined basically as one whose ratio of physicians to population is in the bottom fourth in the nation. There are also accommodations for groups of urban Census tracts, high-risk populations (e.g., migrants), and institutions. Increasingly, states with physician shortages are providing scholarships and loan-forgiveness programs for medical students promising to work in small towns or other underserved populations, and some three-quarters of the states now have agencies dedicated to improving rural health care.

Another problem in North America involves the use and distribution of foreign-trained physicians (or international medical graduates, or IMGs). Aside from the issue of IMG quality of training, are IMGs more likely to be found in underserved areas? Mick, Lee, and Wodchis (2000) analyzed American Medical Association data and discovered that the majority of states had disproportionately high numbers of IMGs. The authors found a positive correlation between IMG disproportions and low doctor-to-population ratios.

There are other within-region imbalances. Research has demonstrated that variations in the practice of medicine, especially surgery, persist from one part of a state to another, or one region of the country to another (Foundation for Health Services Research, 1993). For example, in the 1980s, residents of New Haven, Connecticut, were twice as likely to undergo coronary artery bypass surgery as residents of Boston, which is about a 2-hour drive from New Haven. Eight percent of the children in one Vermont community had tonsillectomies compared to nearly 70% in another community. Women living in the southern region of the United States have a 1.5 times greater rate of hysterectomies than do women living in the northeastern region, and the general rate of gastrointestinal endoscopy is two times higher in the western region than the northeastern. Apparently unable to explain these wide variations in physician practice patterns by patient characteristics or by available medical resources, researchers have concluded that these variations are caused by physician uncertainty and lack of professional consensus about the best method of treatment of many medical conditions. The belief that patterns of surgery are chiefly due to decisions made by providers is the *practice style hypothesis*. To the extent that this thesis is true, fundamental questions must be raised about the efficiency and equity of the medical care system (Bogdanich, 1991). Despite the intuitive appeal and widespread acceptance of this hypothesis, the evidence is not totally supportive (Escarce, 1993). Patient demand variables (e.g., Medicare enrollment, use of preventive services, and method of referral) can influence surgery rate. The geographic research scale may also have a significant effect; different patterns may be found at the metropolitan area level than at the county or smaller area level. Using large areas may underestimate the role of patient preferences, and patient care-seeking behavior can vary more across small areas than among large areas. Further critical research, using other medical procedures or a variety of age, ethnic, and socioeconomic groups, is required to verify this theory.

Microscale studies have usually focused on urban areas. Their results might not generalize to entire regions, but they can provide information for a more detailed analysis. As one would expect, the more deprived urban areas in terms of income and other measures of socioeconomic status are medically under served. In the United Kingdom, for example, the Royal Commission on the NHS reported in 1979 that in parts of inner London, the NHS was failing to provide adequate primary care service because of excess physician caseloads and a variety of problems with medical practice itself (Powell, 1986, p. 1095).

Ethnicity and class differences in the population are important factors. It is not unusual to find large differences in number of primary physicians offices between mostly white and mostly black neighborhoods. Figure 10-5

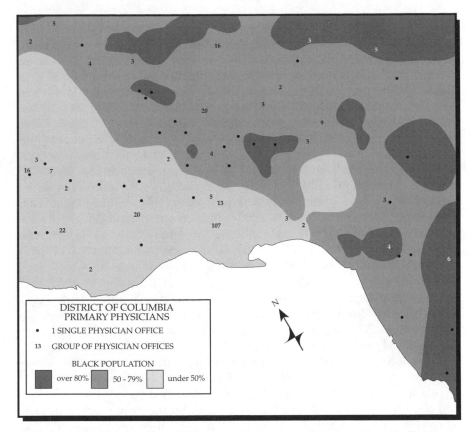

FIGURE 10-5. Distribution of black population, by political ward, and all primary care physicians (general practitioners, pediatricians, and internists) in Washington, DC, in 1991. There appears to be a negative spatial association between the black population distribution and primary care physicians. Data from Washington, DC, telephone directory (classified advertisements), 1991.

shows the distribution in 1991 of the black population and all primary care physicians listed in the classified section of the Washington, DC, telephone directory. The number of persons per primary physician is shown for each of the wards of the city. The population–physician ratio for the entire city, including specialists, is 165 (605 per 100,000 resident persons). The underlying patterns show the proportion of black population by ward and demonstrate the relative paucity of primary care doctors in the nonwhite areas of the city.

In areas where there are few physicians' offices or clinics, primary care might be found only in hospital emergency wards. In 1987, about 14% of all physician contacts in the United States were in a hospital outpatient department (Table 10-2). Blacks and poor Americans were far more likely to visit a hospital for medical care than whites and those with higher incomes.

Central Place Theory

Models of the existing distribution of goods and services are sometimes based on *central place theory*. Basically, this theory states that the quantity and variety of goods and services available to a given population vary with the number of people who have access to these goods and services. A hierarchy of goods and services is established which demonstrates that there are different minimum numbers of consumers and trade area sizes for each level of good. Large populations are offered a wide range of goods and services; small populations have fewer goods and services at their disposal. High-order items (e.g., personal computers) will be found only in larger markets, whereas low-order items (e.g., bread and milk) will be found in virtually everywhere. Low-order goods and services require relatively fewer consumers to be profitable. They also require a smaller market area than do high-order items. Places of each order are distributed across space in a regular pattern, a set of nested hexagons. The theory as Walter Christaller (1966) first formulated it had many simplifying assumptions, such as an isotropic plane and an evenly distributed population with equal purchasing power.

Central place theory can be linked to the functional and spatial organization of an idealized health care delivery system. The levels of the hierarchy range from individual practitioners or paramedics in offices or homes up to large medical centers providing the whole range of health care services. Figure 10-6 illustrates a rudimentary hierarchical health care system for villages in a developing nation (Joseph & Phillips, 1984). Each level is intended to serve a specified number of people within a specified geographic area. Sweden has a hierarchical medical care system, as did the Soviet Union prior to its collapse (Chapter 10). Gesler (1991, Chap. 3) discusses several other instances.

In U.S. metropolitan areas, hospitals are often arranged in a hierarchical pattern on the landscape (Figure 10-7). Typically, the teaching hospital is situated in a university, often in the inner city. This places it strategically in the center of a large potential market. A large veterans hospital may also be located there for the same reason—to take advantage of its central access to the market and to provide its staff with all necessary ancillary goods and services. Neither of these hospital types particularly attract nearby residents, especially if those residents happen to live in low-income neighborhoods. The variety of specialized services offered there are available to patients throughout the metropolitan area and beyond, most of whom are fully insured for medical services. Medium-size (100–300 beds) hospitals, like community shopping centers, are sited in the inner city and inner suburbs and are in somewhat competitive situations, vying for physicians, patients, and funding. Small (100 and fewer beds) hospitals offer the most basic hospital services and are situated throughout the metropolitan area. Satellite hospitals, located beyond the suburban fringe, vary in size from small to medium, depending on the populations they serve and the ability of their founders to raise funds.

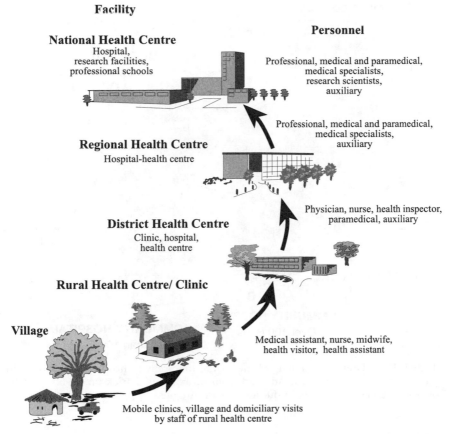

Facility

Personnel

National Health Centre
Hospital,
research facilities,
professional schools

Professional, medical and paramedical,
medical specialists,
research scientists,
auxiliary

Professional, medical and paramedical,
medical specialists,
auxiliary

Regional Health Centre
Hospital-health centre

Physician, nurse, health inspector,
paramedical, auxiliary

District Health Centre
Clinic, hospital,
health centre

Rural Health Centre/ Clinic

Village

Medical assistant, nurse, midwife,
health visitor, health assistant

Mobile clinics, village and domiciliary visits
by staff of rural health centre

FIGURE 10-6. A public health care hierarchy in a developing country. Adapted from Joseph and Phillips (1984, p. 57). Copyright 1984 by Harper & Row. Adapted by permission.

The theoretical central place market area of the hospital resembles a cone, termed a "distance–decay cone" (Figure 10-8). The height of the cone indicates the number of the hospital's patients living at a given distance from the institution. The slope of the cone represents the drawing power of the hospital over distance. Major research hospitals and veterans hospitals are represented by long, gradual slopes, indicating that because there are so few of these comprehensive institutions, patients are attracted from considerable distances. Small hospitals, like small shopping centers, tend to be more numerous and closer together than medium and large hospitals. As a rule, smaller general hospitals offer fewer services and have smaller, less specialized staffs than medium or large institutions.

Applying central place theory must take into account many factors that distort the ideal. These factors include physical barriers, transport networks, and income distribution. The result is a system that usually retains its func-

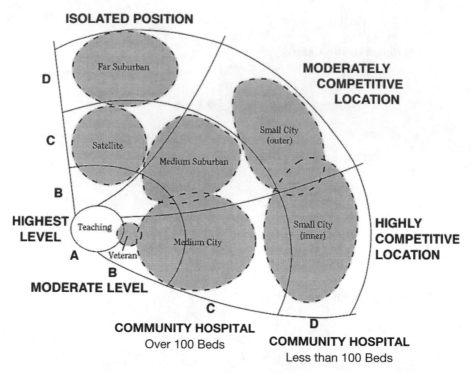

FIGURE 10-7. Graphic summary of the spatial hierarchy of hospital location in the typical eastern American city. Adapted from Morrill and Earickson (1968, p. 233). Copyright 1968 by Health and Education Trust. Adapted by permission.

tional nature but whose spatial configuration rarely resembles nested hexagons. An ideal spatial organization is harder to realize in practice than is a *functional* hierarchy. Some geographers (e.g., Okafor, 1982) contend that central place theory should not be used as an ideal at all. They criticize the theory's claim that market forces should dictate thresholds and ranges for each level of service and argue that social welfare issues should override issues of economic efficiency. Thus, for the good of a population's health, a government might have to establish facilities with smaller minimum populations than central place theory justified. Under a social welfare scheme, providing levels of service in overlapping spatial units is valid and, in fact, occurs in New Zealand, Thailand, and elsewhere. The number of levels and their corresponding populations and service areas will vary according to the type of system. In all but a few nations, the population is so dispersed that a fixed system is not practical and perhaps warrants only occasional visits by a mobile health service team, such as the Unani mobile camp in Tamil Nadu, India (Hyma, Phillips, & Ramesh, 1992). Central place theory ought to be used as one of many explanatory models rather than as a prescriptive model.

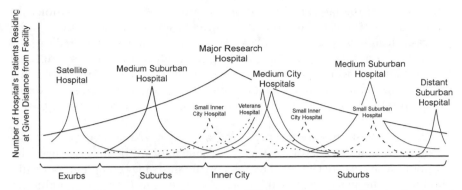

FIGURE 10-8. Distance demand cones for different types of hospitals in the typical eastern American city. Adapted from Pyle (1979, p. 220). Copyright 1979 by John Wiley & Sons. Adapted by permission.

Reasons for Personnel and Facility Location

Given the existence of inequalities in health care resource distribution, no matter how one chooses to measure inequality, the next logical step is to try to devise means to redress imbalances. This requires some knowledge of what caused the inequalities, and many interrelated factors can yield a complex cause and effect scenario.

Two types of analysis have been carried out: macroscale and microscale. Macrolevel analysis concentrates on demographic, socioeconomic, and environmental correlates of location decisions. One of the most consistent findings is that larger populations attract more resources. In both Western and non-Western countries, more health service facilities and higher personnel-to-population ratios are associated with higher levels of urbanization or population concentration. This finding makes sense, particularly in a free-market economy where health care delivery requires a sufficiently large market demand to be viable. As the minimum-service population and market area of a specialty increases, the specialty will be tied more closely to population size: that is, rarer specialties tend to be found in more populous places. Urban places also provide the professional, cultural, and recreational facilities that many physicians and other medical personnel desire. Age structure of the population can be quite important; for example, managed care organizations, such as HMOs, advertise widely to enroll geriatric populations, particularly where they are clustered, as in retirement communities. Highly dispersed populations are problematic, as geographers Cloutier-Fisher and Joseph (2000) have discovered. Other population characteristics that affect health service distributions include social or ethnic composition, educational level, and density.

Macroscale studies, because they deal with aggregates, should be used to describe rather than to explain general patterns of resource distributions. Attempting to extrapolate from the macroscale to smaller areas, and vice versa, can easily lead to an ecological fallacy. Also, some variables associated with resource locations may be correlated among themselves, and it is often difficult to ascertain which variables are the most important ones. Furthermore, the relative importance of these variables may change over time. In some developing countries the data for macroscale analysis are often simply not available.

Microscale studies are the preferred approach to analyzing resource location factors; at the microlevel the actual mechanisms behind resource distribution decisions are clearer. The microscale study may complement results obtained at the macrolevel. A microscale study might focus on practitioner motives for selecting a location. Joseph and Phillips (1984) identified three general reasons why health services are concentrated: economic (i.e., increasingly expensive treatments tend to create centralization of services), professional organization (i.e., increasing specialization and group practices), and government intervention (i.e., attempts to locate health personnel in rural areas). Doctors like to be fairly close to hospitals whose facilities they can use and proximate to colleagues with whom they can discuss cases. They are also influenced by a community's cultural opportunities, age structure, and racial composition. Group practices are common in developed nations because, among other things, they allow professional consultation and flexibility of leisure time. An office in a building with other physicians reduces overhead costs because of shared use of office space, waiting rooms, equipment, and technical and clerical personnel. An important consideration may be where office space is available; medical offices often require special features such as heavy wiring for technical equipment, so that possible sites are limited. Thus doctors tend to practice in professional buildings or in shopping malls rather than in residential areas. Mattingly (1991), in Illinois, and Rosenberg (1984), in Toronto, ascertained that the attractiveness, or the lack of it, of a doctor's office site and of the area around it, nearness to a hospital and adjunct facilities, and access to clientele determined where most physicians located their practices. In a survey of practicing physicians in the Canadian province of British Columbia, Kazanjian and Pagliccia (1996) found that doctors, regardless of rural or urban location, ranked spousal influence to be the most important one when making practice location decisions. Close behind that was the desire to live and/or raise a family in a similar environment to the one the doctor experienced while growing up.

Western-trained doctors in developing countries may have unique criteria for siting their offices. Some doctors use their influence with government health departments to avoid assignments in remote or otherwise undesirable places. Although there has been little investigation of the location decisions of traditional healers, kinship connections and inherited practices probably affect where they locate. Ramesh and Hyma (1981) mapped out the locations of all registered professional traditional healers in Madras City, India. These practitioners of the ayurvedic, siddha, and unani systems tended to concentrate in the older, higher-density residential areas of the city and also in the older, commercial, and manufacturing sectors. New residential areas had fewer of these healers. Phillips (1990, Chap. 3) discusses how traditional beliefs and practices may sometimes be associated with the most serviceable and appropriate features of Western medicine, as in the "doctor monk" schemes using Buddhist priests with basic medical training in Thailand, and the traditional midwives who have been involved in health care since the 1960s in the Philippines, working closely with nurses in locally based primary health care programs.

The type and quantity of health care that is available to a population may be determined by government. In European-controlled colonies, more and better resources were shifted to natural resource production areas and more productive groups of people. A series of maps showing biomedical facility location over time in many developing countries would show a diffusion from the coast inland as the European colonists advanced. The maps would also show concentrations of facilities in places near iron mines and rubber plantations. The owners of plantations and mines wanted to keep their labor forces healthy.

The Appalachian Regional Commission was created by the U.S. government in the 1960s, in part to provide access to affordable, quality health care. In 1994, the U.S. Congress debated the pros and cons of entitling every citizen the right to health care. In that year, about 85% of the population was "covered" by private insurance, Medicare, or Medicaid or by out-of-pocket payment. The cost of covering the remaining population is substantial and would have to be paid either through higher taxes or by requiring employers to help pay for covering their workers, or both.

After a year of congressional hearings and political pronouncements for and against universal coverage, the issue died in committee. Nobody knows when or even whether another attempt will be made to entitle all U.S. citizens the right to basic medical care. Throughout the 1990s, the U.S. Congress was dominated by conservative representatives intent on balancing the national budget by cutting, among other things, social programs. Many of the urban poor have little access to a regular family physician or to community-based preventive and primary care services. Hospitals in poor and minority urban communities have increasingly become providers of last resort for seriously ill patients unable to find care elsewhere (Burns, 1993)

The wishes of individual practitioners and health care planners are often blocked because of various social, economic, and political constraints. To take a simple example, a hospital may be located on a particular site because the land was cheap or was a gift; original capital outlay concerns would override possible long-term inefficiencies (perhaps in transporting supplies to the hospital) and patient and staff accessibility. Power groups other than governments are also involved. Professional medical organizations set standards of admission which control practitioner supply; this, in turn, affects overall distribution. Professional organizations set the tone for the expected lifestyle of their members. Another constraint involves the mix of specialties. A study of Phoenix, Arizona (Gober & Gordon, 1980), showed that specialists, more than primary care physicians, tend to cluster around hospitals. In any system that is top heavy with specialists, patients must travel farther for specialized care.

Another set of constraints, common particularly in developing nations, has been pointed out by Navarro (1985), Curto de Casas (1994), and Scarpaci (1989, 1990). Depending on the social and politicoeconomic ideology of the nation at issue, the maldistribution of health care resources in some developing countries is due to the same factors that help keep these areas underdeveloped: the cultural, technological, and economic dependency of the countries and economic and political control of resources by local elites and foreign interests. As pointed out in the prior chapter, inequalities in the distribution of Western-style health care today can sometimes be traced back to the economic and political structures developed in colonial days. In India, for example, port towns and strategic sites attracted Western doctors to the neglect of the local population in the hinterlands (Akhtar & Izhar, 1986). Navarro's writing suggests that resource imbalances in Latin America have changed little since the 1970s.

Smith (1998) documents inequalities in China, which has spent much more on industrial and military development than on social services compared to most of the world's industrial nations. Urban coastal areas have benefited most from recent economic reforms, and an urban–rural gap in the provision of health care services has been evident for some time. This has been reinforced by two other trends: the preference among trained medical personnel to live and work in cities rather than rural areas and the tendency for individuals who might otherwise have chosen a medical career to choose a more profitable and prestigious form of employment.

Mental Health Services

The delivery of mental health services in developed nations has changed substantially since World War II. Prior to this, many mentally ill patients were incarcerated in asylums and mental hospital wards. The peak rate (498 per 100,000 population) of institutionalization in New Zealand occurred in the mid-1940s and thereafter declined to less than 225 per 100,000 (Hall, 1988). A national policy in the 1970s in the United States to close large and costly mental hospitals had the effect of relocating mental health care services to a variety of community facilities. Besides the financial savings, the goal was to challenge centuries of exclusion and ostracism of the mentally ill from within society's midst. At the time of deinstitutionalization, it was hoped that community mental health centers would become the ambulatory-care version of the older state mental hospitals, focusing on the problems of minorities, the poor, the elderly, and the chronically mentally ill. However, fewer than half of the community centers were actually built, and in 1981 the federal funding for the program was abandoned (Smith, 1989). Deinstitutionalization in New Zealand was attributable more to the medical profession than to a direct out come of central government policy. They had no organization like the community mental health center to absorb hospital patients. As a result, New Zealand now has a highly fragmented and underfunded supply of community mental health services.

Unfortunately, in the United States, there were simply too few formally organized community residential facilities to receive all deinstitutionalized persons. Uncounted numbers drifted into proprietary boarding homes and single-occupancy hotels into a kind of isolation that was little better than that of the now abandoned mental hospitals. Further, a certain proportion of these discharges became homeless in their distrust of any organized living situation (Dear & Wolch, 1987). Mental health care is much more decentralized than the general medical care system both geographically and organizationally in the United States. Mental health services are offered in a wide range of locations and they are administered by a variety of different agencies. Patients are likely to appear in several medical, psychiatric, social service, and criminal justice agencies. In 1988, 60% of mental health care was dispensed as outpatient care, while the remainder was obtained in hospital and other inpatient facilities (Manderscheid & Sonnenschein, 1992). Nonwhite males and females are two to three times more likely to be admitted to mental hospitals than whites, with schizophrenia being the most likely diagnosis (Health Resources and Service Administration, 1990). By far the highest admission rates are found in urban places such as New York and Washington. In many countries, a reported decline in psychiatric hospital admissions is a statistical artifact—the hospital visits are simply shorter and patients have simply been reclassified as "outpatients."

Because of inevitable jurisdictional conflicts, the delivery of adequate public mental health care is less than optimal. In 1975, the U.S. Congress enacted Public Law 94-63, which integrated halfway houses as part of the community mental health center. Such residences became increasingly differentiated, serving persons in large homes and in apartments and caring for patients at different levels of rehabilitation and with different diagnoses. Establishing a residence for the mentally disabled in the community is a difficult and challenging task. To meet this challenge, most states have passed laws allowing their presence in single-family neighborhoods within certain often restrictive guidelines. In Massachusetts, the courts have established that community residences are educational in use, which renders them exempt from exclusionary zoning ordinances.

Whereas siting of mental health facilities is accepted and supported in some U.S. neighborhoods, strenuous local community opposition has become a major problem and an impediment to the establishment of these facilities. In a 1989 national survey in the United States, nearly half of all respondents stated that they would not welcome a group home for the mentally retarded, a homeless shelter, an alcohol rehabilitation center, or a drug treatment center (Borinstein, 1992). Demographically, these respondents tended to be affluent, male, well-educated, professional, married, homeowners, and living in large cities or suburbs. The acceptability of mental health facilities decreased as income increased. That is, respondents with under $25,000 annual household incomes were more accepting than households with $50,000 or more annual income.

Reasons for opposition to mental health facilities tend to focus on a perceived loss of neighborhood property values or potential danger to its inhabitants. However, in comparative neighborhood studies carried out in Chicago, Toronto, Ohio, Massachusetts, and Michigan, no evidence was found that the presence of group homes lowered selling prices, time on the market, ratio of selling price to asking price, or rate of property-value appreciation in these neighborhoods (Budson, 1988). Studies on violence are less conclusive; there is enough material in the media which links the mentally ill to violent acts to cause general public concern. People are cynical about science's ability to treat mental illness, and attempts to reassure them do little to assuage their fear.

One of the difficulties in the mental health field is the decreasing availability of a labor pool of potential counselors and case workers. Caring for the disadvantaged is far less popular and financially rewarding than, say, allopathic medicine, law, business, or computer science. Another problem is that with the rapidly rising costs of health care of all kinds, commercial health insurance carriers are increasingly limiting mental health inpatient benefits. As a consequence, more persons who need hospital care must seek help in the community centers. The funding of community programs has been inadequate to care for the thousands of deinstitutionalized patients from state institutions. There is no question but that some chronically psychotic patients are in personal danger when not protected in an institutional setting, and hospitalization ought to be available for them (Budson, 1988).

Since the mid-1980s, there has been a rapid growth in the provision of private psychiatric hospitals and psychiatric wards in general hospitals. Along with this has come an increased emphasis on preventive mental health services and early detection, community-based services, and programs in the workplace. Many of these services are being provided through preferred provider organizations, health maintenance organizations, and employee assistance programs. Private care is expensive, however, and as we stated previously, it is often beyond the ability of government or insurance companies to pay for this service. The responsibility for mental health care in the United States has fallen mainly on county or city government, whereas funding and planning resides at the federal and state level (Smith, 1989).

Abortion and Family Planning Clinics

Two of the more explosive social issues in the United States in recent decades have been abortion and family planning. There are both resource and access issues inherent in these topics. Rather than split the discussion between this and the following chapters, we have elected to present most of the research findings here. For health geographers, family planning is relevant at several scales, from national to local. At the national level, geographer Patricia Gober asserted that the likelihood of having an abortion in the United States is strongly dependent on where a woman lives (Gober, 1997). Using private and governmental organization data from the early 1990s, Gober discovered that finding abortion services had been growing increasingly more difficult. One reason is that abortion services have been concentrating in metropolitan areas. Clinics dominate the market for abortions in large metropolitan areas, but the presence of a hospital that provides abortion services is the key to access in smaller metropolitan and nonmetropolitan areas. From the supply side, one variable that restricts abortion services is government funding. Public funding for abortions leads directly to higher abortion rates, presumably by making abortions cheaper and easier for poor women to obtain. Public funding also facilitates a medical environment in which more hospitals offer abortion services.

The provision of social services and the NIMBY (not-in-my-back-yard) syndrome are pertinent topics in the location literature. Several geographers have participated in such studies. Chiotti and Joseph (1995) discuss the location of an AIDS hospice in Toronto, noting that such facilities tend to be situated in low-income, largely minority neighborhoods (*service-dependent ghettoes*). Construction of these group facilities has encountered local opposition despite efforts to promote a climate of understanding through the media and public meetings. AIDS was, in the 1980s, a disease that was mainly confined to neighborhoods that contained populations of gay men and intravenous drug users. More recently, however, the disease has diffused beyond these neighborhoods and into other populations. Where will AIDS hospices for these new populations be located? The earlier works of Curtis (1989), Dear and Wolch (1987, 1989), Dear and Laws (1986), and Hall and Joseph (1988) all discuss the difficulty of siting certain health service facilities. Despite evidence to the contrary, there is a strong public perception that such services are "noxious" and thus lead to lower property values and endanger the lives and health of local residents (Dear, 1992).

Location-Allocation Modeling

Just as there are many ways of measuring health resource imbalances, so there are many criteria for locating facilities to try to redress these imbalances. Calvo and Marks (1973) suggest three, based on the three sectors of society involved in location decisions, health care consumers, facility operators (management, practitioners, and staff), and the community (residents and businesses). Each sector is interested in different aspects of the location decision. Consumers would like to have good quality care, short travel times, and low fees; operators desire accessibility to support services, operational freedom, and a guarantee to financial success; and the community is interested in the economic, environmental, and sociopolitical impacts on the area. It is impossible to satisfy all these wishes; what is done in practice is to select a few, often surrogate, variables and try to model them.

Location-allocation modeling is used to locate a set of facilities and allocate groups of people to the facilities, so that selected criteria will be optimized. Model populations are taken as fixed at a particular time, but adjustments can be made if populations shift. Three factors may vary: the number of facilities, their capacity or size, and their location. Solutions depend on whether facilities are constrained to certain places or can be located anywhere and whether populations in certain spatial units will be assigned to a single facility or can be split up among several facilities. Most solutions must be worked out using computer programs. For simple situations there may be unique mathematical solutions, but there are no general mathematical solutions to more complex situations (see Vignette 10-1).

The application of location-allocation models in health service planning has a long geographical pedigree, which dates back to the study of hospital locations in western Guatemala by Gould and Leinbach (1966) and hospital use in Chicago by Morrill and Earickson (1969). Hospital discharge data from the state of Illinois were used to create a computer simulation model that assigned patients to hospitals from their homes in a manner that minimized travel distance. Morrill and Earickson found that reallocating hospital space could substantially decrease patient travel, but they pointed out that the same objective could be achieved by relaxing existing constraints of income and race. One disadvantage of these early models was that they left out nonspatial aspects of health care delivery such as disease diagnosis, population characteristics and health status, not to mention the complicated rules imposed by Medicare and Medicaid. As such, they were too simplistic to be applied to planning applications today. Mayhew (1986) and Thomas (1992) have effectively demonstrated the sophistication that has since evolved in socioeconomic modeling of health service delivery systems.

Mathematical models are employed to rearrange service distributions that were based on criteria that were more expedient than equitable. For example, planners in developing countries often do not consider locations based on accessibility and cost efficiency but respond instead to requests from individual villages. Modeling can produce a plan that is economically efficient or that will overcome resource imbalances. The models' best use is as an aid to planning, and they should not be applied too rigidly. In the final analysis, decision makers (i.e., government officials) will generally opt for a redistribution of resources that purports to improve equity for relatively small relocation costs.

Some attempts have been made to locate facilities within a wider social, cultural, and political context. A good example is the use Bosanac and Hall (1981) made of small-area data to help select feasible sites for primary care clinics in West Virginia. They produced detailed tables and maps of population characteristics and medical data for a variety of spatial units (statewide traffic assignment model zones, minor civil divisions, counties, and the entire state) and used these as a planning guide. In such analyses, geographic information systems (GIS) are useful for linking data to geographic locations, conducting spatial analyses, and producing maps.

Despite the widespread use of classic location-allocation models by both academic and private researchers, there are limits to their efficacy. We first warned against limited models in the beginning of the chapter with a citation from Kearns and Joseph. Rosenberg (1988), in an article that discusses methodologies for analyzing health care delivery systems, is critical of a strategy of evaluating "optimal" solutions to the location of facilities by determining to what extent patients in the system actually benefit by the strategy:

> There is a flaw in this suggestion and it is also a flaw with respect to optimization procedures in general. In testing optimal planning schemes against patient outcomes, implicit assumptions are made about the behaviour of both consumers and suppliers. For example, typical assumptions are that preferences for a service are homogeneous, that individuals will travel to the nearest site to consume a service, that demand in an area can be represented by a point, that services provided at each facility are qualitatively similar, and that all facilities produce services at a particular level at one point in time. These assumptions have little basis in actual consumer behaviour or in how systems of facilities are developed. (p. 180)

Rosenberg goes on to suggest an alternative framework in which the *individual* is placed in a pivotal position being affected on one side by sociocultural influences and on the other side by politicoeconomic influences (Figure 10-9). Individuals make differential decisions to enter the health care delivery system based on a host of sociocultural and politicoeconomic influences. The boxes describing the two sets of influences are organized as nested hierarchies with the central boxes being the points of departure. To some degree, all levels of the two hierarchies exert influence on individuals as they decide to seek health care, or once they are in the system (see Figure 9-1 and associated text). The relative importance of each level varies with the individual's

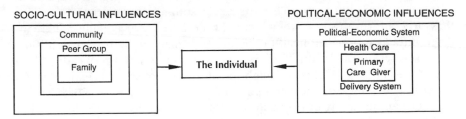

FIGURE 10-9. A framework for analyzing health care delivery. From Rosenberg (1988, p. 181). Copyright 1988 by Elsevier Science. Reprinted by permission.

specific circumstances. Rosenberg maintains that geographical, historical, epidemiological, and environmental factors may enter the analysis in either hierarchy. He uses an example of the delivery of abortion services in Canada to illustrate how sociocultural and political–economic influences affect the individual's decision to seek abortion services. In conclusion, Rosenberg argues that most analyses of health care delivery systems are too narrowly conceived. An economic-based location-allocation model might provide an optimal solution for the allocation of hospital facilities from the point of view of physicians and staff personnel, but such a solution ignores other, equally important factors that have an impact on the population that these hospitals serve.

Regionalization of Medical Service

A region may be defined as a bounded area that is internally homogeneous by one or more criteria. Regions may be precisely defined using numerical measures, or they may be simply mental constructs, such as the perception of the extent of a neighborhood by its residents. Health care regionalization implies an allocation of health services based on geography. Regionalization schemes need not be based solely on geography; they can be based on consciously developed markets. The Kaiser-Permanente Medical Care Program is an example. Kaiser-Permanente was originally established in California for a limited clientele, but it has since expanded virtually throughout the United States and to a wider population base.

Regionalization may recognize that health and social conditions vary among subareas and therefore strive to bring about greater horizontal equity of service. Or, regionalization may be a response to increasing costs. For example, centralizing facilities at fewer hospitals with high patient volumes, rather than offering specialized services at every medical center, may bring about considerable cost savings. A parallel argument may be that by regionalizing hospital care some improvement is made in overall quality of care. Regionalization might appear to be an easy task; however, some basic decisions have to be made. The geographic regions may follow the convenient boundaries of administrative units or may be delineated by function. The second decision, which overlaps with the first, is whether to base regions on existing patterns of patient-to-resource flows or to somehow "rationalize" or alter flows to conform to some scheme based on efficiency or equality. There are three ways to rationalize health care: through management of patient flows (e.g., several hospitals funnel their routine outpatient surgery cases to one large free-standing facility); through the allocation of special services, where expensive high-tech medical equipment is centered in a few major hospitals, or where an hierarchy of clinics and hospitals is established within a region; and by managing the location of health personnel, which follows the same philosophy as the allocation of facilities (Ricketts et al., 1994).

Regionalization decisions and the emphasis placed on regionalization depend on the type of medical system a country has. Welfare state and socialist state systems use regionalization as part of their overall approach. In market economies, management or regionalization is largely controlled or influenced by organized interest groups, such as provider groups and insurance companies, and to a greater or lesser extent by the federal government. Government may see its role as making policy and subsidizing care for part of the population. However, government regulation only works with the cooperation of insurance and provider organizations (Groenewegen, 1994).

In the United States there has been less concern about regionalization than in other developed countries. The free-enterprise system often leads to competition among resources and regional imbalances that are difficult to rationalize. However, a number of attempts have been made to regionalize health care delivery in the United States. A few of these schemes resulted from the legislative acts that were discussed in Chapter 9. Some of the legislation is explicit about the types of units to be used in health care delivery plans; other programs were vague about boundaries or leave such decisions up to the states. Health planners often assess a hospital's performance based on the extent of the institution's catchment, or trade, area. Other planners primarily assume a demand point of view, or how far must prospective clients travel to obtain basic medical services. Still others are concerned with establishing administrative regions, where the goal is to minimize administrative costs.

Regionalization can be attempted for many different kinds of health care resources. The United States has given much attention to delineating hospital service areas since before World War II. The U.S. Hill–Burton Act of 1946 obliged the states to identify general hospital service areas as a condition for funding of hospital construction. Hospitals serving rural areas were at first given priority, although amendments to the Act gradually shifted priority to urban areas. Most hospital service regions consisted of one or more counties. Sometimes, however, regional boundaries cut across political jurisdictions.

In the United States, Title V of the Health Security Act provided for regional professional foundations (RPFs), which are consortia of practicing physicians, academic health centers, medical schools, schools of public health, and other professional organizations. The objectives of RPFs are to develop programs in professional lifetime learning, to foster collaboration among health plans and health care providers within a region to improve the quality and appropriateness of medical care; to participate in outcomes research, and to develop innovative ways to increase patients' participation in their choices of medical care. The spirit of the legislation is to foster collaboration among medical centers, practicing physicians, and other providers to set goals on technical procedures and ethics. Standardization of medical practice quality and style and providing continuing education for practitioners are just some of the possible outcomes. RPFs are organized as not-for-profit corporations in regions as least as large as major academic medical center market areas, but more often within a state. There is a national organization, the Agency for Health Care Policy and Research (ACHPR.gov), which interacts with regional organizations (Wennberg & Keller, 1994).

According to Ricketts et al. (1994), there are several issues to consider when creating regions. Geographic scale is important; regions in densely population areas are necessarily smaller than those in sparsely population areas. In small-area investigations (county or metropolitan area), data may be collected at the block or neighborhood level, whereas in rural areas, only county-level data may be available or meaningful. Theoretically, a region should be geographically contiguous. However, health services supply and demand do not always conform to spatial contiguity. Patients have been known to bypass many providers to seek care with a distant facility or doctor, and indigent patients do not always conveniently live within the same neighborhood or the same city.

Also, using existing political or postal boundaries as medical service regional boundaries is not always realistic. Because demographic data are grouped within political jurisdictions, and taxes collected and funds spent by state and local government also take place within these jurisdictions, there is a tendency to structure service regions within these same borders. However, people often tend to ignore city, county, and state lines in their daily life transactions, and illness and the preconditions for illness certainly are not so constricted. Furthermore, political jurisdictions often lack social and economic homogeneity. One large postal (ZIP) area in the Baltimore, Maryland, metropolitan area, for example, extends from within the city into the county, and contains neighborhoods of different racial as well as economic structure. Chronic disease rates differ significantly in magnitude and kind from one socioeconomic class to another.

Regional schemes should also be subject to adjustment. Census tracts in metropolitan areas are split when their populations become too large, and new post-office subregions are created when populations reach an unmanageable size. As demographic variables shift, and with them health and illness indicators, health service regions may need redefinition.

There are simple and complex methods for constructing service regions. Because the only geographic identifier in patient data is often the postal (ZIP) area of the patient residence, a popular method of regionalizing medical service areas is to consider a medical facility's primary service area as those ZIP areas that contribute the highest proportions of patients to the facility's load (Garnick, Luft, Robinson, & Tetreault, 1987). There are other, more geometric, schemes involving the use of polygons (which roughly delimit the midpoint between cities, towns, or medical facilities), potential and gravity models (which identify clusters of population with specified characteristics based chiefly on where people reside relative to each other and to the facilities they use), and GIS, which combine and analyze all of the information about people and places in a computer mapping environment. There is a large and growing literature on the methodology of regionalization and GIS (see Chapter 13). At every major GIS conference, there is always at least one session on health service applications. Interested readers are advised to consult Ricketts et al. (1994, Chaps. 6, 7) for more details and references.

The distribution and utilization of emergency medical services have a great impact on the well-being of society. They are good examples of hierarchical regionalization. Peters and Hall (2000) demonstrated that ambulance resources, which are an important component of emergency health care, are often insufficient, resulting in performances below those required to respond reliably to emergency calls from demand areas. The authors show how GIS may be used to assess ambulance response performance and its utility as a planning tool in deployment of this service.

CONCLUSION

Analysis of spatial inequalities in health care resources often involves sophisticated mapping techniques and consideration of equality criteria at different scales. The concept of central place theory has shed some light on the organization of facilities in terms of size and specialty hierarchies. Both micro- and macrolevel studies have investigated the reasons why medical personnel and facilities locate where they do. Besides these assessments of existing health care resource distributions, researchers have contributed important insights and practical guidelines to the improvement of health care delivery. One way is location-allocation modeling and another is regionalization. Both of these methods include theoretical models and practical applications.

We should be wary of placing too much faith in sophisticated location-allocation models and regionalization plans as solutions to a nation's health problems. Osleeb and McLafferty (1992) discuss alternatives to providing medical services in developing nations. They say that, whereas

> historically, the greatest improvements in health have come about as a result of improvements in infrastructure, nutrition, and living standards rather than from the provision of medical services, most health care location-allocation planning models continue to focus narrowly on the provision of health services as the primary means of addressing health problems. Even today most health problems require a multifaceted, integrated service-delivery plan that includes investments in education, water supply, housing, and sanitation along with medical services. In general, these diverse services, when combined, coordinated, and mutually reinforced, have the greatest impact on health and disease. (p. 246)

REFERENCES

Akhtar, R., & Izhar, N. (1986). Inequalities in the distribution of health care in India. In R. Akhtar & A. Learmonth (Eds.), *Geographical aspects of health and disease in India*. New Delhi: Concept.

Anderson, M., & Rosenberg, M. W. (1990). Ontario's underserviced area program revisited: An indirect analysis. *Social Science and Medicine, 30,* 35–44.

Bogdanich, W. (1991). *The great white lie: Dishonesty, waste, and incompetence in the medical community.* New York: Simon & Schuster.

Borinstein, A. B. (1992). Public attitudes toward persons with mental illness. *Health Affairs 11,* 187–196.

Bosanac, E. M., & Hall, D. S. (1981). A small area profile system: Its use in primary care resource development. *Social Science and Medicine, 15D,* 313–319.

Budson, R. D. (1988). *Siting community facilities for the mentally ill: Background, issues, and strategies* (Working paper, Lincoln Institute of Land Policy). Cambridge, MA: Lincoln Institute.

Burns J. (1993). Caring for the community: Hospital programs provide a lifeline for the inner cities, but only a few are to be found. *Modern Healthcare, 23,* 30–33.

Calvo, A. B., & Marks, D. H. (1973). Location of health care facilities: An analytical approach. *Socio-economic Planning Sciences, 7,* 407–422.

Chiotti, Q. P., & Joseph, A. E. (1995). Casey House: Interpreting the location of a Toronto AIDS hospice. *Social Science and Medicine, 41,* 131–140.

Christaller, W. (1966). *Central places in Southern Germany.* Englewood Cliffs, NJ: Prentice Hall.

Cloutier-Fisher, D., & Joseph, A. E. (2000). Long-term care restructuring in rural Ontario. *Social Science and Medicine. 50,* 1037–1045.

Curtis, S. (1989). *The geography of public welfare provision.* London: Routledge.

Curto de Casas, S. I. (1994). Health care in Latin America. In D. R. Phillips & Y. Verhasselt (Eds.), *Health and development* (pp. 234–248). London: Routledge.

Davies, B. (1968). *Social needs and resources in local services.* London: Michael Joseph.

Dear, M. (1992) Understanding and overcoming the NIMBY syndrome. *Journal of the American Planning Association, 58,* 288–300.

Dear, M., & Laws, G. (1986). Anatomy of a decision: recent land use zoning appeals and their effect on group home locations in Ontario. *Canadian Journal of Community Mental Health, 5,* 5–17.

Dear, M., & Wolch, J. (1987). *Landscapes of despair.* Cambridge: Polity.

Dear, M., & Wolch, J. (1989). How territory shapes social life. In J. Wolch & M. Dear (Eds.), *The power of geography* (pp. 3–18). Boston: Unwin-Hyman.

Dyck, I. & Kearns, R. (1995). Transforming the relations of research: Towards culturally safe geographies of health and healing. *Health and Place, 1,* 137–147.

Ebdon, D. (1985). *Statistics in geography* (2nd ed.) New York: Blackwell.

Escarce, J. J. (1993). Would eliminating differences in physician practice style reduce geographic variations in cataract surgery rates? *Medical Care, 31,* 1106–1118.

Eyles, J. (1987). *The geography of the national health.* London: Croom Helm.

Fosu, G. B. (1986). Implications of mortality and morbidity for health care delivery in Ghana. *Sociology of Health and Illness, 8,* 252–77.

Foundation for Health Services Research. (1993). *Health outcomes research: A primer.* Washington, DC: Author.

Garnick, D. W., Luft, H. S., Robinson, J. C., & Tetreault, J. (1987). Appropriate measures of hospital market areas. *Health Services Research, 22,* 69–89.

Gesler, W. M. (1991). *The cultural geography of health care.* Pittsburgh, PA: University of Pittsburgh Press.

Gesler, W. M., & Ricketts, T. C. (Eds.). (1992). *Health in rural North America.* New Brunswick, NJ: Rutgers University Press.

Ginzberg, E., Berliner, H. S., & Ostow, M. (1993). *Changing U.S. health care.* Boulder, CO: Westview Press.

Gober, P. (1997). The role of access in explaining state abortion rates. *Social Science and Medicine, 44,* 1003–1016.

Gober, P., & Gordon, R. J. (1980). Intraurban physician location: A case study of Phoenix. *Social Science and Medicine, 14D,* 407–417.

Gould, M., & Moon, G. (2000). Problems of providing health care in British island communities. *Social Science and Medicine, 50,* 1081–1090.

Gould, P., & Leinbach, T. R. (1966). An approach to the geographic assignment of hospital services. *Tijdschrift voor Economische en Sociale Geografie, 57,* 203–206.

Groenewegen, P. (1994). *The shadow of the future: Institutional change in health care.* Paper presented at the Sixth International Symposium on Medical Geography, Vancouver, British Columbia, Canada.

Hall, G. B. (1988). Monitoring and predicting community mental health centre utilization in Auckland, New Zealand. *Social Science and Medicine, 26,* 55–70.

Hall, G. B., & Joseph, A. E. (1988). Group home location and host neighborhood attributes: An ecological analysis. *Professional Geographer, 40,* 297–306.

Hart, L. G., Pirani, M. J., & Rosenblatt, R. A. (1991) Causes and consequences of rural small hospital closures from the perspectives of mayors. *Journal of Rural Health, 7,* 222–245.

Harvey, D. (1972). *Social justice and the city.* London: Edward Arnold.

Health Resources and Services Administration. (1990). *Health status of the disadvantaged.* Washington, DC: Author.

Hemenway, D. (1982). The optimal location of doctors. *New England Journal of Medicine, 306,* 397–401.

Hyma, B., Phillips, D. R., & Ramesh, A. (1992). *Traditional health care delivery through mobile camps: The Unani system of medicine in Tamil Nadu, India.* Paper presented at the Fifth International Symposium on Medical Geography. Charlotte, NC.

Illich, I. (1976). *Medical nemisis: Limits to medicine.* Harmondsworth: Penguin.

Instituto del Tercer Mundo. (1994). *Third World guide, 1993/94.* Bogota: Garamond Press.

Jones, K., & Moon, G. (1987). *Health, disease and society: An introduction to medical geography.* London: Routledge.

Jones, K., & Moon, G. (1991). Progress reports: Medical geography. *Progress in Human Geography, 15,* 437–443.

Joseph, A. E., & Phillips, D. R. (1984). *Accessibility and utilization.* London: Harper & Row.

Kazanjian, A., & Pagliccia, N. (1996). Key factors in physicians' choice of practice location: Findings from a survey of practitioners and their spouses. *Health and Place, 2,* 27–34.

Kearns, R. A., & Joseph, A. E. (1993). Space in its place: Developing the link in medical geography. *Social Science and Medicine, 37,* 711–717.

Manderscheid, R. W., & Sonnenschein, M. A. (Eds.). (1992). *Mental health, United States, 1990.* Rockville, MD: National Institute for Mental Health.

Mattingly, P. F. (1991). The changing location of physician offices in Bloomington–Normal, Illinois: 1870–1988. *The Professional Geographer, 43,* 465–474.

Mayhew, L. D. (1986). *Urban hospital location.* London: Allen & Unwin.

McLafferty, S. L. (1989). The politics of privatization: State and local politics and the restructuring of hospitals in New York City. In J. L. Scarpaci (Ed.), *Health services privatization in industrial societies.* New Brunswick, NJ: Rutgers University Press.

Meade, M. S. (1986). Geographic analysis of disease and care. *Annual Review of Public Health, 7,* 313–335.

Mick, S. S., Lee, S-Y. D., & Wodchis, W. P. (2000). Variations in geographical distribution of foreign- and domestically-trained physicians in the United States. *Social Science and Medicine, 50,* 185–202.

Mohan, J. F. (1998). Explaining geographies of health care: A critique. *Health and Place, 4,* 113–124.

Morrill, R. L., & Earickson, R. J. (1968). Variation in the character and use of Chicago area hospitals. *Health Services Research, 3,* 224–238.

Morrill, R. L., & Earickson, R. J. (1969). Location efficiency in Chicago hospitals. *Health Services Research, 4,* 127–145.

Navarro, V. (1985). The crisis of the international capitalist order and its implications for the welfare state. In J. McKinlay (Ed.), *Issues in the political economy of health care* (pp. 107–140). New York: Tavistock.

Okafor, S. I. (1982). The case of medical facilities in Nigeria. *Social Science and Medicine, 16,* 1971–1977.

Osleeb, J. P., & McLafferty, S. (1992) A weighted covering model to aid in dracunculiasis eradication. *Journal of the Regional Science Association International, 71,* 243–257.

Peters, J., & Hall, G. B. (2000). Assessment of ambulance response performance using a geographic information system. *Social Science and Medicine, 49,* 1551–1566.

Phillips, D. R. (1990). *Health and health care in the third world.* Essex, UK: Longman.

Powell, M. A. (1986). Territorial justice and primary health care: An example from London. *Social Science and Medicine, 23,* 1093–1104.

Powell, M. A. (1990). Need and provision in the National Health Service: An inverse care law? *Policy and Politics, 18,* 31–37.

Pyle, G. F. (1979). *Applied medical geography.* New York: Wiley.

Ramesh, A., & Hyma, B. (1981). Traditional Indian medicine in practice in an Indian metropolitan city. *Social Science and Medicine, 15D,* 69–81.

Ricketts, T. C., & Cromartie, E. (1992). Rural primary care programs in the United States. In W. M. Gesler & T. C. Ricketts (Eds.), *Health in rural North America.* New Brunswick, NJ: Rutgers University Press.

Ricketts, T. C., Savitz, L. A., Gesler, W. M., & Osborne, D. N. (1994). *Geographic methods for health services research.* New York: University Press of America.

Rosenberg, M. W. (1984). Physician location behavior in Metropolitan Toronto. *Canadian Geographer, 28,* 156–170.

Rosenberg, M. W. (1988). Linking the geographical, the medical and the political in analyzing health care delivery systems. *Social Science and Medicine, 26,* 179–186.

Scarpaci, J. L. (1989). Dismantling public health services in authoritarian Chile. In J. L. Scarpaci (Ed.), *Health services privatization in industrial societies* (pp. 219–244). New Brunswick, NJ: Rutgers University Press.

Scarpaci, J. L. (1990). Medical care, welfare state and deindustrialization in the Southern Cone. *Environment and Planning D: Society and Space, 8,* 191–209.

Shapiro, J. P. (1992, August 10). To ration or not to ration? *U.S. News & World Report,* p. 24.

Smith, C. J. (1989). The restructuring of mental health care in the United States. In J.

L. Scarpaci (Ed.), *Health services privatization in industrial societies* (pp. 155–181). New Brunswick, NJ: Rutgers University Press.

Smith, C. J. (1998). Modernization and health care in contemporary China. *Health and Place, 4,* 125–139.

Smith. D. M. (1994). *Geography and social justice.* Oxford: Blackwell.

Sorkin, A. L. (1992). *Health economics.* New York: Lexington Books.

Taylor, P. J. (1977). *Quantitative methods in geography.* London: Houghton Mifflin.

Thomas, R. (1992). *Geomedical systems.* London: Routledge.

Wennberg, J. E., & Keller, R. (1994). Regional professional foundations. *Health Affairs, 13,* 257–263.

World Resources Institute. (1998). *World resources, 1998–99.* New York: Oxford University Press.

FURTHER READING

Agency for Health Care Policy and Research website: *www.achpr.gov*

Appalachian Regional Commission website: *www.arc.gov*

Eyles, J. (1987). *The geography of the national health.* London: Croom Helm.

Foldvary, F. (1994). *Public goods and private communities.* Northampton, MA: Edward Elgar Publishing.

Navarro, V. (Ed.). (1992). *Why the United States does not have a National Health Program.* Amityville, NY: Baywood.

North Carolina rural health website: *www.shepscenter.unc.edu/research_programs/Rural_Program/rhp. html*

Phillips, D. R., & Verhasselt, Y. (1994). *Health and development.* London: Routledge.

Pol, L. D., & Thomas, R. K. (1992). *The demography of health and health care.* New York: Plenum.

Scarpaci, J. L. (Editor) (1989). *Health services privatization in industrial societies.* New Brunswick, NJ: Rutgers University Press.

Smith, C. J. (Ed.). (1988). *Public problems: The management of urban distress.* New York: Guilford Press.

Washington state rural health website: *www.fammed.washington.edu/wamirhrc/*

VIGNETTE 10-1.   Application of Spatial Statistics to Health Care Delivery

In central place theory, the center of a population is the location of a good or service for consumers within some predefined trade area. The trade area may be defined, if there is only one supplier, in terms of how far the average consumer is willing or able to travel to obtain the good or service. If there are multiple suppliers, the consumers must be divided up among the suppliers, and the trade areas will decrease in size as the number of suppliers increases. Suppose there is a large enough population to support a suburban medical center with about 400 beds and a comprehensive clinic. The most equitable location for that center would be one in which the average travel time from the center to the furthest households was the same in all directions.

Assuming that land values, zoning, and other factors were satisfactory, where would the medical center be located to meet the objective of centrality? To illustrate, we arbitrarily choose a county located in the eastern United States, which has been divided into its seven census subdivisions (Vignette 10-1, Figure 1). A coordinate system is superimposed on the map. The spacing on the horizontal and vertical axes produces a 1-mile grid. We make a simplifying assumption that the population of each subdivision is represented by a single "control point" in each area, as shown on the map. The objective is to find the point within the county that lies in the center of the population. This is known as the *bivariate weighted mean center.* The population of this county is not evenly distributed within its subdivisions, as may be seen in Vignette 10-1, Table 1. Because most of the population is concentrated in subdivisions 3, 5, 6, and 7, the bivariate mean should be "pulled" toward this population mass. Note that the target population might consist of particular age groups or might be gender specific. In that case, only the number or proportion of people in the target category would be used to weight each control point.

The weighted mean center of this population can now be found by multiplying the X and Y coordinates for each control point by the population weight associated with that point. The mean of the weighted X coordinates and the mean of the weighted Y coordinates define the position of the weighted mean center. The equations for the weighted mean center are

$$\overline{X}_w = \frac{\Sigma wX}{\Sigma w} \qquad \text{and} \qquad \overline{Y}_w = \frac{\Sigma wY}{\Sigma w}$$

where X and Y are the coordinates of the points, and w is the population weight that is to be multiplied by the X and Y coordinates, respectively. As each wX and

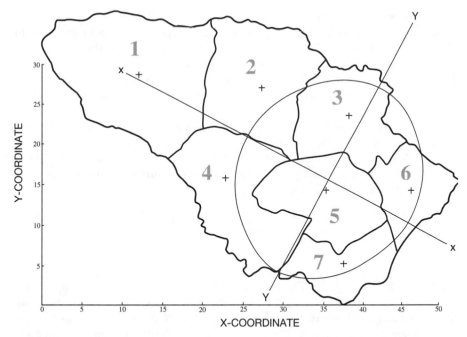

VIGNETTE 10-1, FIGURE 1. A typical U.S. county with seven census subdivisions.

wY operation is completed, they are accumulated to yield the sums that are divided by the sum of the population weights. In our medical center location example, the coordinates of the mean weighted center are $X = 36.13$ and $Y = 16.56$, as shown in Vignette 10-1, Figure 1.

It is also instructive to know how the population is dispersed about the bivariate mean. In the previous example, the district control points are dispersed along a northwest–southeast axis; however, the bulk of the population is concentrated in the southeastern end of the county. To ascertain the distribution of our population, we may employ a *standard deviational ellipse*. This measure, as the

VIGNETTE 10-1, TABLE 1.   County Coordinates and Populations

County subdivision	X coordinate	Y coordinate	Population
1	12	29	11,000
2	27	27	10,400
3	35	22	17,284
4	23	16	7,037
5	36.5	14.5	7,769
6	47	16	7,212
7	42	7	34,800

name implies, summarizes the dispersion of our population in terms of an ellipse, which is balanced on the fulcrum of the mean center, with its long axis in
the direction of the maximum dispersion and its short axis in the direction of
minimum dispersion. Three quantities emerge from the computation of the ellipse: the lengths of the long and short axes and the directional orientation of
the ellipse. It will soon become apparent that this is a complicated process best
suited to a computer.

It is first necessary to *transpose* the coordinate system in terms of the bivariate
mean. This involves subtracting the mean from each of the original X and Y coordinates (Vignette 10-1, Table 2). We may then compute the angle of rotation of
the original axes as it is oriented to the pattern of control points. This is done
with the following trigonometric equation:

$$\tan \theta = \frac{(\Sigma x^2 - \Sigma y^2) + \sqrt{(\Sigma x^2 - \Sigma y^2)^2 + 4(\Sigma xy)^2}}{2(\Sigma xy)}$$

where $\tan \theta$ is the tangent of the angle of rotation, and x and y represent the
quantities $(X - \overline{X})$ and $(Y - \overline{Y})$, respectively. The first two terms in the numerator
of the equation involve summing the squared deviations around the bivariate
mean, but Σxy involves summing the cross product of the deviations around the
mean. Vignette 10-1, Table 2 shows the individual calculations and the sums just
mentioned. Angle θ is measured clockwise from the original Y axis, like a bearing
from north on a map. The angle of rotation equation can produce a negative value of $\tan\theta$. If this occurs, ignore the sign when looking up the value in a table of
tangents. However, the angle found from the tables must be subtracted from 90°
in order to give the correct value of θ. In this case, $\theta = 28°$ for the Y axis. The X
axis is drawn at a 90° angle to the Y axis.

The next step is to calculate standard deviations about each of the trans-
posed axes that will define the shape of the ellipse. Beginning with the X axis,

$$\sigma_x = \sqrt{\frac{(\Sigma x'^2) \cos \theta - 2(\Sigma x'y') \sin \theta \cos \theta + (\Sigma y'^2) \sin^2 \theta}{n}}$$

**VIGNETTE 10-1, TABLE 2. Preliminary Computations for Mean Center and
Standard Deviation**

County subdivision	X coordinate	Y coordinate	$X - \overline{X}$	$Y - \overline{Y}$	x^2	y^2	xy
1	12	29	−24.13	12.44	582.3	154.8	−300.2
2	27	27	−9.13	10.44	83.4	109	−95.3
3	35	22	−1.13	5.44	1.3	29.6	−6.1
4	23	16	−13.13	−.56	172.4	.31	7.4
5	36.5	14.5	.37	−2.06	.14	4.2	−.76
6	47	16	10.87	−.56	118.2	.31	−6.1
7	42	7	5.87	−9.56	34.5	91.4	−56.1
					992.2	389.6	−457.2

where $\cos^2 \theta$ is the square of the cosine of the angle. Similarly $\sin^2 \theta$ is the square of the sine of the angle. The equation for the Y axis is

$$\sigma_y = \sqrt{\frac{(\Sigma x'^2)\sin^2 \theta + 2(\Sigma x'y')\sin \theta \cos \theta + (\Sigma y'^2)\cos^2 \theta}{n}}$$

In this example, $\sigma_x = 11.4$ and $\sigma_y = 13.3$ The resultant standard deviational ellipse is fitted to the county subdivision pattern in Vignette 10-1, Figure 1;. Since σ refers to distance away from the mean, the length of the ellipse along its two axes is $2\sigma_x$ and $2\sigma_y$. For a more complete exposition on the various descriptive measures for spatial distributions, the reader is directed to Ebdon (1985, Chap. 7).

The efficient location of a health care facility should take into account the *relative position* of patients, care providers, and institutions. A technique that is based on the precept that population or activities at one location influences spatial interaction is called *population potential*. Social and economic interaction is substantially influenced by the distance between people and the locations of their activity centers. The notion that a medical center should be placed in the center of its service population is based on the fact that the attraction of a service declines with distance. Furthermore, socially and economically homogeneous communities with larger populations have a greater impact on service centers than do communities with smaller populations. The basic concept of population potential is that the magnitude of spatial interaction is directly influenced by the size of the populations at their origins. In this example, we assume that the seven district control points are the origins of the populations living within their borders. Symbolically, the population potential, V, at any control point i is defined as

$$V_i = \Sigma \frac{P_j}{d_{ij}}$$

where there are n origins influencing location i whose populations are given by P_j and whose distances from i are given by d_{ij}.

Applying this to the medical center problem, we compute for each of the seven districts ($j = 1$ to 7) the ratios P_j/d_{ij} and sum them to yield the potential at i. This result is measured in persons per mile. Vignette 10-1, Table 3 shows the potential computations for the seven county districts. The column labeled "% highest" is the ratio of each potential ($\times 100$) to the maximum potential, which belongs to district 5 in our example.

These potentials were obtained with the help of a computer program written by Earickson. Vignette 10-1, Figure 2 shows an isoline map of the pattern of population potential (in terms of percent highest). The map identifies the population core area of the county. This happens to be the site of the county's major retail center, which was originally constructed in the 1960s. Population potential tells us nothing about the particular characteristics of specific locations. It is a macrospatial concept, just as are mean center and standard deviational ellipse (Taylor, 1977). The potential at any point on the map reflects only the impact of

VIGNETTE 10-1, TABLE 3. Population Potentials for County Districts

District	X coordinate	Y coordinate	Population	Potential	% highest
1	12	29	11,000	120	24
2	27	27	10,400	206	41
3	35	22	54,800	473	95
4	23	16	12,270	186	37
5	36.5	14.5	90,580	497	100
6	47	16	34,800	300	60
7	42	7	31,750	310	62

control-point populations and their relative distances to other control points. In effect it tells us how close (relatively) we are to large population clusters. We could, instead of population, substitute income, disease incidence, ethnic population, or any other characteristic. Potential maps of these variables would have obvious utility to business or government decision makers.

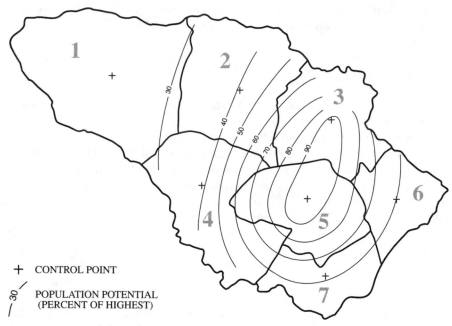

+   CONTROL POINT

30 POPULATION POTENTIAL
(PERCENT OF HIGHEST)

VIGNETTE 10-1, FIGURE 2. Isolines of population potential around the population center of a county.

11

Accessibility, Utilization, and Health Services Planning

The most important link or interaction in any health care delivery system is that between consumer and provider. An optimal distribution of health care resources is possible only if this relationship is understood. Beyond that, many actors become involved. Institutions that manage the finances for health care providers can facilitate or hinder the provision of services, and government and the courts have been called on to set policy and adjudicate conflicts between consumers, providers, and financial managers. Improving access to health care ultimately involves issues of allocation: matching resources to needs, setting priorities among treatments to be offered, and establishing criteria for the selection of patients.

Academicians in public health and also government policymakers have paid considerable attention to the concept of *access* since the 1960s. Access to health care is the product of four sets of variables: the availability of services, the possession of the means of access (money or insurance, transportation), the nondiscriminatory attitudes of health care providers, and the failure of the ill themselves to cope with their situation, such as their ability to recognize symptoms, communicate with health professionals, and navigate the health care system (Lee, Wolch, & Walsh, 1998). For many, the cost of health care reduces or blocks accessibility to care providers. One out of every six people in the United States, for one reason or another, has inadequate health insurance or none at all. Much political pressure has been brought to bear on the U.S. health care industry to improve accessibility with the goals of improving health and reducing mortality for the general population. The problems of cost, inflation, and uninsured persons have led to numerous proposals for some form of national health insurance, such as the programs found in Canada or western Europe (Chapter 9).

In the world's affluent nations, much lip service has also been paid to a policy of service *equity*, with attempts to effect a sense of social responsibility to the economically disadvantaged. The question of what is equitable in terms of the provision of health care is a complex one. Starr (1993) suggests that inequality situations fall somewhere in a continuum between mass exclusion of populations to health care and the universal right of populations to health care. He suggests the following four-stage hierarchy:

> *Stage 1: Mass exclusion from basic coverage.* Under mass exclusion, only a minority in a society have access to health care services and health insurance generally regarded as standard and basic. The majority of the population are, by common definition, underserved and unprotected.
>
> *Stage 2: Minority exclusion from basic coverage.* Under minority exclusion, the mass public has some reasonable level of standard coverage, but a minority of the population still does not. Where the excluded minority consists of well-defined groups, we can speak of "concentrated minority exclusion." Where the excluded minority consists of diverse and disorganized individuals, we can speak of "dispersed minority exclusion."
>
> *Stage 3: Two- or multitier coverage.* Under a multitier system, the entire population has basic coverage, but some have additional coverage and perhaps privileged access. For example, the wealthy may "opt out" of a public insurance system into a more comprehensive or generous private alternative. A key factor here is the relative size of the upper tier and the base: The politics of a system that is 90 percent public and 10 percent private are profoundly different from the politics of a system that is 90 percent private and 10 percent public. The former we can describe as a system of "broad-based, two-tier coverage;" the latter as "narrow-based, two-tier coverage."
>
> *Stage 4: Broad-based universalism.* Under a broad-based, universal system, there is essentially one level of coverage for the entire population (although this may or may not mean equally effective access to health care for all segments of society). (pp. 22–23)

Researchers in the United States have yet to attempt to classify geographic variations in equity and access based on this hierarchy. With the nationwide emphasis in the 1990s on cost containment and shifting funding of health care for the poor and aged from the federal to the state and family levels, the geographic variations in access among states and population groups would help to focus public attention where it might make the greatest difference.

Two aspects of the consumer–provider interaction have been intensively examined: accessibility and utilization. Access is an important concept, one that has much to do with the way health care is delivered. Accessibility can be thought of as a *potential* link. In a study of urbanization from the late 19th to the early 20th century, Shumsky, Bohland, and Knox (1986) argue that scientific advances, medical technology, and the influence of doctors were less important in determining access to care than economic, political, social, and spatial changes in the structure of cities. For example, physician home visits or a short journey to a family doctor gave way to a longer journey to hospitals or specialists because services were more spatially concentrated. On the positive side, quality services have expanded to cover some, if not all, people and areas that were poorly served before.

Since the 1960s, health policymakers in the United States have attempted to understand those aspects of accessibility that could be altered administratively or through policy action to improve health care for the citizenry. This has not been achieved, primarily because access is a complex set of characteristics and behaviors which is not fully understood, and whose principles have not been agreed on by all participants in the health care delivery process. Of course, this position may not lead to utilization of resources (the *actual* link). Both accessibility and utilization are influenced by the same factors, and their patterns are often quite similar.

The following discussion assesses the part distance plays in accessibility and utilization. A variety of nonspatial factors are discussed. The interaction of distance and other factors is examined and utilization processes and models are discussed.

FACTORS IN PROVIDER–CONSUMER CONTACTS

The Role of Distance

Studies have often determined that physical proximity is an important factor in accessibility and utilization of health care resources (Mayer, 1983; Powell, 1995). Closeness to a particular doctor or facility is one of the main reasons for using that resource. Chapter 10 discussed the role of distance in the size of the market area of a health care facility. The importance of distance seems obvious, but, unfortunately, it has often been overlooked in planning decisions.

The provider–consumer link weakens as distance increases, following a distance decay curve. Distance decay derives from the gravity model, which states that the attractional force between two objects is directly proportional to their masses and inversely proportional to the square of the distance between them. Distance decay is usually a concave curve that demonstrates a decline of attraction to a facility as distance to the facility increases. When distance decay is applied to health care resources, it usually measures the interactions between a single facility or practitioner and people at varying distances from this resource.

Distance decay has been studied in connection with the use of mental health facilities. Hunter, Shannon and Sambrook (1986), using data compiled by Edward Jarvis in the mid-19th century in the United States, discussed universality of distance decay around mental hospitals. Jarvis demonstrated that patients in "lunatic hospitals" were far more likely to have been committed from places near the hospital than far from the hospital. This distance decay was so pervasive that the phenomenon became known as *Jarvis's law*. Subsequent studies have confirmed the distance decay principal but have found that the distance patients travel to mental institutions is affected by other important factors, such as type of mental problem and the degree to which families and the community are willing to assume the burden of care for the mentally ill (Hall, 1988). The phenomenon has weakened considerably since the deinstitutionalization movement of the 1970s (see Chapter 10, this volume).

The actual form that the distance decay function should take has been widely debated. There are several possibilities. One of the simplest equations that has been applied is the concave function, $f = kd^{-b}$, where f is the frequency of consumer–resource contact, d is distance, and k and b are parameters that must be determined for any particular situation. There is no single formula that fits all interactions, which means that the best fitting equation can only be determined empirically.

Of particular interest is the "friction of distance," or how rapidly interaction decreases as distance increases. If the previous equation were used, friction could be measured by the size of the distance exponent, b. If b is relatively large, there is a rapid dropoff of contact. The slope of the distance decay lines represents the b parameter. For mental hospitals in Hunter's study, the slope of the distance decay function varied from –2.6 to –17.9. The average slope for eight long-established asylums was –9.2 (Figure 11-1). Patterns of admission rates to mental hospitals in the eastern United States reflect this

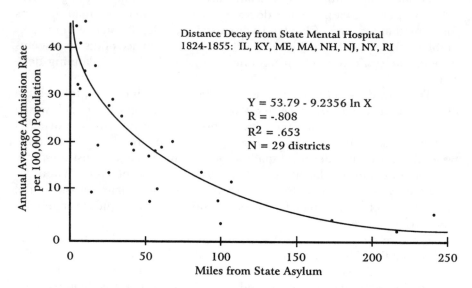

FIGURE 11-1. A distance decay curve of admissions to state mental hospitals in selected states in the 19th century. From Hunter, Shannon, and Sambrook (1986, p. 1046). Copyright 1986 by Elsevier Science. Reprinted by permission.

distance decay (Figure 11-2). There is a consistent pattern of concentric rings around hospitals with peak admission rates in home counties and diminished rates in the more remote districts

Distance decay, or friction of distance, is useful in determining central place hierarchies and functional regionalization (Chapter 10). If distance appears to be a factor in provision of a certain level of health care service, this service should be decentralized and locally accessible. This usually applies to low-order services such as first aid. High-order services, such as the treatment of rare diseases or heart transplants, are not as sensitive to distance. People are willing to travel farther for these services, so resources can be centralized. Friction of distance can establish threshold distances for levels of service. For example, a distance decay curve shows that people in low-income countries will normally walk up to 3 kilometers (1.86 miles) to a primary health care clinic. A low-level clinic beyond this threshold has limited usefulness.

There are many ways to measure distance. *Map distance* from a patient's residence to a health care resource is commonly used because it is relatively easy to determine, and when distances are short, as they often are in metropolitan study areas, map distances coincide with physical distances. Other distance measures may be more meaningful in certain situations, however. *Road distance* takes into account the actual or supposed route taken from home to practitioner. This measure can be weighted by road quality. In their investi-

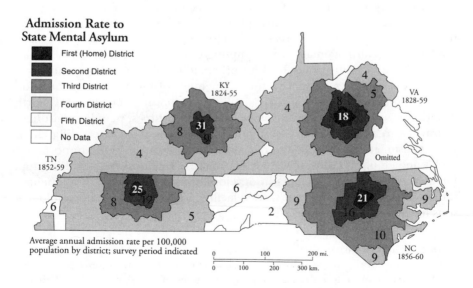

FIGURE 11-2. The effect of distance on state mental hospital admissions in selected northeastern states in the 19th century. From Hunter, Shannon, and Sambrook (1986, p. 1041). Copyright 1986 by Elsevier Science. Reprinted by permission.

gation of access to health services in Grenada, Poland, Taylor, and Hayes (1990) scored accessibility as "average" or "poor" on the basis of topography, particularly slope, and vehicle traffic volume, which was a surrogate for the ease in hitching a ride.

In societies in which time is often more important than distance, the time it takes to reach a facility, *time distance*, may be the best measure. The degree of patient *mobility*, which involves the type of transportation available, is also implicated in distance measures. Harder to determine accurately, because it is subjective, is *perceived distance*, a patient's idea of how far away health care resources are. Some important distance measures that do not involve distance in the geographic sense are sociocultural distances. *Social distance* is the gap between consumer and provider in terms such as social status or illness beliefs. *Economic distance* is the ability to pay for services.

These sociocultural types of distance measures can be used in accessibility and utilization studies through such techniques as multidimensional scaling (MDS). With MDS, the researcher must have a table of "proximity" measurements between, say, all pairs of providers and consumers in a study area. These measurements represent the characteristics of both providers and consumers that would tend to attract or repel one from the other. Clearly, some form of distance is one of these characteristics; income and social class are also useful in such an analysis. The technique partitions the providers and consumers according to their characteristics and shows clusters of relatively homogeneous subgroups. Statistical techniques such as MDS provide useful ways of testing theories related to distance decay or social class attraction, for example.

According to Rushton (1984) and others, research reveals that because of poor geographical accessibility, primary health care does not reach the majority of people in rural areas in developing countries. As a result, many government health agencies are attempting to expand the number of health service sites and to distribute health workers to remote areas. In some developing areas, facilities located within a few miles of most of the population may be rarely used because their quality is so poor. Even in rural North America, where there are relatively few health resources, people might have to travel a great distance for treatment. Distance is not the overriding factor in all consumer-resource situations, and sometimes it is of little importance. Bailey and Phillips (1990), in a study of the use of health services in Kingston, Jamaica, found that consumers in developing nations do not always behave rationally by using the nearest service facility. There are several possible reasons for this:

Doctors' offices vary in their attractiveness, convenience and location; doctors' services vary in real or perceived quality, and in costs and convenience in terms of a number of factors such as time and attitudes of ancillary staff. In Third World cities, social factors and costs as well as local reputation, physicians' attitudes, and the like seem to vary considerably in reality and also in the public estimation. (p. 9)

Geographers should be aware of the danger of a narrow focus on distance; it can mask other factors (Jones & Moon, 1993). Most social scientists are aware of this and consider distance in relation to other variables.

Nonspatial Factors

In Chapter 9 we made the point that analysis of health care delivery systems requires a multidisciplinary approach. Cultural, social, economic, and political constraints on health care–seeking behavior require a similar approach to understanding client–provider interactions.

As a policymaking tool, one approach to analyzing access would be to look at the *continuum of coverage* (Ricketts, Savitz, Gester, & Osborne, 1994). At the lower end of this continuum it is useful to specify what proportion of any population in fact has available health care. The next step involves estimating what proportion of that population actually can use (has access to) these services; then, we need to know what proportion are willing to make use of these services; next, we must determine what proportion actually use the services; finally, at the top of the continuum, we might ask what proportion received effective care. Whereas the conceptual scheme seems plausible, difficulties arise when we attempt to define such terms as "available," "access," "willing," and "effective." Clearly, this is not a simplistic approach.

Population subgroups differ in terms of accessibility and utilization according to their age, sex, social class, and ethnicity. For example, elderly people typically use health care resources more often than other age groups. Women in the United States appear to require more hospital care than do men. Lower social status and minority populations often have relatively less access to health care.

In the United States, elderly persons who cannot finance their own medical care may apply for a joint federal–state program called Medicare. Besides the services provided for illness, Medicare may also pay for disease-preventing vaccinations. During 1993, for example, almost 10 million persons received Medicare-reimbursed influenza vaccinations (Centers for Disease Control and Prevention, 1995). However, eligible black people were far less likely to receive inoculations than were whites. In 33 states and in the District of Columbia, vaccination rates for blacks were below 60% of the rates for whites. To reach greater numbers of minority elderly people with potentially life-saving vaccinations, we need to know what socioeconomic and access barriers might exist.

Indigent persons who are too young to qualify for Medicare may apply for Medicaid. Families that receive welfare benefits are automatically eligible for Medicaid. Some persons or families who are poor enough to qualify for welfare but are excluded for other reasons may be qualified for Medicaid. Still others have incomes above the public assistance eligibility level, but their medical expenses are so high that they qualify for Medicaid coverage. While the federal government defines the groups that qualify for federal matching funds, the states determine what minimum income levels and other categories are allowed to be included in Medicaid. There are substantial differences in variability among the state Medicaid programs. States along the Pacific coast, in the upper Midwest, and in the Northeast have higher proportions of eligible Medicaid recipients than do the other states (Bohland, 1990).

In the 1994 general election, California voters passed by a margin of 3 to 2 an initiative called Proposition 187, which barred access to welfare services, nonemergency medical treatment, and public schooling to foreigners living illegally in the state. Prior to the election, there had been widespread complaints from health, education, and welfare agencies that they could scarcely afford to provide services to citizens, much less noncitizens. Passage of the referendum triggered public demonstrations throughout the state by the large Hispanic community. So draconian was this measure that its enforcement was delayed by federal and state judges, and several lawsuits were filed immediately by ethnic organizations.

In 1993, a health research team decided to find out how access to health care differed among white, black, and Hispanic adolescents (ages 10–17) in the United States (Lieu, Newacheck, & McManus, 1993). They found that black and Hispanic adolescents made fewer visits to doctors or clinics for routine care than did their white counterparts. Compared with over 80% of whites, only 59% of black adolescents and 58% of Hispanic adolescents cited a doctor's office, private clinic, or HMO as their source of routine health care. Alternatively, they used neighborhood or hospital clinics. This was partly due to lack of insurance or other financial resources. What people believe about the causes of illness and the appropriate treatment of illness also affects the kinds of help they will seek. Lieu et al. (1993) argued that the worse health status of their black and Hispanic adolescents could be the result of cultural differences in disease perception. They cited several references that gave evidence that different beliefs regarding health have been found to influence the use of health care among adults of different races. The research did not rule out the possibility of discrimination in either institutional access or physician behavior.

Economic constraints on health care access may display unexpected complexity. Pyle and Lauer (1975) investigated disease rates and hospital service use in Akron and Summit County, Ohio. They found a consistent progression from high to low mortality, from heart disease, strokes, and cancer, that was associated with low to high income groups. However, a consistent relationship was not found between income and use of hospitals. The poorest people, who received Medicaid payments, demanded services at higher levels than did the marginally poor, who could not claim these benefits.

Provision of care involves the level and quality of care, staff attitudes toward patients and the possible religious affiliation of hospitals. In addition, health-seeking behavior has a political and cultural context. There is some evidence, for example, that there may be cultural barriers to health care utilization and access among non-Anglo immigrants to the United States (Gellert, Maxwell, Higgins, Mai, & Lowery, 1995). Based on a sample survey of Vietnamese Americans in Southern California, researchers found that 21% of respondents reported difficulty in communicating with medical staff in hospitals. Clearly, women in particular were significantly more apt than men to cite fear, cost, lack of time, transportation, child care, and companionship as barriers to utilization of health care facilities. It appears that the *ability to communicate*, which may be related more to organizational and cultural issues, is a more critical problem than language differences per se. Certain respondents, for example, were more inclined than others to believe in fate or destiny as an important component of health. Whereas surveys of this kind help to identify barriers to access, their findings have limited generalizability to immigrants. The level of income and education of the residents certainly would affect the findings. Also, respondents who participated in interviews may be more likely than others to be acculturated into U.S. society.

The system of government and the actions of power-wielding groups are important also. For example, most people living in a welfare state will have access to a minimum level of health care but little access to top-quality care. Also, there are numerous examples in which public health facilities in developing countries are underutilized because of the poor quality of service rendered (Haddad & Fournier, 1995; Bailey & Phillips, 1990). Health care facilities operated by religious orders are often preferred to public facilities because they offer better quality services, though their fees are often higher. People are sometimes prepared to travel much greater distances to visit a missionary doctor than they are for government-run clinics. The researchers admit that they do not know exactly what changes in public health facilities might reverse this pattern of underutilization, but they suggest that the balance of use would begin to shift toward public health facilities if the government would provide more technically competent personnel and increase the availability of drugs.

Distance as It Interacts with Other Factors

Distance can be combined with nonspatial variables to aid in understanding consumer–provider contacts. Distance is distorted by political, cultural, and economic considerations; it may be a surrogate for other variables or a mask for the importance of other variables. Economic studies show that low household income is often a barrier to the use of health services, both physical and mental, even when these are universally available (Feinson & Popper, 1995).

Most research has looked at distance and at least two other factors. Weiss and Greenlick (1970) investigated the behavior of members of a prepaid group practice, the Kaiser Foundation Health Plan, in the Portland, Oregon, standard metropolitan statistical area. All the patients they studied were treated in a uniform way at three clinics and a hospital. Subjects were classified as either working or middle class, based on the occupation of the household head. Distance was measured along the best route from home to facility. People approached the medical care system in four ways, by telephone, previously scheduled appointment, walk-in, and emergency room use. Use of these four approaches varied by distance and social class. For example, scheduled appointments by middle-class patients dropped substantially at distances over 15 miles from a facility. Overall, social class was more important than distance as an influence on the likelihood of contact.

Some of the earliest studies of patient travel distance was done by Morrill, Earickson, and Rees (1970) in Chicago. One important factor that is often overlooked is that physicians, and not patients, usually choose the hospital a patient will use. Patients often travel beyond their closest facility because their doctor is affiliated with, or closer to, a different hospital. Doctors' offices were closer to hospitals than patients' homes were to either doctors or hospitals. A patient might go to a more distant facility for one of two sociocultural reasons. They traveled farther because of attractive features of certain hospitals (e.g., the religious affiliation of the hospital was especially important to Jews and Catholics). Some people were denied access to certain hospitals because of admission or referral practices; this was most often true for blacks and lower-income people.

Other Geographic Considerations

Residential location affects aspects of health care delivery other than overall utilization rates. Lasker (1984) found that rural versus urban residence could be an important factor in illness behavior among subjects in the Ivory Coast. When both traditional and biomedical healers were available, villagers used native healers first, and urban people used biomedical practitioners first.

Cunningham and Cornelius (1995) used data from the Survey of American Indians and Alaska Natives to demonstrate that persons who are eligible to receive health care free of charge from the Indian Health Service were less likely to use ambulatory care and had considerably longer travel times than did those living in metropolitan areas. American Indians and Alaska Natives live in some of the most remote and sparsely populated areas in North America and depend more than other populations on publicly provided health services. Part of the explanation for nonuse of services had to do with the shortage of medical personnel and long travel distances involved for isolated communities. Also, given the variation in cultural practices between different tribes, patterns of health care–seeking behavior are believed to vary considerably, although this was not tested in the present research.

For the poorest populations in the United States, place of residence is a significant factor in the access and utilization of health services. As potential beneficiaries of the Medicaid system, the poor are governed by the disparate policy approaches of the 50 state governments. These sometimes extreme differences in provision of health care often reflect the political culture and traditions of the states. States' provision of Medicaid benefits spans an enormous range:

> Income levels for basic eligibility—the state definition of "poor"—vary sixfold (and help to explain the differences in uninsured numbers). Rationing of services is by no means restricted to the controversial and infamous case of Oregon [see Chapter 10]. In some 31 states Medicaid beneficiaries cannot obtain occupation therapy; in 23 and 15 states heart and liver transplants, respectively, are excluded. Patients can receive no more than a limited number of physician visits in 29 states. Only 19 states include clinical preventive services among the benefits provided to adult Medicaid recipients. Seven states will not even provide hearing aids! . . . 22 state Medicaid systems were not utilizing HMOs [which are purported to contain medical care costs through careful management of patient care]. . . . And the inter-state variation in physician fees is almost beyond belief. The 27 states that lay down fee schedules have set them at, on average, just under half the amounts private physicians would charge. But 19 states still allow physicians to set their own fees, on the basis of their usual rates. Consequently the examination of a new-born baby attracts Medicaid fees ranging from $10 to $236. (Wood, 1965, p. 62)

People living in certain sections of urban areas have more difficulty than others in reaching health care. Students of the social geography of the city have identified areas of deprivation where the residents do not receive their fair share of services, including health care. Residential relocation affects the relative location of people and practitioners. In his study of patient behavior in West Glamorgan, Wales, Phillips (1979) discovered that some people traveled quite far to general practitioners (GPs). This was due to historical inertia. These people went to certain GPs before moving away and maintained a strong enough allegiance to their GPs to make the long trip back to consult them.

Recall the study involving the location of a controversial AIDS hospice reported by Chiotti and Joseph (1995) in Chapter 10. Toronto's Casey House was in an area characterized as representative of *service-dependent* neighborhoods: places where other controversial facilities are located and with a history of institutional use. It is convenient for neighboring disease victims to have access to facilities to ameliorate their illness, but what about access for victims who live at a distance from a facility? When mental hospital patients are discharged into the community and need institutions for counseling or drug treatment, community residents resist siting of institutions in their neighborhoods, claiming potential loss of property value or bodily danger. Often, the institutions are relegated to the neighborhoods where there is the least political resistance, and the victims must either find transportation or move closer to the facility.

Another geographic consideration is the link between disease and its treatment. Girt (1973) asked a sample of adults in rural Newfoundland several questions about their attitudes toward disease and health care. He found that people who lived farther away from health care resources were more aware of the development of disease but less likely to consult a physician for treatment. The balance point between awareness and consultation varied by type of disease.

Utilization Models

Faced with the wide variety of spatial and nonspatial variables that are associated with patient–practitioner contacts to varying degrees in various situations, how can one make any useful generalizations? Models of health care utilization behavior assess the relative importance of different factors and try to arrange these factors in ways that demonstrate causal relationships.

Different disciplinary perspectives have different approaches to utilization. The *sociocultural* approach emphasizes factors such as family structure, religion, economic status, health beliefs, and friendship networks. *Sociodemographic* studies deal with population characteristics such as age, sex, education, occupation, ethnicity, and health status. Knowledge, beliefs, and attitudes about disease and health care are the focus of the *social–psychological* approach. Those who take the *organizational* approach believe that utilization is mainly determined by the structure of the health services system; they look at things such as government policies and payment plans. The *social systems* approach (and the approach of this text) attempts to fuse the other approaches by considering health care a system with various components and interrelationships

Another popular approach was introduced by Aday and Andersen (1974). This is a model that seeks to explain variations in use. The model classifies determinants of health care use into predisposing, need, and enabling components. *Predisposing* characteristics include demographic and other variables that predispose one to use of health services, including age, gender, where one lives (*geographic access*), attitudes toward health care, having a regular source of care, knowledge of treatment possibilities, and so on. *Need* variables would include self-reported indicators of health status, such as number of days spent in bed the past year. Finally, resources are required to obtain care. *Enabling* variables such as income, health insurance status, education of the head of household, and availability of transportation are measurements that are employed by health care researchers.

Accounting procedures and access and utilization modeling are facilitated by geographic information systems and affordable desktop computer mapping software. Albert (1994), for example, examined the geographic patterns of physicians who work out of two or more medical practice locations in North Carolina, using a personal computer and MapInfo mapping software. Albert's research addressed the problem of a medical distribution system that appears to result in some places suffering a shortage of doctors while other places enjoy more than adequate numbers of physicians. It comes as no surprise that there are more doctors in urban areas with affluent populations.

CURRENT TOPICS

Health care delivery and accessibility are continually developing areas of research for medical geographers. Two areas in which investigation has begun but which would benefit from further study are the process of change in a medical system and the integration of traditional health care and biomedicine.

Change in Medical Systems

Disease and health care delivery are embedded in the social fabric of a group of people; therefore a cultural system will elicit change in its medical systems. Because disease patterns change, technologies are improved, and perceptions change, health care systems are bound to change as well. Examples of this are fluctuations in public and private support of health care in Australia, the changing roles of groups in Democratic Republic of Congo's medical system, and changes in accessibility to doctors in urban areas of the United States. For this section, readers are reminded of the parallel material in Chapter 9.

The temporal shifts in health care subsystems have their spatial parallels. The modern system of biomedicine did not diffuse uniformly over space. There were areas of both acceptance and rejection, areas where it was more or less profitable to practice biomedicine. The beginnings of holistic health care (HHC) were in Virginia and Florida in the 19th century. In the 20th century the system spread slowly at first. By 1950 it had reached New York, Maine, Wisconsin, Illinois, North Carolina, and Louisiana. In the 1950s organized groups appeared in California, Oregon, Missouri, and Pennsylvania; in the 1960s Kansas, Colorado, Arkansas, and Maryland became involved; and in the 1970s there was a proliferation of HHC establishments throughout the country. The diffusion of HHC has hierarchical aspects; it tends to begin in larger cities first and spreads to smaller places. There is also a distinct element of resurfacing or readoption of older folk methodologies in some relatively remote areas of the United States.

Chiropractic, another important alternative to biomedicine, began around the turn of the century in the Midwest. Records from 1965 show that chiropractor-to-population ratios were highest in the North Central, northern Mountain, and West Coast states. Between 1965 and 1978, chiropractic made some gains in several states but showed losses in others. No clear spatial pattern of change is evident, however. There is some evidence to suggest that relatively more chiropractors are found in states where there are low doctor-to-population ratios; perhaps they "fill in" for doctors in these states. Chiropractors tend to compete with osteopaths (doctors who deal with musculoskeletal problems) over the same territory.

An important development in the United States in the 1990s is the conversion of hospitals from nonprofit to investor owned (Whiteis, 1998). One organization alone has ascended to the most powerful medical care conglomerate in the nation. As of 1996, the firm controlled nearly half of all for-profit hospital beds and 7% of all beds in the United States. This was accomplished by purchasing community hospitals, closing or consolidating facilities deemed unprofitable, developing monopolistic local referral networks, and cutting staff. The effect on access to citizens is that while corporate activity has been on the increase, there has been an unprecedented withdrawal of support from public and community-based health care providers.

Integrating Traditional and Modern Medicine

In most countries, traditional (professional and nonprofessional) and biomedical systems coexist. In most instances there is little cooperation between these two systems. Some Western-trained personnel feel that there is no place for traditional medicine at all. However, traditional healers are accessible to most of the world's population, and it will be a long time before the same can be said of Western practitioners. Although the integration of the two systems would be a good idea in wealthy societies, the benefits of integration would be even greater in low-income countries.

Several policy options are open to those in charge of health delivery systems that have traditional and modern components. One is to make traditional medicine illegal, as the Ivory Coast has tried to do; this is not a realistic approach. Some places, such as Hong Kong and Singapore, have informally recognized traditional medicine, but healers have no legal status, and the government is only concerned that they obey the laws of medical practice. A third approach has been to pass simple legislation to license traditional healers, as Nigeria and Ghana have done. However, the license is no guarantee of good quality traditional practice, and there are few attempts at integration under this option. A fourth tactic is to gradually increase cooperation between modern and traditional practitioners. This approach is supported by the World Health Organization (WHO) and, if done intelligently, offers the best solution. It takes advantage of medical pluralism and is ecologically sound, providing system diversity and maturity.

An essential part of the integration process is a rational examination of the strengths and weaknesses of different medical systems. Western medicine, especially following World War II, has brought mortality and morbidity rates down dramatically around the world. Immunizations, antibiotic injections, and various drugs have been effective against many infectious diseases. Western medicine can also boast a systematic body of scientific knowledge, great advances in surgical techniques, and the effective use of high technology.

On the negative side, biomedicine's emphasis on cures and costly technology is not suitable to areas where prevention would solve far more health problems and where people are very poor. Most doctors trained in biomedicine, whether in their own countries or abroad, are not trained to deal with local health problems. They know little about the cultural, political, and economic environments in which disease is experienced and help is sought. Indigenous doctors trained in Western medicine often are reluctant to serve outside sites. Some leave their countries for more lucrative jobs in industrialized countries, where they can use the technology they have studied. In addition, the elite (which includes doctors) in many poor countries control ministries of health and perpetuate the hegemony of biomedicine; building a prestigious teaching hospital may take precedence over providing a minimum level of health care for all the people.

The main positive quality of traditional medicine is that it is part of the culture of the people it serves. Thus traditional healers can convey social and psychological benefits through sympathy for a patient's beliefs and feelings. Traditional medicine is holistic; that is, it treats body and mind and attempts to integrate the person, society, and physical environment. Some of the drugs developed by traditional healers over many centuries are very effective, and specialists such as bonesetters and traditional birth attendants may be very effective.

Indigenous healers can be criticized for several possible shortcomings. Many of their herbs may be ineffective, and cures are often based on trial and error. Ignorance of proper drug dosage can be dangerous. Witchcraft and sorcery practices are potentially harmful. Western medicine is quite expensive, but indigenous healers have likewise been known to have their eye on the marketplace. Both systems attract quacks.

Successful integration of modern and traditional practice is most likely if it follows the goals of primary health care (Chapter 10, this volume). These goals include an emphasis on self-reliance and decision making at the local level, the use of paramedical personnel for lower levels of care, appropriate technology, and geographic, financial, cultural, and functional accessibility to prevention and treatment.

According to Hyma and Ramesh (1994), the interaction between traditional and modern medical systems has been rather poorly researched and understood (see Chapter 9, this volume). Good (1987) suggested some necessary steps to achieve integration: (1) systematically evaluate the knowledge and skills of practitioners of both systems; (2) identify and train traditional healers as health aids for each basic spatial unit, defined by community social boundaries; (3) identify and train traditional birth attendants; (4) identify and use selected traditional healers as psychiatric aides; (5) supply communities with small stocks of drugs; and (6) establish a simple, flexible, referral system. Figure 11-3 diagrams Good's proposed cooperative health care system. Hyma and Ramesh (1994) feel that this model represents a type of integration that is probably appropriate for agrarian communities in countries such as Kenya, where one is likely to find community-based preventive and curative care. More research is needed on referrals and linkages between traditional and modern medicine in other cultures.

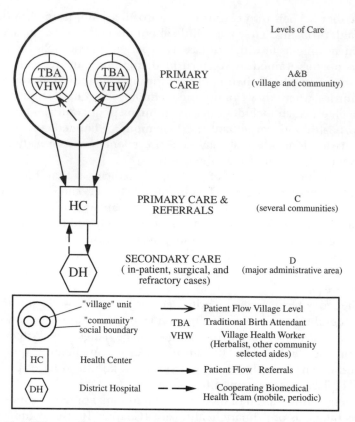

FIGURE 11-3. The structure of a proposed cooperative health care system that integrates traditional and biomedical practices. Adapted from Good (1987, p. 313). Copyright 1987 by The Guilford Press. Adapted by permission.

One of the difficulties of improving accessibility to health facilities in the Third World, according to Phillips (1990) and Oppong and Hodgson (1994), is that health care delivery systems often evolve in a fragmented manner, provided by government, private, missionary, and other sources, and they have frequently been redundant and competitive in their services and locations.

There is evidence that traditional healers are becoming somewhat accepted by biomedically trained people in some societies. Two examples show what can be done in small ways. In the United States, the Internal Revenue Service accepts payments to Navaho medicine men as legitimate medical expenses. In Zambia a traditional healer has made powdered milk part of his pharmacopoeia; he dissolves his own herbal remedies in the milk, and thus his patients receive the benefits of two medical systems. If integration is to succeed, however, it must do so on a large scale.

Until recently, China had gone farther along the route of health system integration than any other nation (Ru-Kang, 1994), but Phillips maintains that traditional medicine, with its rich clinical experience and ancient theoretical system, has been somewhat favored over modern medicine. Smith (1998) maintains that it has been documented that access to quality social services has always been determined more by politics than by considerations of need: "In comparison to the 'productive' sectors of the economy and other privileged groups, most notably the Party and the Army, social service agencies and their clients were treated as second class citizens" (p. 126). Furthermore, Smith maintains that rural women have significantly less access to health care services than do men, particularly prenatal care. Much of this bias has to do with the Chinese culture, which favors those who do "productive" or economically gainful work in the household. But, inequality goes beyond gender. There is continuing concern in China about declining access to health care in some of the poorer rural areas. Health care facilities are much less accessible in the rural areas than in cities.

CONCLUSION

The work of medical geographers and others using geographic techniques has made a clear contribution to our understanding of accessibility and utilization, which are measures of the vital links among health care providers and consumers. The concept of distance decay, although its exact form may be difficult to determine, has played an important role. However, medical geographers have become aware of the limitations of an overemphasis on distance measures alone and have proceeded to the far more important task of determining how distance interacts with nonspatial factors in utilization and accessibility. Other geographic contributions in this area have included the concept of the spatial location of consumers and providers and attempts to encompass the factor of illness in research. Finally, medical geographers have become involved in up-to-date issues such as how medical systems change over time and space and how the integration of traditional and modern medicine might be achieved to improve health care delivery in many countries of the world.

This chapter reviews some of the research on access and utilization of health care facilities. Implicit in much of the discussion are the goals of greater equity and improving the health of societies through more and/or higher-quality health services, but these goals are at odds with cost containment and reduction in the health care industry. There is also conflict between populations based on class and socioeconomic status. Most people agree that it is desirable to pay attention to smaller but vulnerable populations—minorities, youth, the elderly, and the chronically mentally ill. Readers are urged to revisit the conclusion to Chapter 10, which presents the case for a radically different approach to the improvement of the health of populations.

REFERENCES

Aday, L., & Andersen, R. (1974). A framework for the study of access to medical care. *Health Services Research, 9,* 208–220.

Albert, D. P. (1994). Physician office locations and land use planning: Asheville, North Carolina, 1948–1993. *The North Carolina Geographer, 3,* 31–46.

Bailey, W., & Phillips, D. R. (1990). Spatial patterns of use of health services in the Kingston Metropolitan Area, Jamaica. *Social Science and Medicine, 30,* 1–12.

Bohland, J. (1990). State variations in the distribution of the medically vulnerable: The impact of health policy. In J. E. Kodras & J. P. Jones (Eds.), *Geographic dimensions of United States social policy.* New York: Edward Arnold.

Centers for Disease Control and Prevention. (1995). Race-specific differences in influenza vaccination levels among Medicare beneficiaries—United States, 1993. *Morbidity and Mortality Weekly Report, 44,* 24.

Chiotti, Q. P., & Joseph, A. E. (1995). Casey House: Interpreting the location of a Toronto AIDS hospice. *Social Science and Medicine, 41,* 131–140.

Cunningham, P. J., & Cornelius L. J. (1995). Access to ambulatory care for American Indians and Alaska Natives: The relative importance of personal and community resources. *Social Science and Medicine, 40,* 393–408.

Feinson, M. C., & Popper, M. (1995). Does affordability affect mental health utilization? A United States—Israel comparison of older adults. *Social Science and Medicine, 40,* 669–678.

Gellert, G. A., Maxwell, R. M., Higgins, K. V., Mai, K. K., & Lowery, R. (1995). Barriers to health care access and utilization among Vietnamese Americans in southern California. *Health and Place, 1,* 91–99.

Girt, J. L. (1973) Distance to general medical practice and its effect on revealed ill-health in a rural environment. *Canadian Geographer, 17,* 154–166.

Good, C. M. (1987). *Ethnomedical systems in Africa: Patterns of traditional medicine in rural and urban Kenya.* New York: Guilford Press.

Haddad, S., & Fournier, P. (1995). Quality, cost and utilization of health services in developing countries. A longitudinal study in Zaire. *Social Science and Medicine, 40,* 743–753.

Hall, G. B. (1988). Monitoring and predicting community mental health centre utilization in Auckland, New Zealand. *Social Science and Medicine, 26,* 55–70.

Hunter, J. M., Shannon, G. W., & Sambrook, S. L. (1986). Rings of madness: Service areas of 19th century asylums in North America. *Social Science and Medicine, 23,* 1033–1050.

Hyma, B., & Ramesh, A. (1994). Traditional medicine: Its extent and potential for incorporation into modern national health systems. In D. R. Phillips & Y. Verhasselt (Eds.), *Health and development* (pp. 65–82). London: Routledge.

Jones, K., & Moon, G. (1993). Medical geography: Taking space seriously. *Progress in Human Geography, 17,* 515–524.

Lasker, J. M. (1984). Choosing among therapies: Illness behavior in the Ivory Coast. *Social Science and Medicine, 15A,* 157–168.

Lee, J., Wolch, J. R., & Walsh, J. (1998). Homeless health and service needs. In R. A. Kearns & W. M. Gesler (Eds.), *Putting health into place* (pp. 120–142). Syracuse, NY: Syracuse University Press.

Lieu, T. A., Newacheck, P. W., & McManus, M. A. (1993). Race, ethnicity, and access to ambulatory care among U. S. adolescents. *American Journal of Public Health, 83*(7), 960–965.

Mayer, J. D. (1983). The distance behavior of hospital patients: A disaggregated analysis. *Social Science and Medicine, 17,* 819–827.

Morrill, R. L., Earickson, R., & Rees, P. (1970). Factors influencing distances traveled to hospitals. *Economic Geography, 51,* 50–68.

Oppong, J. R., & Hodgson, M. J. (1994). Spatial accessibility to health care facilities in Suhum District, Ghana. *Professional Geographer, 46,* 199–209.

Phillips, D. R. (1979). Spatial variations in attendance at general practitioner services. *Social Science and Medicine, 13D,* 169–181.

Poland, B., Taylor, S. M., & Hayes, M. V. (1990). The ecology of health services utilization in Grenada, West Indies. *Social Science and Medicine, 30,* 13–24.

Powell, M. (1995). On the outside looking in: Medical geography, medical geographers and access to health care. *Health and Place, 1,* 41–50.

Pyle, G. F., & Lauer, B. M. (1975). Comparing spatial configurations: Hospital service areas and disease rates. *Economic Geography, 51,* 50–68.

Ricketts, T. C., Savitz, L. A., Gesler, W. M., & Osborne, D. N. (1994). *Geographic methods for health services research.* New York: University Press of America.

Ru-Kang, F. (1994). Health, environment and health care in the People's Republic of China. In D. R. Phillips & Y. Verhasselt (Eds.), *Health and development.* London: Routledge.

Rushton, G. (1984). Use of location–allocation models for improving the geographical accessibility of rural services in developing countries. *International Regional Science Review, 9,* 217–240.

Shumsky, L., Bohland, J., & Knox, P. (1986). Separating doctors' homes and doctors' offices: San Francisco, 1881–1941. *Social Science and Medicine, 23,* 1051–1057.

Smith, C. J. (1998). Modernization and health care in contemporary China. *Health and Place, 4,* 125–139.

Whiteis, D. G. (1998). Third world medicine in first world cities: Capital accumulation, uneven development and public health. *Social Science and Medicine, 47,* 795–808.

Wood, B. (1995). Federalism, implementation and equity: the importance of place in American health care reform. *Health and Place, 1,* 61–64.

FURTHER READING

Health Affairs. A multidisciplinary, peer-reviewed journal dedicated to the exploration of American and international health policy and system change. Established in 1981.

Joseph, A., & Phillips, D. (1984). *Accessibility and utilization: Geographical perspectives on health care delivery.* London: Harper & Row.

Kearns, R. A., & Gesler, W. M. (1998). *Putting health into place: Landscape, identity, and well-being.* Syracuse, NY: Syracuse University Press.

Liska, D. W., Brennan, N. J., & Bruen, B. K. (1998). *State level databook on health care access and financing.* Washington, DC: Urban Institute Press.

Mechanic, D. (1994). *Inescapable decisions: The imperatives of health reform.* New Brunswick, NJ: Transaction.

Phillips, D. R. (1981). *Contemporary issues in the geography of health care.* Norwich, UK: Geo Books.

Phillips, D. R., & Verhasselt, Y. (Eds.) (1994). *Health and development.* London: Routledge.

Ricketts, T. C., & Savitz, L. A. (1994). Access to health services. In T. C. Ricketts, L. A. Savitz, W. M. Gesler, & D. N. Osborne (Eds.), *Geographic methods for health services research.* New York: University Press of America.

Rogers, D. E., & Ginzberg, E. (1992). *Medical care and the health of the poor.* Boulder, CO: Westview Press.

Smith, D. B. (1999). *Health care divided: Race and healing a nation.* Ann Arbor, MI: University of Michigan Press.

12

Data, Measures, and Methodologies

Although many health scientists speak about studying and promoting health, it is usually disease and the risk of disease that gets measured, discussed, and portrayed in charts and graphs. This may be done through individual fieldwork participation and interviews or through massive government surveys, or commonly through routinely collected vital statistics. Many books and courses are available on methods of spatial analysis, epidemiological research design, and statistics; this book does not attempt to emulate or replace them. Our intent is to promote awareness of why they are important and to provide the basic means for understanding the descriptions and analyses commonly encountered in research articles and even newspapers. The sections that follow on data, age structure and standardization, epidemiological methods, and statistics start with basic information but become rather technical. People have different backgrounds and purposes for reading this book, and they may find different levels appropriate for them in the following material.

TYPES OF DATA AND TERMINOLOGY

Research findings cannot be discussed or questions be clearly posed if one is unfamiliar with how available or limited medical data and statistics are. This section describes the main sources of medical information and discusses some of the problems with using them.

Historical information on specific diseases is difficult to obtain. John Graunt, often called the father of demography, first used tombstones and bills of mortality in London in 1632 to analyze age, sex, and cause of death. Although he did record that of 9,584 total deaths, 1,797 were from consumption, 531 from smallpox, and 15 from suicide, most deaths were ascribed to symptoms or to conditions that are totally unrecognized today: bloody flux, colick, dropsie, fever, grief, jawfain, impostume, lethargie, rising of the lights, livergrown, palsie, tissick, and so on. Even old records that are otherwise useful for demographic statistics are seldom helpful for disease-specific information because there have been such major changes in beliefs about disease etiology and classification. Until a century ago illness was often ascribed to imbalance in body humors. Fever or diarrhea, which today are considered merely symptoms of entities usually identified by the microorganism that causes them, were discussed as though they were the disease. Even the best physicians, for example, might have written that malaria "became typhous in its course" or might have failed to distinguish between yellow fever and cholera. One can search the medical descriptions to see whether particular diseases might have been present in certain times and places, and then say that syphilis was not known in medieval Europe or that smallpox was introduced to the Aztecs by the Spaniards. Total deaths can sometimes be collected from church records or private journals, and these sources are also used to estimate mortality from malaria, scarlet fever, and other diseases that can be identified. However, for most diseases, disease-specific mortality rates cannot be estimated, except possibly for the catastrophic epidemics; and even then several diseases may have been occurring concurrently.

Registration of vital statistics provides the most important single source of data. In 1842, Massachusetts became the first state to enact legislation requiring the systematic registration of vital events. In 1880, the U.S. Census Bureau established a national registration area for deaths. Initially only Massachusetts, New Jersey, the District of Columbia, and a few large cities were included. It was not complete in coverage until the last southern state achieved standards in 1932. During the latter part of the 19th century, as the New York City Board of Health codification of cause of death spread and was more widely used, it became possible to study patterns of mortality. The 1890 Census of Population (U.S. Census Bureau, 1890) included survey questions on cause of death that, although subject to much error, provide landmark coverage for the entire population.

There is great variation internationally in the reliability of cause-of-death data. In many countries the World Health Organization maintains special registration areas in which cause of death is better diagnosed and reported than elsewhere in the country. The organization's statistics are often based on these areas, which may not be typical of rural areas or remote regions with different ethnic groups. Nevertheless, there is extensive reporting of cause of death in most countries according to the categories of the *International Classification of Diseases* (World Health Organization, 1993).

Even in economically developed countries where mortality is well reported, the only really accurate data are those derived from autopsies. Autopsy surveys have demonstrated that cause of death is inaccurately diagnosed much of the time—as much as 20% or 30% for some causes. It is difficult, for example, to determine cause of death from cancer of the pancreas, the stomach, or other internal organs without an autopsy. In recent years cancer registries have been created for a few countries (e.g., Singapore) and several states, provinces, and cities. Quality varies greatly depending on the registries' completeness of coverage and basis of diagnosis, but they provide the basis for promising new research. At the other extreme, the worst reporting is evident when a large proportion of deaths are ascribed to "senility and ill-defined symptoms." As a general guide, the larger the proportion of deaths in this category, the poorer the statistics in general.

Morbidity data are more difficult to obtain and less reliable. There are a variety of sources including surveys, registers, physician reports, and hospital data. Many developed countries, including the United States, maintain national morbidity surveys in which samples of the population are given clinical exams and interviewed at length. It is from such surveys that the prevalence of diseases such as arthritis or lower back pain is estimated. Such surveys, however, are sampled on the basis of demographic and socioeconomic groupings across the nation. Data for specific geographic areas cannot be derived from them. National and usually state reports on morbidity are available for reported diseases. Such morbidity data, however, need to be regarded with suspicion and interpreted cautiously. For some diseases, such as plague, the data are probably complete, but for many diseases, such as those that are sexually transmitted, they are notoriously inaccurate. Hospital discharge data collected for governmental oversight and payment have become an important new source, although sometimes limited for geographic research because of the lack of geographic detail in the aggregated data released.

There are several levels of reportable diseases. Three—plague, yellow fever, and cholera—are quarantinable diseases under the International Health Regulations and reporting is universally required. Smallpox is also in this category but has been eradicated from the earth. Even "mandatory" reports, however, are sometimes not sent because the economic cost can be so severe—from loss of tourism, for example. Case reporting is also required for the diseases under international surveillance: louse-borne typhus and relapsing fever, paralytic poliomyelitis, viral influenza, and malaria. Beyond these, each nation and usually its states or local communities determine which diseases are important enough, or possibly controllable enough, to be reported. Thus, in the United States, AIDS, typhoid, or rabies are nationally reportable, but individual cases of food poisoning or strep throat are not.

Geographers interested in specific diseases or in determining health care needs for a variety of diseases sometimes have recourse to the records of private physicians or hospitals. For some diseases these records can be good sources, if the geographer can get past the confidentiality problems posed by the need for addresses. Some geographers conduct their own surveys and base their studies on the subjects' self-reporting, which is relatively accurate for some conditions and useless as a source for others.

RATES AND RATIOS

Rates give the frequency of one thing (numerator) relative to another (denominator) within a given period. In demographic studies such as health studies, the numerator is the event happening to the population and the denominator is the population at risk for the event. As an equation, the rate is expressed in the following manner:

$$\text{Rate} = \frac{\text{Number of events in a given population for specified time and place}}{\text{Total population at risk during the specified time in that place}}$$

The better one can specify the population actually at risk for the event, the more accurate and informative the results. When one must use the total population, the rate is referred to as crude. With reference to natality, for example, one may calculate the

$$\text{Crude birth rate} = \frac{\text{Number of births during year}}{\text{Total midyear population}} \times K$$

or the better specified

$$\text{Fertility rate} = \frac{\text{Number of births during year}}{\text{Midyear number of women ages 15–45}} \times K$$

Rates are often multiplied by a constant, K (usually 100, 1000, or 100,000), to facilitate comparisons among places and time periods and, in some cases, to produce whole numbers. It is more comprehensible to speak of 11 babies dying per 1,000 born alive than of .011 deaths per baby.

Specific rates present a more accurate picture of what is occurring, but they require specific categories of data that are not always available. When considering birthrates, for example, it is obvious that men, children, and old people do not give birth—they are not at risk for the event. A change or difference in the proportion of the population constituted by old men or by preschool children would change the crude birth or death rates (because they are part of the total population) without reflecting any change in conditions or behavior or experience. Specific rates are always preferred.

Ratios describe the proportion of one quantity as compared to another, at a given point in time. Commonly absolute quantities are compared but relative rates may also be used. A ratio is said to be "dimensionless" because the magnitude of the phenomenon is lost, that is, the proportion is not "per thousand" or "per" anything. If the standard mortality ratio in place 1 80 and that of place 2 is 160 for a disease, one knows that there is twice as much of it in place 2, but one still does not know whether it is rare or common.

The following rates and ratios are among the most frequently used in medical geography.

Rates

- *Crude death rate (CDR):* The number of deaths in an area during some time period divided by the total population of that area.
- *Age-specific death rate (ASDR):* The number of deaths of people at a certain age (year or group of years) in an area during some time period divided by the population of that age category in that area.
- *Standard (age-adjusted) death rate:* What the crude death rate would be if the age structure of the population being studied were the same as the age structure of the standard, or reference, population (see age standardization). The standard death rate can be adjusted not only for differences in the proportion of the population at various ages but also for different proportions of sex, ethnicity, income, or other classifications.
- *Infant mortality rate (IMR):* The number of deaths occurring to children under 1 year of age in an area during some time period, divided by the number of births during that period. The infant mortality rate is frequently used and is valid for comparison among places for three main reasons: (1) It is an age-specific rate and so is not affected by differences in the age structure of various populations; (2) the numbers of births and deaths to infants under 1 year are some of the most widely collected and available data; and (3) infant mortality is highly sensitive to conditions of both the social and natural environment and rapidly reflects deterioration or improvement of health conditions.
- *Incidence rate:* The number of cases diagnosed in an area during some time period divided by the total midperiod population of that area.
- *Prevalence rate:* The proportion of a population that is affected by a disease at a given point in time. Prevalence rates may be high for a disease, such as arthritis, that have low mortality and accumulate over years; prevalence may be low even for diseases with high incidence rates if they are quickly fatal.
- *Case mortality (fatality) rate:* The number of people who die from a disease divided by the number of people diagnosed as having that disease, all within a certain time period. It is usually expressed as a percentage and applied to a specific outbreak of a disease in which all patients have been followed for long enough to include all attributable deaths. The agent causing a disease with a high fatality or case mortality rate (not general mortality rate) is often referred to as "virulent." This rate says nothing about how common a disease is in a population.
- *Attack rate:* The incidence rate for a disease in a particular group of people during a limited period, as during an epidemic. It tells what proportion of the population becomes sick with the disease. The *secondary attack rate* expresses the number of cases occurring within the incubation pe-

riod of the first case among the sick person's contacts—a measure of how contagious it is.

Ratios

• *Population per bed:* The number of people in an area, usually an administrative unit, for each bed in a hospital in that area.

• *Population per physician (or specialist):* The number of people in an area, usually an administrative unit, for each physician located there. This ratio is often calculated in reverse manner, that is, as physicians per (1,000 or 100,000) population.

• *Relative risk:* The incidence of a study variable (disease) in one group divided by the incidence in another group, when the groups are classified according to certain exposures, such as those who smoke a pack of cigarettes a day or who do not, or those who live within 1 mile of a smelter and those who live further away. The absolute effect is the difference between the two incidence rates. The relative effect generally is a better indicator of the strength of an association and so is used for etiological research. Usually the relative risk is given as a simple ratio of rates, but sometimes, as when expressed as percentage of greater risk, "1" is subtracted in the calculation.

• *Standard mortality ratio (SMR)* or *standard rate ratio (SRR):* The proportion of observed deaths in a unit compared to the proportion of deaths that would be expected there if the age distribution were the same as that of a standard population. Although the SMR is more commonly used, the SRR is the measure that is truly standardized to a common standard and so suitable for comparison (see age standardization).

• *Life Expectancy:* Neither a rate nor a ratio, *life expectancy* is a mathematical construct. It represents the mean number of years a person would live if he or she were in a hypothetical group (cohort) of people born at the same time and proceeding through life subject to all the age-specific mortality rates existing at the time of birth. The cohort of population may be started at any age to determine the remaining years of life that can be expected, as in life expectancy "after retirement." Because so much mortality befalls small children, a population has a longer life expectancy when the cohort is started at 5 years of age rather than at birth. Life expectancy is a valid measure for comparison among places, as it is based on age-specific rates. It is a hypothetical measure, however, because the age-specific rates change with time as real people go through their lives, and no one person could actually experience all the present mortality conditions that affect people of every age. The argument for life expectancy is as follows: Under existing mortality conditions, if 100,000 people were born, what proportion would survive to be 1 year old; and so how many people-years would they have lived? Of the number who lived to be 1, how many would live to be 2; and how many people-years was that? This continues until all the people are deceased; the total number of people-years lived year by year can then be added up and divided by 100,000 to yield the average number of years lived: life expectancy at birth. Because people die at various points throughout a year, the craft of demography is to calculate how many people-years are actually being lived by the cohort.

Problems with Reported Rates

The casual reader as well as the researcher needs to be aware of the many sources of error within the neat, authoritative, published morbidity and mortality statistics that have just been defined. These are discussed next in terms of numerator problems, denominator problems, and scale problems.

The numerator of a rate is composed of events, for our purposes, the number of deaths or cases of illness from specific diseases. Problems crop up because diagnosis varies over space and time. The types of laboratory tests or special equipment that are available to one physician but not another can result in different diagnoses. The school at which a physician is trained inculcates its own procedures and definitions. The degree to which laws mandate or permit autopsies varies. All these things have spatial bias. In some states the coroner must be a physician, but elsewhere coroners are popularly elected and may have no medical background at all. In some states reports of deaths due to ill-defined symptoms or senility are rejected and autopsies are ordered; in others, even large numbers of such reports from certain counties will be accepted without notice.

There are also biases in diagnosis that result from changes in classification over time. The greatest classification change in the United States occurred in 1949. Until that time, cause of death was statistically classified according to the "lethal importance" of the conditions the physician reported to be present. After that year, the "underlying cause" of death was specified by the physician. For example, after 1949 emphysema leaped into importance in the United States, in a seemingly terrible epidemic, when in fact its significance had been repressed previously by a "nonlethal" designation. Reporting of emphysema also exhibits spatial bias; there is great variation in its diagnosis internationally. Most British physicians diagnose "bronchitis" whereas U.S physicians find "emphysema."

The denominator of a rate represents the population at risk of an event. Arriving at a fair count of people presents spatial and time biases. Consider a place in which there are 1,000 people living on January 1; 30 die during the year, 20 are born, and 5,000 tourists come to spend the summer. If there were five deaths from motor vehicle accidents, what is the appropriate denominator for determining the death rate from that cause? Conventionally, demographers use the estimated midyear population to balance deaths and births, and this is reasonably accurate if deaths occur evenly throughout the year and not in one disastrous period. But the tourists were part of the population at risk for several months, and a death rate attributed to the resident population alone would be inflated. Furthermore, even an excellent census has its undercounts, overcounts, and biases. A *de jure* census, such as most developed countries use, attempts to reassign people from where they were at the time of the census to where they habitually and legally reside. Inevitably some people get counted twice. Some people, especially minority ethnic groups in young, mobile categories, escape being counted altogether. Illegal aliens may be counted in one place and not another, but they are at risk of those automobile accidents.

The ages that people report to the census exaggerate the age of older people. In some cultures sometimes respondents forget to report the existence of people under age 5. Everyone, furthermore, seems to like to "round to zero," so there is a general phenomenon of "age heaping" at 20, 30, 50, and so on. Death rates could be higher for 31-year-olds as a group because many of them declared themselves to be 30-year-olds, whose rates consequently go down (because the denominator population of those who are 31 is reduced and that of those who are 30 is enlarged while the number of deaths remains unchanged). Demographers use a variety of multipliers and smoothing indexes to remove these distortions, but often for calculation of disease rates health researchers use the reported census population without adjustment as a denominator.

The distortions of scale stem from small populations, geographical variations among areas of data collection, and modifiable units of observation. When a particular population is very small, such as the number of old black males in Appalachian counties, disease events occurring to them result in enormous fluctuations and extremes of rates. For example, consider a small town that has 20 18-year-olds. Five of them are killed in 1 year in a single car accident. The accident rate is 250 per 1,000, enough to raise any mean or distort computerized map intervals. Yet, the next year the accident rate may be zero. For this reason it is important to aggregate enough data for small populations to stabilize the fluctuations. The data can be aggregated over time by using 5-, 10-, or 20-year periods or creating running averages. Alternatively, data can be aggregated over space by adding enough small units together to create a stable population. When there is a lot of spatial variation, aggregation over time is better; when there is rapid change, aggregation over space is better. When there is rapid change and diverse conditions spatially, the area must usually be excluded from the larger study.

Another problem with aggregation is related to the existence of spatial variation in conditions. Data are usually available for units that serve administrative convenience but that may mask material geographic difference. Imagine two adjacent counties through which a river flows. Encephalitis is epidemic to an equal extent in both counties among the people living in the river lowland. One county, however, has a large urban population and the other is not only mainly rural but three times the size. The encephalitis cases and the populations are totaled by county unit, giving different rates of occurrence with no etiological information and misleading information for public health intervention. The alternative to using such conveniently aggregated data, however, is often expensive fieldwork for which funding is scarce.

These terms, measures, and sources of data are the common property of all who investigate health-related topics. Geographers need to be thoroughly familiar with them and their pitfalls if sound research is to be promoted or appreciated. Further issues of scale are discussed later in this chapter.

Getting at Multiple and Complex Causes

Just as "lethal importance" once distorted "cause of death" and suppressed understanding, so it can be argued that using the one cause that a doctor designates as "underlying" can distort and suppress important information. Multiple conditions are listed on a death certificate, but in the past only one has entered statistics and analysis. Perhaps that one condition would not have caused death without the presence, or complications, of any others. Understanding about combinations and synergisms in cause of death were suppressed by this classification system. Much of the reduction in mortality that took place in the 1970s was due to declines in mortality from circulatory system diseases. Because diabetes, hypertension, and arteriosclerosis are all background risk conditions for stroke or heart disease, changes in their treatment or progression that have resulted in their shifting from "underlying" causes of death in their own right to "associated" (also on the death certificate) causes. This makes it difficult, for example, to forecast or assume that trends in mortality from circulatory diseases will continue. Often information on the prevalence of other present conditions is simply lost. Determining the "cause" of death for purposes of vital statistics can be complicated or arbitrary. If someone with emphysema is frightened by a near collision with an automobile, suffers a heart attack with hypertension and arteriosclerosis present, and after being hospitalized develops pneumonia in her compromised and infected lungs, what is the cause of death for the statistics?

"Multiple-cause-of-death" reporting systems and recent demographic techniques of "decomposing" changes in life expectancy and reallocating causes of death (supposing a cause of death to have been eliminated, for example) have allowed mortality differentials to be examined by sex, ethnicity, region, and other subpopulations. Targeting specific conditions or behaviors in specific populations for intervention or special service may thus become possible. Epidemiological models of multiple causes continue to develop, using advanced techniques of logistic regression and structural equations that will allow much more relative and complex information to be teased out of vital statistics.

AGE STRUCTURE AND ITS COMPLICATIONS

In the triangle of disease ecology, age is an intrinsic characteristic of people, and age structure is an intrinsic characteristic of the population. This section discusses how age structure can be visualized, how it relates to many health conditions, how it confounds efforts at causal analysis by affecting causes and results so constantly, and how its effects can be controlled in analysis.

Age directly affects the likelihood of mortality, fertility, and mobility. One useful way of visualizing the impact of age structure is to construct *population pyramids* of it. These are simply a kind of bar graph. The convention is to represent males on the left of a center line and females on the right, and to stack the bars representing the percentage of population in each age category, whether for individual years or 5-year groupings. For traditional populations in which fertility and mortality are both high, the size of the young age groups is so much larger than that of the older groups that the stack of bars takes on the form of a pyramid. As a diagram of age structure for populations in economically advanced countries, the form usually looks more like a rectangle. Pyramids often show clearly, by gouges in the appropriate age bars, the effect of such past events as wars, which kill mostly young men and prevent babies from being born during their absence, or mass famines, which kill both genders. More usefully for health planners, pyramids also show the effects of in- or outmigration and of changed fertility rates. The simplest kind of population projection is to look at a pyramid and mentally move the bars up the desired number of years. Figure 12-1 illustrates a county in Wyoming, in which energy development attracted young laborers, who a few year laters had children, and also a county in Florida, which is attractive to retirees and to younger families that provide goods and services to retirees.

The cumulative human experiences and needs that are expressed in morbidity, mortality, and health service demand can be conveniently summarized in terms of "stage of life." Infancy, childhood, young adulthood, maturity, seniority, and old age each have their separate characteristics for health (Meade, 1992).

Stage of Life

• *Infancy.* The greatest risk of dying short of age 60 occurs in the first year of life, and within that in the first month after birth (neonatal) or the first month both before and after birth (perinatal). The chief components of this risk in developed countries are respiratory conditions and disorders related to short gestation, low birthweight, and congenital abnormalities. Sudden infant death syndrome, accidents, and pneumonia complete the top five causes of death. Infections pose the greatest risk in developing countries, as discussed in Chapter 4.

• *Childhood.* When fatal infectious diseases have been largely eliminated by vaccination and antibiotics, the major cause of death is accidents and even these occur rarely. Leukemia does occur, and congenital abnormalities still take their toll, especially in heart disease. In the United States, murder and suicide have become more common than death from pneumonia and meningitis. The biggest racial difference is that among African Americans

SWEETWATER COUNTY, WYOMING, 1990

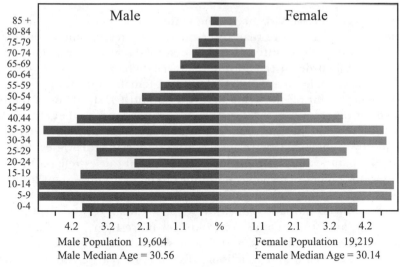

Male Population 19,604
Male Median Age = 30.56

Female Population 19,219
Female Median Age = 30.14

Total Population 38,823
Median Age = 30.35

MARION COUNTY, FLORIDA, 1990

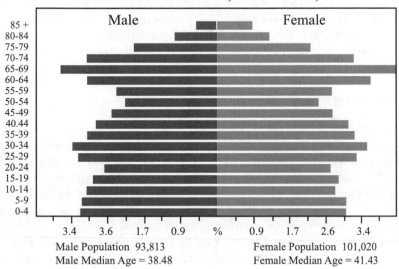

Male Population 93,813
Male Median Age = 38.48

Female Population 101,020
Female Median Age = 41.43

Total Population 194,833
Median Age = 39.96

FIGURE 12-1. Population pyramids of 1990 population in two counties.

and Hispanics, infection with HIV has become one of the top 10 causes of death.

• *Young adulthood.* Violence in the United States—accidents, homicide, suicide—accounts for more than three-quarters of deaths among those ages 15–24. The overall death rate of barely 1 in a 1000 conceals great gender differences in violent death (e.g., white male accidents 2.7 times white female accidents; black male homicide 8.4 times black female homicide).

• *Maturity.* during the years between 25 and 64, death rates increase ninefold, degenerative diseases rise to dominance, and gender, racial, and ethnic differentials increase. Although chronic pulmonary obstructive disease (mostly emphysema) is relatively more important for whites, liver disease for Hispanics, and AIDS for blacks, the top 10 causes remain the same for all groups except that suicide continues to be more important for whites and murder for blacks and Hispanics.

• *Seniority.* As mortality increases steeply between 65 and 74, heart disease, cancer, and stroke come to account for more than 75% of all deaths. Kidney disease, liver cirrhosis, and diabetes as well as emphysema become major causes of death and functional disability increases. Although three-quarters of seniors have no trouble with such personal care activities as walking, dressing, or bathing, the need for home help becomes more common. Blacks continue to have death rates half again as high as whites, and male deaths continue to exceed female.

• *Old age.* In old age, the causes of death in seniority escalate and pneumonia becomes a common threat. Morbidity increases greatly. More than half the population suffers from arthritis, and a third from serious impairment of vision and/or of hearing. Mental illness increases steeply. In this group there are high rates of institutionalization, lower proportions of minorities, and a uniquely low sex ratio. The population over 85 is the most rapidly growing group in the population structure.

The ability, noted earlier, to decompose risks of mortality from specific disease by sex, ethnicity, region, education, occupation, and other groupings has made it clear that there are strong cohort effects for mortality and morbidity. As conditions of poverty and education, behaviors, and environmental exposures change in the future, some of these stage-of-life associations will certainly be altered. It is obvious, however, that the effect of age through both biology and experience pervades the experience of health and disease. Those counties represented by the population pyramids in Figure 12.1 have different incidences of heart attacks, accidents, ear infections, pregnancy, mental illness, AIDS, and every other condition and health service need merely because of their differences in age structure. The causation of any of those conditions, furthermore, cannot be studied or addressed through any comparison of those places without controlling somehow for those differences in age structure. The ubiquitous presence of age as a confounding influence is routinely handled by standardization.

AGE STANDARDIZATION

Few things can be so misleading as comparisons between populations with different age structures. Because the very old and the very young have particularly high mortality rates, differences in the proportion of the population in these categories alter the number of deaths occurring in the population and so alter the crude death rates. Differences in the possibility of disease occurring are not accurately reflected, as discussed previously.

Consider the crude death rates in three countries: Country A has 4.3 deaths per 1,000; B has 6.0 per 1,000; and C has 4.3 per 1,000. It would appear that the population of country B is far worse off. Table 12-1 also shows the age

TABLE 12-1. Age-Specific Death Rates for Three Hypothetical Counties

Age	Population	Deaths (per 1,000)	Age-specific death rate
County A			
0–1	300	15	50.0
1–9	2,250	11	4.8
10–19	1,700	5	2.9
20–29	1,400	2	1.4
30–39	1,350	1	0.7
40–49	1,200	1	0.8
50–59	1,000	2	2.0
60+	800	6	7.5
Total	10,000	43	CDR = 4.3/1,000
County B			
0–1	600	30	50.0
1–9	3,500	17	4.8
10–19	1,950	6	3.0
20–29	1,400	2	1.4
30–39	1,050	1	0.9
40–49	700	1	1.4
50–59	500	1	2.0
60+	300	2	6.7
Total	1,000	60	CDR = 6.0/1,000
County C			
0–1	300	4	13.3
1–9	2,250	2	0.9
10–19	1,700	1	0.6
20–29	1,400	2	1.4
30–39	1,350	3	2.2
40–49	1,200	5	4.2
50–59	1,000	10	10.0
60+	800	16	20.0
Total	10,000	43	CDR = 4.3/1,000

structure and the age-specific death rates, however, and it can be seen that country *B* has the same mortality experience as country *A*. The difference is the proportion of its population that is at risk of the higher rates because of age structure. In contrast, country *C* has the same crude death rate as country *A*, and an identical population structure, but its health conditions are characterized by higher mortality rates for the elderly and lower ones for infants.

One can compare mortality among these three countries by using the age-specific death rates. If individual years of age were used instead of 10-year groupings, however, or if more countries were involved, the tables would soon become too complex for comprehension. A single, summary figure is needed, one similar to the crude death rate but which takes into account differences in age structure.

This summary, comparative figure is the *standardized death rate*. To calculate it, a standard population is needed. The age-specific death rates for all the populations are then applied to the age structure of the standard population. This answers the question, "How many deaths would there be if the study populations, given their separate mortality experiences, had the same age structure?" The total number of expected deaths is then divided by the total standard population to create a summary death rate that is valid for comparison.

Sometimes it is difficult to identify an appropriate standard population. Usually if one is comparing subdivisions of a whole, such as states of the union or counties of a state, the total population by race or sex, as appropriate, is used. A world standard and separate regional standards are used by the World Health Organization. Sometimes geographers engaged in fieldwork find no appropriate standard population available, and recourse is made to adding the village or other studied populations together and using the total as a standard. The choice of a standard population needs to be carefully considered with respect to the research question.

Table 12-2 illustrates the calculation of standard death rates. In this example the three populations were added together to make the standard. If *B* had been standardized on *C*'s population or by some other combination, the result would have been different. The general formula for direct age adjustment is

$$\frac{\Sigma M_x \times P_x^s}{\Sigma P_x^s}$$

where *M* is the mortality rate, *P* is the population at risk, *x* is the age category, and *s* is the standard population. For example, M_x is the mortality rate of population age *x* of the study population, and P_x^s is the population of age *x* in the standard population.

To calculate the directly adjusted death rate, one needs to know the age-specific death rates of the study population. It sometimes happens that one knows the total number of deaths, but not the ages of the deceased, and thus

TABLE 12-2. Direct Age Standardization for the Death Rates of Table 12-1

Age	Standard population $(A + B + C)$	Population A		Population C	
		Age-specific death rate	Expected deaths	Age-specific death rate	Expected deaths
0–1	1,200	.0500	60.0	.0133	16.0
1–9	8,000	.0048	38.4	.0009	7.1
10–19	5,350	.0029	15.5	.0006	3.2
20–29	4,200	.0014	5.9	.0014	5.9
30–39	3,750	.0007	2.6	.0022	8.2
40–49	3,100	.0008	2.5	.0042	13.0
50–59	2,500	.0020	5.0	.0100	25.0
60+	1,900	.0075	14.3	.0200	38.0
Total	30,000		144.		116.

Note. Total population crude death rate per 1,000 = 146/30,000 = 4.87.

Standard death rate per 1,000: population A = 144/300,000 = 4.8.
population B = same ASDR = 4.8.
population C = 116/30,000 = 3.8.

Standard rate ratio   population A = 4.8/4.87 = 1.
population B = 4.8/4.87 = 1.
population C = 3.87/4.87 = 0.8.

the data cannot be directly standardized. In that case, if age-specific deaths are available for a standard population, the death rates may be indirectly standardized. The direct process is then reversed. The age-specific death rates of the standard population are applied to the study population's age structure to answer the question, "How many deaths would there be if the study population, given its age distribution, had the mortality experience of the standard?" The observed deaths are then compared with the expected deaths to create the standard mortality ratio. If this ratio of mortality experience is multiplied by the crude death rate of the standard population, a standardized death rate results. The indirectly standardized death rate is commonly used by geographers because age information for death is often not available at the microscale. The SMR, which is calculated by the indirect method, is also convenient for comparing the spatial patterns of common and rare diseases in the same place as it lends itself to mapping. The direct method of age standardization is statistically more valid, however, and should be used whenever practicable.

In fact, despite the widespread usage of SMRs in both geography for mapping and in epidemiology, biostatisticians find indirect standardization so clearly invalid that the equation is not presented here. The problem is that the SMR is actually a weighted average in which the weights are derived from the study population, and so the standard is always the experience structure of the study population. The idea that indirect standardization is based on the nonstudy population as the common standard is a misconception which results in a common methodological error: mapping SMRs for comparison, although they do not share a standard population. Whenever age-specific rates are available, which is almost always the case today, a mappable ratio can be easily developed: the standard rate ratio. As the table shows, the standard rate ratio results from dividing the standard death rate (directly calculated) of the study population by the crude death rate of the standard population, in the same way that the SMR was calculated from indirect standardization.

EPIDEMIOLOGICAL DESIGN

Age standardization of rates, often sex or race standardized as well, is usually the first step for comparison and pattern discernment among differences in risk and exposure. Etiological analysis, however, often involves analyzing developments over long periods or among people with diverse behavior and habitats. Determining the cause of an acute infectious disease can often be helped by interviews and by the small numbers and specific nature of the cases involved. Determining the cause of a disease with a long latency period can be even more difficult, but the same logic is followed as for infectious or acute diseases (Susser, 1973). Four of the logical canons developed by John Stuart Mill (1856) underlie most causal reasoning in health studies.

1. *Difference.* When all conditions among the study populations are alike except for one, it is implicated as either causal or preventive of the disease. This is the classic logic of laboratory experimental studies. Rats with the same inheritance are kept under identical conditions, except for exposure to the chemical that is being studied. The best application of such experimental design to study of human populations can be found in the clinical trial, in which one group of people is given a new drug and another group is given a placebo, such as a valueless sugar pill. In this way psychological attitude as well as the healing or exposure risks of time are the same for both groups except for effects of the drug being studied.

2. *Agreement.* When all circumstances are different except for the variable being studied, it is implicated as causal.

3. *Concomitant variation.* When a factor varies systematically with the frequency of the disease, it is implicated as being causal. When more or less of the variable is associated with more or less of the disease, it is varying systematically.

4. *Residue.* When the effect of the known causal factor is removed in order to isolate and measure the variation remaining, successful explanation of the remainder supports factor causality. This is the method that geographers use when they map the residuals of a regression or the factor scores of a factor analysis in order to see whether the pattern of unexplained variation remaining elicits any further hypotheses.

When repeated studies support these logical canons, causation is gradually established. Studies of cigarette smoking, for example, have found that when groups are matched for age, sex, ethnicity, income, education, occupation, personality, and activity and differ only in smoking cigarettes or not, there is a great difference in the incidence of cancer between them (difference). If people are studied who live in totally different cultures and environments—if they are Moslems and Buddhists and Christians, poor and rich, literate and illiterate, if they do and do not eat meat, it they live in cold, dry places and hot, wet places or in urban places and rural places—always the smokers have a higher incidence of lung cancer than do the nonsmokers (agreement). When populations of smokers are subdivided according to how many cigarettes they smoke, at every increment there is associated greater risk of getting cancer (concomitant variation). When the effect of cigarette smoking is statistically removed, it is possible to identify patterns of exposure to air pollution. Thus, although statistics cannot prove anything, the accumulated and consistent evidence along different logical paths makes doubt that cigarette smoking causes lung cancer unreasonable.

It is difficult to be sure, however, that all other factors are the same. Many early animal studies of the dietary effects of water hardness, for example, had to be redone when scientists learned how to measure trace elements. The water had not only differed in calcium carbonate, as intended and measured, but also in the trace amounts of molybdenum, cadmium, selenium, and other elements. The amounts of trace elements had not been held constant and plausibly were causally related to the outcome.

A *confounding variable* is one that varies in a systematic way with the hypothesized causal relationship being studied. Although *A* seems to cause *B*, in fact another variable, *C*, is affecting both *A* and *B*. The relationship between *A* and *B* is therefore spurious. Sometimes one is aware of a confusing interaction. For example, soft water has been associated with higher risk of stroke. In the United States, soft water occurs in the Southeast on the coastal plain, which, of course, is a little above sea level. When researchers study stroke in soft water regions and hard water regions, they also find strong associations with altitude and with the range of temperature changes. Which is truly causal? Or do these characteristics (variables) affect each other and merely happen to vary in the same way as stroke, perhaps because of still another variable that has yet to be identified? One of the most difficult tasks of social science research on health is identifying which variables need to be controlled so that they will not confound the relationship being studied. This, of course, is the role of theory, but at early levels of understanding of disease etiology, theory may be inadequate.

Confounding can be controlled by both analysis and by research design. The most confounding variable of all, as discussed earlier, is age. Whether one studies the prevalence of antibodies to a virus, life stresses, activity pattern, cholesterol deposition, or public health knowledge, one needs to know the age of those involved. We have seen how analytical technique can control for age by standardizing data. The devilish thing about confounding factors, however, is that the researcher may not know they exist. One of the major purposes of epidemiological research strategy is to control for confounding factors even when they are not clearly specified.

The ideal epidemiological evidence is to find that the different disease frequencies in two populations are dependent on a difference in a certain factor, and that, furthermore, within each of the populations, that factor is more common among those with the disease than those without it. Two broad strategies address these questions: cohort studies and case-control studies, both diagrammed in Figure 12-2. In a cohort study, a population is studied. It is divided into those with and without a particular exposure, and the frequency of the disease outcome is noted. When this study is started before the exposure and people are followed forward in time, it is called a *prospective study*. When the disease outcome has already happened and the history is reconstructed through interviews and records, it is a *retrospective*

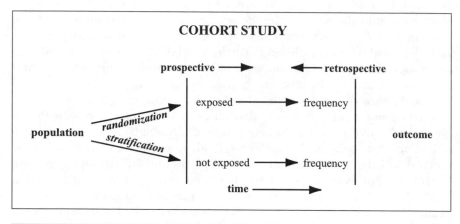

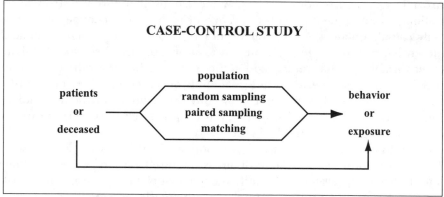

FIGURE 12-2. Epidemiological design.

study. The case study starts with people who have the disease or who died of it and compares their behavior and exposures with those of the rest of the population. Although all the nondiseased population may be used, usually it is sampled. The whole population may be sampled randomly, or cases may be paired in a systematic way with people from the general population. One may interview the neighbor next door to the right, for example, or the next patient admitted to the hospital for a nonrelated reason. Alternatively, one may pair the sample deliberately by matching the patient on a series of criteria such as age, sex, ethnicity, income, education, and so on.

Each of these research strategies has advantages and disadvantages. A prospective cohort study has the great value of allowing direct estimation of the risk associated with causal factors. As one follows the population through time, for example, one can measure how many times they ate a certain food or drank a certain source of water and how long they spent in a certain occupation. There are no spurious relationships added by the means of collecting data, such as a bias introduced when people who are suffering are motivated to remember events more carefully. The great disadvantage of such a study, however, is the cost in time, skilled personnel, and money. Following a population is laborious, time-consuming, and expensive, especially if the disease is not too common and large numbers of people must be involved in order to get enough data for a definitive analysis.

A case–control study is relatively quick and inexpensive, and these characteristics make it easily repeatable and able to include large numbers of people. There can be certain biases introduced to data collection, however, and researchers are less likely to find things they did not set out to find. Questions are formed by researchers, and people recall their specific experience in reaction to the question.

In both strategies of study, randomization and stratification are used to convert confounding variables into control variables. When a population is randomly assigned to two groups or individuals are randomly chosen for comparison, the effects of the confounding variable are converted into residual variation equally distributed between groups, so there is no need for analytic control of it. For example, consider a test of a new vaccine. Some children are naturally resistant to the disease, and some may have had it already. Some children are more in contact with other children, some have better diets, some have more psychological stress. All these things might affect whether or not a child gets the disease. One wants to compare the proportion of children given the vaccine who contract the disease with the proportion of unvaccinated children (given a placebo) who contract the disease, in order to assess the vaccine's effectiveness. By assigning children randomly, the difference in contracting the disease that is due to relative natural resistance or to differences in exposure is converted into unexplained variation common to both groups equally, and so is removed as a confounding factor. Matching cases or stratifying the population with regard to certain characteristics has the same effect of making sure those characteristics do not introduce confounding variance. Stratifying or matching by ethnicity or education, for example, eliminates variance due not only to those characteristics but to every variable associated with them, such as diet, home environment, and neighborhood influences. These epidemiological methods of analysis have been developed and standardized over decades (MacMahon, Pugh, & Ipson, 1960; Kleinbaum, Kupper, & Morgenstern, 1982; Rothman, 1986).

Geographers have implicitly used such causal logic in several of their methodologies (Amedeo & Golledge, 1975). *Analog area analysis*, for example, matches characteristics of regions so that they are as similar as possible except for the variable being studied. The method of agreement is frequently used. Japanese and Icelanders are different in almost every respect, except that both populations have a high incidence of stomach cancer and both populations consume large quantities of smoked fish. Therefore, other populations that consume large quantities of smoked fish should have a high incidence of stomach cancer. The research question is posed. Similarly, in an old but conceptually important study Girt (1972) explicitly based a sampling frame on theories of urban structure. He used knowledge of how the location of neighborhoods is related to the age of structures, economic activity, ethnic composition, sex ratio and age structure, income and commuting, and land value to stratify his sample population. Instead of stratifying by socioeconomic groupings as other social scientists would do, he stratified by structural location within the city and sampled within areas. The use of theoretical understanding of the environmental, economic, and demographic development of cities over time should be especially important for studying those degenerative and chronic diseases that take decades to develop.

STATISTICS

Although this chapter has tried to introduce basic measures and procedures, it has assumed that many students using this book are unfamiliar with statistics. Most of the problems of research design and interpretation of research findings can be comprehended without understanding the statistics involved. Knowledge of statistics for geographical study of health and disease needs to be pursued elsewhere (see Earickson & Harlin, 1994). As one reads about risk and relative risk and significant differences and such, however, whether in journals or newspapers, two statistical tests, chi square and regression/correlation, are so basic, widely used, and generally useful that we have elected to explain them using simple examples (Vignettes 12-2, 12-3), so that students may actually calculate them with the help of a hand calculator.

Chi-Square Statistical Test

A common problem faced in the health sciences involves comparison of sample frequencies and some specified theoretical distribution of frequencies to ascertain how closely their distributions match. This is what is known as a *goodness-of-fit* test. It is applied to problems in which sample data are analyzed with statistics, such as chi-square or Kolmogorov–Smirnov, and the resultant statistic is tested for significance. (The symbol for chi-square is χ^2, where the Greek lowercase letter chi is pronounced as the "ky" in "sky.") For example, it is common to test a hypothesis using sample data drawn from a population with a *normal* frequency distribution; another common test distribution is the *Poisson*, which assumes events (diseases or accidents) that are rare and random (Figure 12-3).

For the uninitiated, it often comes as a surprise that most statistical methods are designed for a certain form of data. Chi square is intended for testing hypotheses about *nominal* data (frequency) distributions. For example, the number of cases of influenza represents nominal measurement. Suppose a list of influenza frequencies for all the counties (the *population*) of the United States in a given year was sorted from smallest to largest. Assume that the average frequency of all U.S. counties was 139.5, and that these frequencies ranged from 0 to 280. If we divided this range into seven equal (40 case) *class intervals*, then counted the number of counties in each interval, we might discover that the middle interval (121–160 cases) had the highest frequency of counties; the intervals on either side of this (81–120 and 161–200 cases) had the next smallest frequencies, and so forth. We could then state a hypothesis that annual influenza frequencies in the U.S. counties were normally distributed about their mean.

Using a deductive approach, we might posit that a sample county frequency distribution from another year was not significantly different from frequencies that were normally distributed. What does it mean to say that an obtained result is "statistically significant," or that it departs "significantly" from chance expectation? Most statistical tests are based on the outcomes of a large number of experiments using random samples. For the chi-square test the differences between observed frequencies (f_o) and theoretical fre-

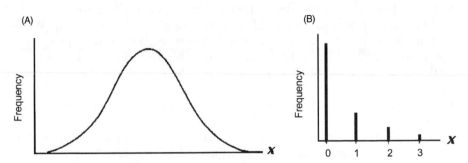

FIGURE 12-3. Statistical distributions. (A) Normal. (B) Poisson. Normal distributions are continuous whereas Poisson distributions are discrete.

quencies (f_e) for class intervals should be relatively small if the distributions are to be judged insignificant. How much variation is considered "too much" is a function of sample size and how much variation one assumes in sample data. In any case, the number of small differences should be far greater than the number of large differences $(f_o - f_e)$.

In the chi-square test, the sum of the term $(f_o - f_e)^2 / f_e$ for all class intervals may be compared with established χ^2 values expected for various numbers of classes, and one can then state the probability that a computed sum of that magnitude could have occurred simply by the coincidence. In the U.S. influenza example stated earlier, suppose the sum of terms $(f_o - f_e)^2 / f_e$ for seven class intervals was, say, 20.0. Based on a table of chi-square distribution in any standard statistics text, we could state that there is only about one chance in a thousand $(p = .001)$ that the difference between our sample frequencies and a normal distribution of frequencies could be due to chance alone. The difference is highly significant. Based on this experiment, we cannot accept our hypothesis. In Vignette 12-2, we work through two chi-square problems to further illustrate the utility of the technique.

Regression–Correlation Statistical Test

For the family of statistical tests that may be referred to as regression and correlation, the principle is that the relationship between characteristics may be one of functional dependence of one on the others. Here, we focus on the simplest of these forms, using only two variables. In this *bivariate linear* model, the magnitude of one characteristic (so-called dependent variable) is assumed to be determined by (i.e., is a function of) the magnitude of a second characteristic (so-called independent variable).

The calculations required to produce regression and correlation statistics take a bit more effort than for a chi-square problem that has only a few classes. If one has access to a computer with appropriate statistical software, it is advisable to use it for any regression or correlation problem involving more than a handful of observations.

As an example of a simple two-variable relationship, consider the maps in Figure 12-4, showing the distributions of families living in poverty and the rate of low birthweights (below 2,500 grams) in the U.S. capital city, Washington, DC. Low birthweight is an established surrogate for teen pregnancy and inadequate prenatal care. In the relationship between poverty and low-birthweight births, low-birthweight births may be considered the dependent variable and poverty rate the independent variable. We may reasonably assume that although low birthweights might be a function of poverty, poverty is not determined by poor prenatal conditions among women. Clearly poverty is not the only determinant of poor prenatal care, but it is considered to be one explanatory factor. The maps in Figure 12-4 show that the area on the east side of the city appears to have both higher proportions of the popula-

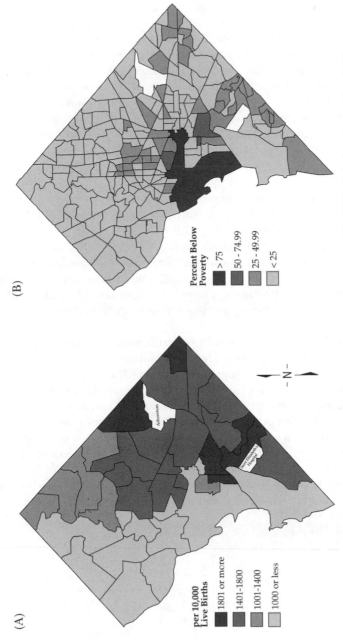

FIGURE 12–4. Maps of low birthweight rate (A) and percentage of individuals below poverty level (B).

tion below the poverty level and higher low-birthweight births. The fact that high values of the independent variable are associated with high values of the dependent variable, and similarly for low values, indicates that this is a *direct,* or *positive,* correlation.

Regression and correlation statistics usually are calculated from *metric* or *ratio* data. The resulting predictive equation, $Y = a + bX$, produces coefficients, a and b, based on the assumption that both variables may have fractional parts. One form of correlation, called rank correlation, actually produces a statistic based solely on the relationship between the ranks of two variables. Referring to the poverty and birthweight problem, the U.S. census routinely reports the proportion of individuals and families whose income places them below the federal dollar value specified as the poverty level. Thus, the independent variable is a ratio measure—percentage. Low-birthweight births are usually reported per 1,000 live births, another ratio measure.

One important statistic produced by correlation–regression analysis is the bivariate coefficient of correlation, which uses the symbol r. Potential values of this coefficient range from -1.0 to $+1.0$. A value of $r = 0$ means that there is effectively no measurable correlation between the variables. The closer r is to 1.0 (in either direction) the greater is the association between the variables. If the coefficient for two variables was 1.0, we would be able to predict the exact value of Y for every known value of X within a given geographic area. Another way of putting it is to say that there would be no error term in the model.

Geographers are interested in *place* differences. Depending on the scale at which we are working, our places (observation points) may range from city blocks to nations. In U.S. cities, the units of observation are usually census tracts (districts). The objective is to attempt to explain some of the spatial variation in low-birthweight births with the spatial variation in the proportion of families below the poverty line. Working deductively, we might posit that the simple correlation between low-birthweight birth rates (Y) and percentage of population below the poverty line (X) in a sample of census tracts in any Eastern U.S. city in a given year was positive and significantly greater than zero. Any such sample is assumed to have been drawn at random from the population of tracts in the city, and these populations are assumed to be normally distributed.

To test this hypothesis, it is first necessary to calculate

$$r = \frac{\Sigma XY - \dfrac{\Sigma X \Sigma Y}{n}}{\sqrt{\left(\Sigma X^2 - \dfrac{(\Sigma X)^2}{n}\right)\left(\Sigma Y^2 - \dfrac{(\Sigma Y)^2}{n}\right)}}$$

where r is the coefficient of correlation, n is the sample size, X is the poverty variable, Y is the birth variable, and Σ is the symbol for summation; XY refers to the cross product of X and Y, and X^2 or Y^2 refers to the square of the values of X or Y. If a table is initially established listing X, Y, X^2, Y^2, and XY for the sample tracts, then it is a relatively simple matter to sum these columns. Vignette 12-3 explains the procedure for computing correlation and regression statistics, using a pocket calculator, for the Washington low-birthweight problem.

The correlation coefficient that is calculated from a sample is an estimate of a population parameter, in this case the correlation coefficient in the population from which the sample was drawn. Recall that our hypothesis is that there is a significant positive correlation between Y and X. Symbolically, that is $r > 0$. There are ways of testing the significance of the value of r. It is, however, necessary to have a basic level of understanding of inferential statistics to determine the significance of values computed in statistical tests.

To gain more realistic insights into the nature and degree of human disease and health relationships, multivariate statistics and/or mathematical models are far superior to simple univariate or bivariate statistics. One would be severely challenged to identify any measurable population characteristics or behaviors that could be satisfactorily explained by just one or two independent variables. Since the 1960s, the increasing power and availability of computers, coupled with the increasing sophistication of statistical software packages has put complex statistical analysis capabilities within the reach of spatial analysts in many fields. A few useful multivariate techniques include regression, canonical correlation, factor analysis, discriminant analysis, analysis of variance, and cluster analysis. A good reference to multivariate statistical analysis is that of Griffith and Amrhein (1997). Recently, a useful technique called multilevel modeling has enjoyed success in spatial studies which allows for simultaneous evaluation of phenomena at different scales (e.g., local, regional and national). When we add the capabilities of geographic information systems (GIS) software to our arsenal, geography indeed has powerful analytical tools for the identification of and solutions for problems involving disease and health services.

CONCLUSION

The careful and accurate specification and analysis of disease data are complex undertakings. Confounding, misrepresentation, and distortion can easily happen without any but the best intent. There may be errors in the data itself, distortions from the age structure, and unrealized influences from other variables that systematically affect the outcome of cause-and-effect analysis. There are also, however, well-developed methodologies for adjustment and randomization and comparison of significance. Simply looking for whether these have been properly employed can raise confidence in results.

Much of the most important analysis in geography is of patterns and dynamics "in space" or over distance. Spatial analysis has some special complications of its own but also some of the most powerful methods of portrayal and communication. The following chapter is concerned with the analytical issues of scale, and with the ancient methodologies of cartography and their evolution through computers into GIS for spatial analysis.

REFERENCES

Amedeo, D., & Golledge, R.G. (1975). *An introduction to scientific reasoning in geography.* New York: Wiley.

Arriaga, E. E. (1984). Measuring and explaining the change in life expectancies. *Demography, 21,* 83–92.

Bailey, A. J., Sargent, J. D., Goodman, D. C., Freeman, J., & Brown, M. J. (1994) Poisoned landscapes: The epidemiology of environmental lead exposure in Massachuesetts children 1990–1991. *Social Science and Medicine, 39,* 757–766.

District of Columbia (1990).

Earickson, R. & J. Harlin. (1994). *Geographic measurement and quantitative analysis.* New York: Macmillan.

Girt, J. L. (1972). Simple chronic bronchitis and urban ecological structure. In N. D. McGlashan (Ed.), *Medical geography: Techniques and field studies* (pp. 211–231). London: Methuen.

Griffith, D. A., & Amrhein, C. G. (1997). *Multivariate statistical analysis for geographers.* Upper Saddle River, NJ: Prentice Hall.

Kleinbaum, D. G., Kupper, L. L., & Morgenstern, H. (1982). *Epidemiologic research.* Belmont, CA: Wadsworth.

MacMahon, B., Pugh, T. F., & Ipson, J. (1960). *Epidemiologic methods.* Boston: Little, Brown.

Manton, K. G., & Stallard, E. (1982). Temporal trends in U.S. multiple cause of death mortality data: 1968–1977. *Demography, 19,* 527–547.

Meade, M. S. (1992). Implications of changing demographic structures for rural health services. In W. M. Gesler & T. C. Ricketts (Eds.), *Health in rural North America* (pp. 69–85). New Brunswick, NJ: Rutgers University Press.

Mill, J. S. (1856). *A system of logic.* London: Parker, Son & Bowin.

Misch, A. (1994). Assessing environmental health risks. In L. R. Brown, et al. (Eds.), *State of the world, 1994.* New York: Norton.

Pollard, J. H. (1988). On the decomposition of changes in expectation of life and differentials in life expectancy. *Demography, 25,* 265–276.

Rothman, K. J. (1986). *Modern epidemiology.* Boston: Little, Brown.

Susser, M. (1973). *Causal thinking in the health sciences.* New York: Oxford University Press.

U.S. Census Bureau. (1890). *1890 census of population.* Washington, DC: U.S. Government Printing Office.

U.S. Census Bureau. (1990). *Census of population.* Washington, DC: U.S. Government Printing Office.

World Health Organization. (1993). *Basic tabulation list.* Geneva: World Health Organization.

FURTHER READING

Eyles, J., & Wood, K. J. (1983). *The social geography of medicine and health.* New York: St. Martin's Press.

Lilienfeld, A. M., & Lilienfeld, D. E. (1980). *Foundations of epidemiology* (2nd ed.). New York: Oxford University Press.

McGlashan, N. D., & Blunden, J. R. (1983). *Geographical Aspects of health.* New York: Academic Press.

Pyle, G. F. (1979). *Applied medical geography.* New York: Wiley.

VIGNETTE 12-1.   Data on the Web

In the past decade there has been a revolution in the availability of data in processed or unprocessed form. The explosion in digital data and GIS is partly driving this change. Software is available for mapping, age adjusting, even matching with census geography units and population. Maps that could not be made from data that could not be analyzed a decade ago are now free to download and print out in color. Vital statistics and national/international survey data collected by governments, the United Nations, and the World Health Organization are available in short, long, raw, and analyzed forms. There are a plethora of health information and support groups, newsletters, international reporting, and government and foundation reports free for the contact. There are also a lot of junk, misleading analysis, distortions, and commercial hype available.

A textbook cannot be a vehicle for presenting such a dynamic and proliferating medium. Serious web pages appear and disappear continually. Following are a few of the most important sources of information, data, and interpretation which are structurally likely to continue and which offer a wide variety of links to new sites.

For the following, begin **<http://>**. Bullet address follows/then target site/

- **www.who.int**   World Health Organization

  /whosis   Statistics and Information System

  Statistical information on cause of death, burden of disease, AIDS; socioeconomic indicators; health care resources and expenditures; summaries of countries' 1997 Health for All strategy evaluations; links to the world.

  /ctd/html/   Control of Tropical Diseases

  Description, data, maps, control efforts, GIS examples for dengue, onchocerciasis, malaria, Chagas, etc.

  /outbreak/   Monitoring of epidemics

  Information on active international outbreaks of hanta virus, DHF, cholera, meningitis, everything hot.

  /emc-hiv/fact sheets/   Most recent data on HIV/AIDS prevalence and incidence

  /peh-emf   Program on Environmental Health, including electromagnetic frequency

- **www.cihi.com**   Center for International Health Information

  Country health profiles and health care resources.

- **www.macroint.com/dhs** Demographic and Health Surveys

  Search engine provides country data on fertility, contraception, childhood and infant mortality, and other survery response of these landmark international surveys, including sample sizes and information on respondents.

- **www.census.gov**   United States Census Bureau

  Population data and current projections, plus complex linking to all manner of data and reports, from job opportunities in the 2000 census to

  /sdc/www/   state census web sites

- **www. census. gov/ipc** U.S. census bureau's international data base containing demographic and socioeconomic data and projections from more than 200 countries: life tables, vital rates, marital status, employment, income, and more. At ipc/www/idbpyr.html for example, users can generate population pyramids for selected countries.

- **www.undp.org/popin/popin.htm** United Nations Population information network (popin)

- **www.popnet.org/maps/maps.htm** PopNet is a global directory of web sites related to population and health maintained by the Population reference bureau.

- **www.prb.org**   Population Reference Bureau data, estimates, and current events.

- **www.cdc.gov/** Centers for Disease Control and Prevention

  U.S. government public health site with links to all major data reported, government publications, and policy organizations; online journal (/EID) Emerging Infectious Disease.

  /ncid/   National Center for Infectious Disease (CDC)

  Disease description, data, pictures of vectors, summary of prevention or treatment; latest information on risk of Lyme, Dengue Hemorrhagic Fever, Japanese encephalitis, tiger mosquitoes, and more!

  /nchswww/data   National Center for Health Statistics

  Publications and data: vital statistics, surveys, reported morbidity, birth information, special surveys and studies

  /nchswww/products

  Get surveys, books, cdroms, reports, such as the National Atlas of Mortality; see it presently at www.cdc.gov/nchsswww/products/pubs/pubd/other/atlas/hdwm.htm

  /hazdat   hazardous waste data

  /travel   latest advice for medicine, prophylaxis, and vaccination for international travel

- **www.epa.gov**   U.S. Environmental Protection Agency, with links to state agencies and reporting

  /enviro/html/   National Geographic Information System

  GIS and links; map your watershed, look at the National Spatial Data Infrastructure (/nsdi), access census block tiger files.

- **www.unep.org**   United Nations Environment Program

  Health-related data on global emissions, uv light, global warming\

- **www.gateway.ciesin.org**   Center for International Earth Science Information Network

  Climate change models, world population gridded, land use and agricultural production in China, Mexico, and many places.\

- //**quest.arc.nasa.gov**/ltc/special/disease   NASA Learning Technology Channel

  Site for showing use of GIS and satellite imagery for, especially, forecasting and modeling vectored diseases: MARA (Mapping Malaria Role in Africa)—climate-based models for predicting malaria transmission and developing spatial models of risk; Center for Vector-borne Diseases, North America—methodology to predict mosquito-borne encephalitis in California; Forecasting Rift Valley Fever epidemic in Kenya; epidemic early warning for dengue in Bangkok.

VIGNETTE 12-2.   Chi-Square Statistical Test

A common problem faced in the health sciences involves comparison of two sets of frequencies to ascertain how closely their distributions match. This is what is known as a goodness-of-fit test. It is applied to problems in which sample data are analyzed with statistics, such as chi-square (χ^2) or Kolmogorov–Smirnov, and the resultant statistic is tested for significance. What does it mean to say that an obtained result is "statistically significant," that it departs "significantly" from chance expectation? As a simple example, consider the following situation: The environmental health literature tells us that one of many health problems associated with living in industrialized nations may be due to the presence of heavy metals such as lead or mercury in the human environment (Misch, 1994). Lead is a by-product of the manufacture of batteries and with the burning of fossil fuels, and its presence has been associated with certain illnesses, particularly among children under 7 years of age (Bailey, Sargent, Freeman, & Brown, 1994). Based on a large number of pediatric blood-lead tests, we expect that in any sample of blood tests from that population, the number of individuals in each of seven categories of blood-lead concentration should not deviate significantly from the curve of Vignette 12-2, Figure 1. If the results do deviate substantially, then the sample individuals are either at much higher or much lower risk than is typical. As the figure shows, just over half the children should be expected to have fewer than 10 micrograms of lead per deciliter of blood, just under a quarter of them should have between 10 and 14 micrograms per deciliter, and so forth. If too many children in a sample have higher than expected levels of lead in their blood, the sample distribution will deviate significantly from that shown in the figure. Some deviation might be expected by chance, because no two samples are likely to produce exactly the same results. So, how much deviation in a sample distribution is considered significant?

To answer this question, a statistical test known as one-sample χ^2 is performed. A table is set up to obtain the necessary terms for the computation of χ^2 (Vignette 12-2, Table 1). The term f_o means "frequency observed" and f_e means "frequency expected." Remember that the function of this statistical test is to compare observed results with those to be expected on the basis of an empirically derived distribution. Thus we compare the frequencies in seven categories of a sample of 15,077 Baltimore, Maryland, children's 1991 blood-lead levels with expected frequencies. The expected frequencies are derived using the proportions for each category shown in the figure (e.g., 53% of 15,077 is 7,991). The differences between observed and expected frequencies vary more in some categories than others. The biggest difference occurs in the 25–34 mg category, and the smallest difference is found in the 50+ mg category. Could either or all of these differences have happened just by an accident of sampling (chance variation)? And, do the row differences matter, or is it just the total amount of variation that matters? The χ^2 test is computed with the equation

$$\chi^2 = 3\left[\frac{(f_o - f_e)^2}{f_e}\right]$$

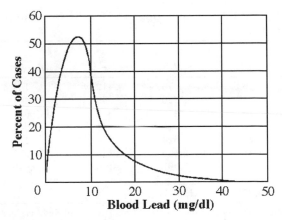

VIGNETTE 12-2, FIGURE 1. Distribution of blood-lead levels.

VIGNETTE 12-2, TABLE 1. Blood-Lead Frequencies for Baltimore City and Maryland Rural County Children, by Lead Content Category, 1991

Blood lead (mg/dl)	Baltimore City f_o	Rural counties f_o	Totals
50+	63	7	70
35–49	275	9	284
25–34	792	34	826
20–24	951	23	974
15–19	1,768	64	1,832
10–14	3,414	202	3,616
<10	7,814	1,099	8,913
Totals	15,077	1,438	16,515

which simply says: subtract each expected frequency from the comparable observed frequency, square this difference, divide the difference squared by the expected frequency and then add up these quotients. This is done in Vignette 12-2, Table 2.

What does $\chi^2 = 283.3$ mean? The larger χ^2 is, the greater the observed frequencies deviate from the expected frequencies. Chi-square ranges from 0, which indicates no departure of observed v expected frequencies, through a large number of increasing values. A large value of χ^2 indicates that there is a large variation between one or more of the categories in the observed and the expected frequencies. This would suggest that the variation was due to more than just an accident of sampling. Statisticians have determined empirically and tabulated the probabilities that any computed χ^2 value with a given number of categories could have occurred by chance. It is now necessary to consult this χ^2 table, which may be found in almost any statistics book, together with instructions on how to use it. For this particular problem the table reveals that the value of $\chi^2 = 283.3$ could

VIGNETTE 12-2, TABLE 2. Computation of χ^2 for the One-Sample Blood-Lead Problem

Blood Lead (mg/dl)	f_o	f_e	$f_o - f_e$	$[f_o - f_e]^2$	$\dfrac{[f_o - f_e]^2}{f_e}$
50+	63	75	−12	144	1.9
35–49	275	226	49	2,401	10.6
25–34	792	452	340	115,600	255.8
20–24	951	920	31	961	1.0
15–19	1,768	1,824	−56	3,136	1.7
10–14	3,414	3,589	−174	30,276	8.4
<10	7,814	7,991	−176	30,976	3.9
Totals	15,077	15,077			$\chi^2 = 283.3$

Note. Observed frequencies are from the Maryland Childhood Lead Registry, Maryland Office of the Environment, 1991.

have occurred by chance alone less than 1 time in 10,000 (written $p < .0000$). Suppose we had specified beforehand that in order for the computed value of χ^2 to be considered insignificant, it must not have occurred by chance more than once in 100 samples of this size ($p \times .01$). According to the χ^2 table, the computed x— would have to have been less than 16.8. As we can see in the last column of Table 12.2b, the difference in the 25–34 mg category alone would have been enough to lead us to conclude that the two distributions varied much more than could have been accounted for by chance. Apparently, Baltimore City has an unusually large number of children with blood-lead levels in that range, and a somewhat excessive number in the 35–49 mg category as well. Thus we may state that the differences in categorical frequencies between Baltimore children and a set of expected frequencies are too great to attribute to chance.

A Two-Sample Case

The chi-square test can also be used as a test of whether there is a difference between two samples of data expressed in frequency form. Vignette 12-2, Table 3 shows a two-sample contingency table. The Maryland Childhood Lead Registry for 1991 is again used to show the numbers of Baltimore City children with blood-lead levels distributed in seven categories. This is compared with the frequencies of rural Maryland county children in the same seven categories. Because there is generally less industry and fewer motor vehicles in the rural counties, we might expect lead levels to be lower there. The questions to be asked are whether or not the differences are significant and what the probability is that such differences could be attributable to chance. The χ^2 test can be applied to these data to find out whether there is a significant difference between rural and city children in terms of their blood-lead levels in 1991.

From the table, it may be readily seen that the proportions of children in most of the categories differ between the city and the rural counties. City children are only about 7 times as likely to have the lowest blood-lead levels as the rural counties, but they are about 17 times more likely to be in the 10–14 mg category and over 30 times more likely to be in the 35–49 mg category. Are these differences due to chance in the sampling process, or are they representative of the blood-lead situation in the total population of city and rural children? The test statistic for this situation, where there are more than two categories, is the same as that for the one-sample test. However, in a one-sample test the expected frequencies are known at the outset; in the two-sample case they must be calculated.

From the information given in the contingency table, it can be stated that 15,077 ÷ 16,515 of the total set of children are from the city and 1,438 ÷ 16,515 are from the rural counties. If there were no difference between the blood-lead levels of city and rural children, these same proportions should be expected to apply to both samples. In other words 15,077/16,515 of the 70 children in the 50+ mg blood-lead category (i.e., about 64 of them) should be city children. Similarly 1,438/16,515 of these 70 children (i.e. about 6 of them) should be rural children. Vignette 12-2, Table 3 shows all the expected frequencies, and in brack-

VIGNETTE 12-2, TABLE 3. Computation of Expected Frequencies for χ^2 Test on Two-Sample Blood-Lead Problem

Blood lead (mg/dl)	Baltimore City f_o	Rural counties f_e	Totals
50+	63.9 $\left[\dfrac{15{,}077 \times 70}{16{,}515}\right]$	6.1 $\left[\dfrac{1{,}438 \times 70}{16{,}515}\right]$	70
35–49	259.3 $\left[\dfrac{15{,}077 \times 284}{16{,}515}\right]$	24.7 $\left[\dfrac{1{,}438 \times 284}{16{,}515}\right]$	284
25–34	754.1 $\left[\dfrac{15{,}077 \times 826}{16{,}515}\right]$	71.9 $\left[\dfrac{1{,}438 \times 826}{16{,}515}\right]$	826
20–24	889.2 $\left[\dfrac{15{,}077 \times 974}{16{,}515}\right]$	84.8 $\left[\dfrac{1{,}438 \times 974}{16{,}515}\right]$	974
15–19	1672.5 $\left[\dfrac{15{,}077 \times 1{,}832}{16{,}515}\right]$	159.5 $\left[\dfrac{1{,}438 \times 1{,}832}{16{,}515}\right]$	1,832
10–14	3301.2 $\left[\dfrac{15{,}077 \times 3{,}616}{16{,}515}\right]$	314.8 $\left[\dfrac{1{,}438 \times 3{,}616}{16{,}515}\right]$	3,616
<10	8,137.9 $\left[\dfrac{15{,}077 \times 8{,}913}{16{,}515}\right]$	776.1 $\left[\dfrac{1{,}438 \times 8{,}913}{16{,}515}\right]$	8,913
Totals	15,077[a]	1,438[a]	16,515

[a]Columns may not sum to totals shown due to rounding.

ets beneath each one the calculations required. The effective assumption is made that the proportion of children in city and rural environments should be the same for all blood-lead categories. Thus the expected frequency for any cell can be calculated by a simple mechanical rule:

$$f_e = \frac{\text{Column total} \times \text{Row total}}{\text{Grand total}}$$

Having computed the expected frequencies, the value of χ^2 can be calculated using the equation shown in the one sample case above. In this case, there are

14 cells each of observed frequencies and expected frequencies. Differences must be obtained between each f_o and each f_e and these differences must be squared and divided by f_e. Again, a table of χ^2 must be consulted. A summation of this yields a value of 336.5. The probability that a value this large could have occurred by chance alone is minuscule ($p < .000$). We may declare this a statistically significant result. Clearly, rural children are much more likely to exhibit the lowest levels of blood lead. In order for this difference to be considered insignificant at $p \times .01$ ($df = 6$), the computed χ^2 should fall below 16.8.

VIGNETTE 12-3.   Bivariate Regression and Correlation

Figure 12-4 shows maps of the phenomena low-birthweight rates and proportion of population below the poverty line in Washington, DC, as a 5-year annual average around the year 1990. As we described in the chapter, the assumption is that higher levels of health problems for mothers and their offspring are expected in neighborhoods with low family incomes. Using data from the city department of vital statistics and from the 1990 census, we produce Vignette 12-3, Table 1 (U.S. Census Bureau, 1990).

From the data of Vignette 12-3, Table 1, it is convenient to graph the relationship between the two variables (Vignette 12-3, Figure 1). The line of best fit, the so-called least-squares regression line, may be fit to the scatter in Vignette 12-3, Figure 1. To compute the correlation coefficient (r), we substitute data from the row labeled "totals" in Vignette 12-3, Table 1, into the equation found in this chapter:

$$r = \frac{\Sigma XY - \dfrac{\Sigma X \Sigma Y}{n}}{\sqrt{\left(\Sigma X^2 - \dfrac{(\Sigma X)^2}{n}\right)\left(\Sigma Y^2 - \dfrac{(\Sigma Y)^2}{n}\right)}}$$

$$= \frac{44,946 - \dfrac{284(2,528)}{18}}{\sqrt{\left(6,546 - \dfrac{80,656}{18}\right)\left(385,912 - \dfrac{6,390,784}{18}\right)}}$$

$$= \frac{5,059.8}{7,984.1}$$

$$= .63$$

VIGNETTE 12-3, TABLE 1. Data for Computing a Correlation Coefficient for (Y) Low Birthweight Rate per 1,000 Live Births, and (X) Percentage of Families Below Poverty

Census Tract	Y	X	Y^2	X^2	XY
5.1	62	9	3,844	81	558
16	120	2	14,400	4	240
28	106	27	11,236	729	2,862
45	178	20	31,684	400	3,560
61	119	3	14,161	9	357
74.5	182	35	33,124	1,225	6,370
79.1	174	21	30,276	441	3,654
89.3	173	18	29,929	324	3,114
96.1	145	10	21,025	100	1,450
8.1	49	3	2,401	9	147
19.2	134	6	17,956	36	804
33.2	182	16	33,124	256	2,912
52.1	122	15	14,884	225	1,830
64.1	204	43	41,616	1,849	8,772
76.3	103	11	10,609	121	1,133
83.1	147	9	21,609	81	1,323
92.3	153	20	23,409	400	3,060
98.4	175	16	30,625	256	2,800
Totals	2,528	284	385,912	6,546	44,946

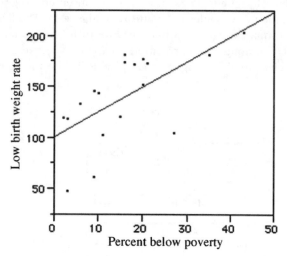

VIGNETTE 12-3, FIGURE 1. Regression line for low birthweight births and percentage of families living below poverty line. The greater the proportion of families living below the poverty line, the greater the rate of low-birthweight births is expected.

As confirmed by the scatter diagram, the coefficient is positive. But, given the size of the sample, is r significantly greater than zero? One test of significance for this is known as the Student t test:

$$t_r = r \sqrt{\frac{n-2}{1-r^2}}$$

Substituting for calculated values of r, r^2 and n, we obtain a value (3.26) that may be compared with a standard table of t values for any size sample and any level of significance.

$$= .63 \sqrt{\frac{16}{.598}} = 3.26.$$

This value has a probability ($p = .005$) of about 5 chances in 1,000 of being due to sampling variation alone. Thus, we can be reasonably certain that, in Washington, DC, the more birthweights below 2,500 grams in a neighborhood, the more likely we will find families earning below the poverty level of income.

13

Scale, Spatial Analysis, and Geographic Visualization

Geography has a fundamental interest in variation over space and in how things are put together at different scales of thinking about them. Its ancient tool in addressing issues of scale and spatial variation is the map. As historians are concerned with actions and influences considered over time, analyzed in periods of various length, so geographers are concerned with actions over distance and interrelationships considered across space, analyzed at various scales. The capabilities of computers and the capacity for digital transmission of information available today have transformed not so much the questions geographers ask as their ability to address them. Although, like other social scientists, geographers have for decades used statistics, only recently have technological developments allowed the power of the computer to be directed at spatial data management through new software packages. The map has become the tool known as a geographical information system (GIS).

The purpose of this chapter is to increase awareness of the ways things can be analyzed spatially and across scale, the ways queries and findings can be portrayed and presented, and the potential for error and abuse that lurks in computerized analysis. There is not enough space to review all the ways spatial analysis has been applied to measuring disease distributions, and we could not do such a review as well as the tour de force of Cliff and Haggett (1988). Nor will we attempt to explain how to make maps or conceptualize and manage a GIS. Those specialized kinds of knowledge have many sequential courses and texts of their own (Clarke, 1995; Davis, 1999; Burrough & McDonnell, 1988; Hohl & Mayo, 1997; Monmonier, 1993, 1997). Some readers will learn new questions they can ask and ways that these can be addressed. Whether or not we do research, we all see some maps and research results in journals, books, and papers. These will proliferate as GIS spreads

(Clarke, McLafferty, & Tempalski, 1996; Openshaw, 1996). People dealing with health and disease matters today need to become more spatially sophisticated. This chapter is intended to help them do that.

SOME ISSUES OF SCALE

Scale is most simply thought of as the amount of area being considered, while realizing that the area under consideration is at once a component of a larger area and is itself made up of smaller areas: Space is a continuum. The word itself originates from the Latin word for ladder, which was both a means of ascent and descent and a set of marks used for measuring. A scale is the proportion a map, or other model, bears to the thing it represents.

A scale can be a ratio between the dimensions of a representation and those of the object being represented, as in "one inch to a mile." Its technical terminology in geography, through cartography, is sometimes at variance with common usage. This can be a source of confusion. If one centimeter on a map represents 100,000 centimeters on the earth's surface, the scale is 1/100,000; if one centimeter represents 1,000 centimeters, the scale is 1/1,000. Because the former fraction is a much smaller number than the latter, it is referred to as "small scale" and the latter as "large scale." Note, however, that the small-scale map covers a much larger area, and the large-scale map covers a smaller area. Thus, a map of the United States is small scale, and a map of a house's interior is large scale. To avoid confusion, it is not uncommon today to speak of "macro" and "micro" studies, referring to the area covered in terms more familiar to common usage (large areas or populations being macro, and small populations or areas being micro).

Things vary over space. The amount of that variation that can be captured and studied is necessarily dependent on the proportion being represented (i.e., on the scale of analysis). This causes both the fascination and the frustration, the inherent challenge, of spatial analysis.

The Ecological Fallacy

The infamous ecological fallacy has bedeviled geographic comparisons for a long time. It crops up when statistics are compared across scale. We cannot use a state-level risk factor to predict what will happen to specific individuals, and we cannot interview friends and neighbors to predict national opinion. Even given bona fide cause and effect, measurable association varies differently at different scales. Sociologists first confronted this issue by aggregating population but trying to analyze its groups. Geographers also confront it by aggregating area to different scales and trying to analyze zones: the modifiable areal unit problem.

Variance changes with scale. If information is based on individual questionnaires, we are aware of the diversity of response. When these answers are aggregated to county level, central tendency leveling takes place. There will be less variation among 100 counties in a state than there was among the millions of individuals who contributed the information. There is less variance among state economic areas than among counties, and less among states than among state economic areas. These changes in variance have little to do with cause and effect and a lot to do with the way we can measure and generalize our findings.

Cleek (1979) and others have pointed out that correlations are especially affected by changes in aggregation. Data are often aggregated by an independent variable. This inflates correlation coefficients but usually does not affect regression coefficients. For example, as the individuals are aggregated into the county in which they live, socioeconomic measures are generalized. Several adjacent counties are likely to be more similar with regard to such generalized characteristics as median income than are the thousands of individuals who compose them. (In Cleek's example, the coefficient of variation [standard deviation/mean] for mortality rates from leukemia was 7.0% comparing states at the national level and 20.9% comparing counties within the state of Wisconsin. Similarly, the coefficient of variation of mortality rates for cancer of the nasopharynx is 188.9% for Wisconsin at county level and 24.4% for the United States at state level. Colon cancer, however, has higher state-level variation, 25.8%, than county-level variation, 17.3%. The message, Cleek says, is clear: Report regression coefficients, and treat correlation coefficients with care.)

What this all means is that patterns of association are different at different scales of analysis, and it is an error to take an association that is true at one scale and infer that it will be true at any other scale. On the other hand, the change in pattern of association can itself sometimes be used as an etiological clue to separate the expression of different causal factors. In one case there may be great between-state variation but little within-state, between-county variation; in another there may be great local variation but little state-level variation. These patterns can be used to address different possible causes that relate to individual behavior, broader patterns of water sources or occupations, or still broader regional patterns of atmospheric pollution or population migration.

Scale of Analysis and Units of Observation

One of the first things a researcher must decide is the scale at which a question will be addressed and the units of observation that will be used. Individuals may be a source of information, but their information must be merged and aggregated. Socially, people may be grouped into families, play or work groups, ethnic groups, and so on. Spatially, people may be aggregated into households (which occupy a living space), census blocks, census tracts, cities or minor civil divisions, counties, state economic areas (which are merely groupings of counties that create a larger areal aggregation), states, regions, and so on. Such units of observation, or data collection, may be split up or put together to make other units. This may be done either deliberately, as when regions are defined for a specific research purpose, or inadvertently, as when census tract boundaries are altered from one decennial census to the next. Regions can be defined that cut across borders, raising an issue that is sometimes referred to as *modifiable units*. Changes in boundaries often alter the level of analysis, make comparisons difficult, and affect the interpretation of results, as illustrated in the following examples.

The first example shows what might happen when one is looking for the cause of a disease (Figure 13-1). Suppose an industrial chemical is being dumped into a river. This causes people who live along the river and drink its water to contract a certain disease. This disease can also be contracted by breathing car emissions or by breathing the chemical put into the air by a smelter. Because people who live near the smelter, along the river, or in congested parts of this town tend to have common socioeconomic characteristics, ethnicity, income, and race may be associated with this disease. As discussed in Chapter 12, these associations can be confounding. If one were to study this disease of unknown etiology at different scales (i.e., using different geographic units of analysis), different associations would be identified.

Study 1 focuses on a minor civil division where people breathe the air of a smelter (*a*) and car emissions (*b*), and so *a* and *b* are found to be associated

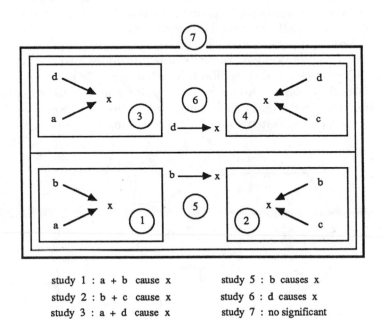

study 1 : a + b cause x   study 5 : b causes x
study 2 : b + c cause x   study 6 : d causes x
study 3 : a + d cause x   study 7 : no significant
study 4 : c + d cause x   association with x

FIGURE 13-1. Disease causation factors at different scales of analysis.

with the disease. Study 2 examines another minor civil division where people drink water from a stream (*c*) and breathe car emissions (*b*). Study 3 is carried out in a rather rural minor civil division wherein people work in a smelter and breathe its air (*a*) and are German in ethnic origin (*d*). In study 4 the rural minor civil division has ethnic German people (*d*) who drink the stream water (*c*). These associations are found at the microscale, but they are puzzling because there is so little consistency. Suppose that study 5 looks at county data, combining areas 1 and 2, and finds that car emissions (*b*) are important. Study 6 also examines county data, combining areas 3 and 4, and finds that being German (*d*) is important. Finally, study 7 uses state data and combines all these areas but finds no important associations.

The second example of modifiable units deals with health care delivery. Suppose a health systems agency (HSA) consists of 10 counties, as shown in Figure 13-2. Table 13-1 shows the number of physicians and total population for each county. Planners in the HSA might wish to organize their counties in different ways and then compare groups of counties to determine whether they were relatively well or poorly served by physicians. Suppose they compare a "northern tier" (counties *A–E*) with a "southern tier" (counties *F–J*). The northern tier would have an overall physician-to-population ratio of 128.8 and the southern tier one of 171.2. Now suppose that there is an interest in comparing the Standard Metropolitan Statistical Area (SMSA) (counties *D*, *F*, and *G*) with the other, more rural counties. The SMSA has a physician-to-population ratio of 187.5 and the other seven counties a ratio of 84.9. Choosing the way one groups the counties clearly changes the assessment of the resource situation. Urban–rural investigations (see air pollution in Chapter 6) confront this issue constantly. Do we use the metropolitan statistical area, urban area, political city, central county, or minor civil division in the analysis? The results can vary significantly. Whatever scale of unit is used for analysis faces this problem: Even census tracts, for example, have spatial variation within them such that values may be more similar between two blocks across the tract border (often a street) than across the census tract unit of ob-

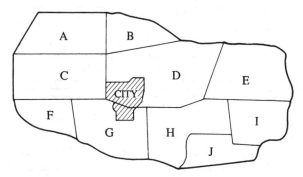

FIGURE 13-2. Counties within a health systems agency jurisdiction.

TABLE 13-1. Health System Agency County Physician-to-Population Ratios

County	Number of physicians	Population	Physician-to-population ratio (per 100,000)
A	12	19,122	62.8
B	15	25,639	58.5
C	2	4,553	43.9
D	126	62,798	200.6
E	10	16,014	62.4
F	40	29,528	135.5
G	74	35,670	207.5
H	22	9,608	229.0
I	5	5,926	84.4
J	8	6,321	126.6
Totals	314	215,179	145.9

servation. A technique called the spatial filter/monte carlo approach can be helpful with these problems (Openshaw, Charlton, Wymer, & Craft, 1987; Rushton, 1998).

Because these units of observation exist in spatial relationships with each other (adjacency, distance, etc.), another issue that needs to be addressed is *spatial autocorrelation.* That is, census tracts or counties when used as units of observation may not be truly independent of each other as most statistical procedures require. Adjacent territories usually influence each other, as the property value of one house affects that of property adjacent. Times-series analysis also has to confront this problem, as the value of something in one year usually affects the value in the next year, so that using sequential years as units of observation can be statistically invalid because of autocorrelation. Because more scientists worry about time than about space, statistical procedures have been developed to "remove" or adjust for the autocorrelation in time periods and geographers usually adapt these techniques to their study in space.

These issues of *scale dependency* are complex but critical to spatial analysis. What are the range of scales at which relationships are alike, and at what scale do things appear and act differently? That is, at what scale does spatial autocorrelation break into randomness and scale independence occur? There are a variety of specialized techniques, using such things as semivariograms to analyze scale relationships and fractal analysis to describe the nature and degree of the spatial relationships. Vignette 13-1 presents one example of the way units can be "joined" and tested for spatial autocorrelations, and its usage is discussed in Chapter 8 (on diffusion). The very extent of the spatial associations, whether limited just to adjacent units or extending over broad regions, can be used to illuminate etiology. Just as change in variability through scale can be usefully or fallaciously used, so the phenomenon of spatial autocorrelation can be used.

Microstudies

Aggregate studies fill most of the journals and are the source of most of the statistical associations and "proofs." There is a long tradition in geography of fieldwork, however, and this finds expression in studies of disease ecology based on population mobility and circulation, among other things. Studies of individuals and households as they move through and among specific habitats can identify the nature, extent, and duration of exposure to risks. As discussed and referenced in Chapter 4, by collecting detailed field information on the micromobility of people and specific habitat conditions, points of exposure, types of change in risk, and points of intervention can be studied. Vignette 13-2 explains one way to measure specific circulation through recall of 24-hour mobility. Vignette 10-1 presents a way of aggregating population circulation/exposure by delimiting activity areas measured in a standard deviation ellipse. Such microstudies require detailed mapping.

MAPPING

Cartography is a field highly developed as both an art and a science. It has advanced through the centuries along with the mathematics, astronomy, and technology of navigation. It has invoked the curiosity and imagination of countless minds. It has been computer automated, and is currently being revolutionized by satellites and their beacons and cameras. Even cartography textbooks cannot do justice to all of this, and this book certainly will not try. People working in health sciences, however, need to become aware of more and different ways they can spatially analyze and portray their data, and of the ways such maps not only can be used but can be abused to lie and distort, or simply to err.

This section is an introduction to the complexity and opportunity embodied in mapping. After briefly considering some historical roots, we describe several issues involved in choosing maps and presenting data. We discuss the crucial determination of intervals in mapping and present less familiar kinds of mapping, such as probability, demographic base, and trend surface. Finally, we consider the changes brought about by computerized mapping and how they lead toward GIS.

Historical Roots

The beginnings of medical geography in the United States lie in mapping, specifically in Jacques May's project of mapping major vectored, parasitic, and nutritional diseases at the world scale for the American Geographic Society in New York. Between 1950 and 1954 he produced a series of 17 maps which were published with limited commentary as supplements to the journal, *The Geographic Review* (see May references). Several maps were later reduced and published in May's *Ecology of Human Disease* (1958). These were for most geographers the first time that distributions of disease and their ecological relationships with cultural patterns and physical environments had ever been brought to their attention. A few years later, Rodenwaldt and Jusatz (1952–1961) edited the more comprehensive, three-volume *Welt-Seuchen Atlas* (*World Atlas of Epidemic Disease*) in German and English. This atlas includes global and regional maps (with a special emphasis on Europe) and a commentary on the diseases. It had a wide impact in public health and international medical and development centers. The *Atlas of United States Mortality* (National Center for Health Statistics, 1997) now present color maps, text, and adjustment methods in book, CD-ROM, and excerpts online (Vignette 12-1). It makes widely accessible in the public domain maps and data that could not be created at the time of this text's first edition.

As an abstraction of reality, a map is a distillation of complex interrelationships which the map maker *chooses* as important to represent. That is, all of reality cannot be put on a map. The cartographer must *generalize.* The teacher or researcher must decide which elements to represent: If roads, what type; if vegetation, how specific; if water courses, what size or permanence; if houses, what type, what detail. Although disease data are usually collected according to administrative organization, such as counties, a map can portray the patterns of habitat, wind-borne pollutants, or water sources and flows that render the administrative borders dangerous irrelevancies. A map is a model of what a map maker believes crucial for analyzing etiology or communicating important relationships.

Geographers sometimes forget the power of a simple map. Yet much of the early geographic disease studies' impact on our understanding of health stems from the use of maps. To quote an 1852 cholera study,

> Geographical delineation is of the utmost value, and even indispensable; for while the symbols of the masses of statistical data in figures, however clearly they might be arranged in the Systematic Tables, present but a uniform appearance, the same data embodied in a Map, will convey at once, the relative bearing and proportion of the single data together with their position, extent, and distance, and thus, a Map will make visible to the eye the development and nature of any phenomenon in regard to its geographic distribution. (Petermann, 1852, cited in Gilbert, 1958, p. 178)

Modern medical geography (frequently called *medical topography* during the 1800s) began in Europe during the late 18th century when most of today's disciplines were not separately defined. Investigators, who were usually medical practitioners, described a place's topography and climate as they related to health and disease. This, of course, was in the Hippocratic tradition as exemplified in this book's frontispiece. Although disease distributions were often described in detail and the reports sometimes did contain detailed topographic maps, they did not contain disease maps.

The yellow fever epidemics of the late 18th and early 19th centuries and the cholera outbreaks of the 19th generated the first disease maps. Dot maps of the distribution of yellow-fever victims (which were clustered in the filthy port and sailor lodging area) were used by both contagionists and anticontagionists in their argument over the nature of what caused that dread disease. Contagionists considered it a single disease brought by travelers from places already afflicted with yellow fever, whereas anticontagionists thought that it simply emerged from crowded, filthy urban areas. Apparently the first such map was produced by Dr. Valentine Seaman in his anticontagionist treatise on yellow fever in New York City in 1798. His work was continued over the next half century by many other people.

In 1852, Heinrich Berghaus published his *Physikalischer Atlas.* One of its eight sections included a number of medical maps and charts. These were the first medical maps included in an atlas, the first to show the distribution of a variety of epidemic and endemic diseases, and the first published by a major cartographer. The extraordinary quality of these maps represents a singularly important development in medical cartography.

The most famous 19th-century disease map, used to argue the contagionists' analysis, was John Snow's 1854 dot map of cholera around Broad Street water pump in London (Figure 13-3). The clustering of cholera in the vicinity of the well supported Snow's contention that cholera was a waterborne disease, with the pump the local source of infection. He urged that the handle be removed and the pump shut down. It was, and the local incidence of cholera declined quickly.

Some Issues in the Type of Map

Although a map can be visually effective and authoritative, it really can be no better than its data. The importance of political or administrative borders for the collection of data and their frequent irrelevance to the patterns of distributions on the surface of the earth has been intensely spotlighted by the availability of digitized satellite imagery of such distributions. The effort to reconcile this difference is at the core of much research in GIS systems and medical geography today. The origins, however, lie in the basic question of scale of analysis and of how different types of information are portrayed.

Map Scale

The type of projection used to portray the round globe on a flat sheet of paper remains important for global mapping of distributions or diffusion. Most

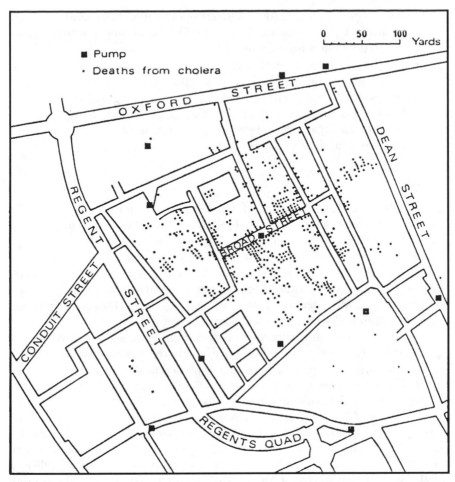

FIGURE 13-3. Snow's map of cholera. The affected well is clearly identified by the concentration of cases in its vicinity. From Howe (1972, p. 178).

health researchers of course will—and can—just use the base maps of the city blocks, counties, or countries that are readily available to them. It may be, however, that the most convenient map is not of the best scale and the easiest route will not yield the best outcome. Base maps, blank maps waiting for data, need to be sought out for the scale most appropriate for aggregation and analysis of the topic at hand.

- *Small scale:* 1:250,000 to 1: 1,000,000 or more; continents, realms, large regions
- *Medium scale:* 1: 25,000 to 1: 250,000; states—state economic areas— health service areas—standard metropolitan statistical areas—coun-

ties—minor civil divisions—cities; topographic maps and coverage from the U.S. Geological Survey satellite vegetation coverage, water sheds, geological formations

- *Large scale:* 1:200 to 1:25,000; minor civil divisions—cities—census tracts—blocks-building interiors; satellite imagery of transportation routes, buildings, agricultural fields and local vegetational features; USGS topographic coverage; air photography special coverage; Census Bureau Tiger Files; engineering blueprints (of electrical, sewerage, water, and other infrastructure)

Type of Data

Point data represent information that has no spatial dimension, but of course this is a matter of scale. An individual with a case of tuberculosis may be represented by a point on a city map; a city's population can become a point on a smaller-scale national map. These kinds of data are most commonly presented in *dot distribution maps* (like Snow's). The dots can become quite elaborate. A graduated circle indicating population or incidence size, a pie graph with proportions for outcomes or types of people, even a climagraph showing seasonal distribution of data can all be used as point symbols.

Lines are used to show direction of movement (*flow maps*), often with the thickness of the line being scalar (proportional to the amount that is moving). Most commonly, lines are used to connect points and so portray new information. *Isolines* (also known as *isopleths,* or *isarithms*) can connect points of equal data value. These are most familiar as lines of equal altitude on topographic sheets or lines of equal atmospheric pressure on weather maps. In potential maps, lines connect points of equal *population potential* (Vignette 10-1, Figure 2); in diffusion maps they connect equal times of arrival; in health service maps they can connect equal proportions of population using a facility or equal distances traveled to the facility. Isolines are two-dimensional representations of three-dimensional reality, because they have both extension in space and a value (i.e., an X, Y, and Z axis). The area that lines separate into different spaces is continuous, and points are discrete. To connect the points with a line through area with no data points, values are *interpolated.* For example, a line connecting points of value 10 could be drawn midway between points of value 5 and value 15 as well as through points of value 10 itself. This used to be a laborious as well as specialized art, but many computer programs do the calculations routinely now. Careful inspection and human art are still required, however, as there can be more than one way to configure such interpolated line patterns and the simplest computer solution is not always the most sensible. Figure 13-4 illustrates an isoline map of blood lead levels determined by laboratory screening tests allocated to the residential location of the children. The pattern of distribution identified is much richer and more intricate than a mere dot distribution of cases that exceeded a certain limit.

Area information is symbolized on thematic maps by shades, patterns, or

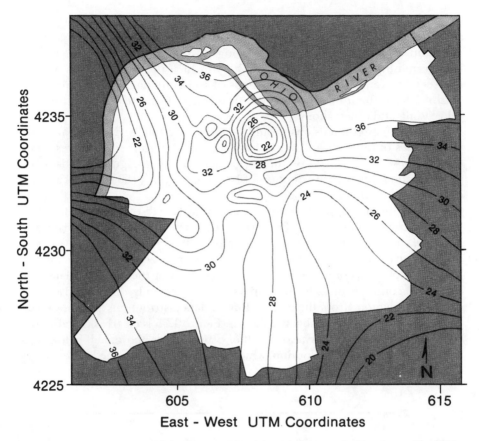

FIGURE 13-4. Lines of equal pediatric blood lead levels, Louisville, Kentucky, 1979. Values are micrograms per deciliter of blood.

colors covering the area and symbolizing the class, or category, to which the information value belongs. This kind of map is known as a *choropleth map*. Choropleth maps are the familiar maps of data distribution by county or state or nation, but the areas do not have to be politically delimited. Vegetation regions, soil regions, activity areas, or population circulation regions—any areas that can be discretely defined—may be appropriate units for choroplethic thematic mapping.

Critical Intervals: Mapping Pattern

Choropleth maps are the most commonly used maps for presenting disease or health service information, and they are the most readily available type on commercial computer mapping programs. A remarkable number of people accept the patterns that are produced on maps in black and white as true, even authoritative, and never give a thought to the role of the cartographer in determining those patterns by the way in which the data are classified. In this section, we present a series of maps of the same data, each mapped according to a different method of classification, to illustrate the need for critical reading and observation.

Basically, two dimensions should be considered here: data can have different types of distribution, and intervals can be determined to represent either the *area/range covered* or the *observations included.* Figure 13-5 is a bar graph of the frequency distribution of North Carolina's 100 counties according to their infant mortality rates.

When the mean, median, and mode of a data distribution ordered by the frequency of observation of different values are the same, the distribution is *normal,* and the data distribution is said to "follow a normal curve." Normal distributions are featured in many statistical procedures because of the known proportions of observations in any portion of the range of data (the curve). A common measure of dispersion for normally distributed data is standard deviation (from the mean). But all data distributions are not so symmetrical. The infant mortality graphed in Figure 13-5 is clearly skewed to the left, with the median observation (half of observations above, half below) less than the mean of the distribution, which has a long "tail" to the higher values

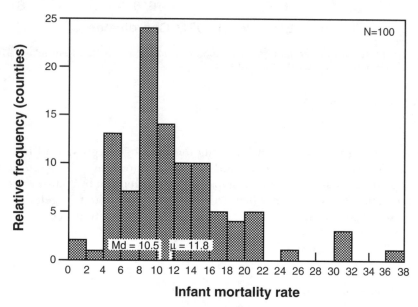

FIGURE 13-5. Frequency graph of infant mortality rates by county in North Carolina, 1991.

on the right. The question is how to divide this data distribution into intervals (i.e., create classes) to be symbolized with different shading on a choropleth map of North Carolina.

A map made well can communicate a lot of information. The information, however, can be distorted if the intervals are not appropriate to the data distribution. First, there can be too many intervals. Students sometimes think there will be more detail in the distribution if they map 10 or 15 categories, but cartographic research has determined that the mind can only differentiate pattern from six or seven categories in black and white, and fewer in color. Too few categories, of course, will lose detail and information. However many categories are used, selecting shading, colors, or patterns to grade continuously from one class to another will eliminate the need to consult the key for every observation and will allow whatever pattern there is to appear. When a series of maps compares distributions over time periods or different areas, consistent class selection is necessary for comparison; otherwise, clusters and patterns will seem similarly significant even though actual prevalence varies enormously. A variety of data categorizations can be used: geometric (2, 4, 16, 256), logarithmic, and so on. The most popular method in health sciences is to map quantiles (quantitative divisions), especially quintiles (20% categories) or quartiles (25% categories). There can be confusion about whether the data range (from the lowest point to the highest) or number of observations (i.e., geographical units) is being so divided and classified. Sometimes the default option of computer mapping programs does the former (i.e., divides the range of data into five categories) whereas the researcher intends the latter (i.e., to divide the number of observations into five groups).

Figure 13-6a illustrates the most intuitive way of categorizing classes of infant mortality rates: division by natural breaks. When a frequency distribution is plotted with the values on one axis and the number of observations accumulated on the other, "breaks" usually appear in the curve; that is, many observations accumulate over a range of values and then the rate of accumulation slows and even levels out until a new range of values is reached. These natural breaks in the data distribution can sometimes be more interesting in an etiological sense than the standardized breaks are; the problem with this method is the difficulty of comparing the patterns on one map with another done the same way.

Figure 13-6b shows the classification of infant mortality rates into five equal divisions of the range of the data from lowest to highest value. These equal divisions are a common default on commercial mapping programs and are easily interpreted if the data distribution is normal. Otherwise, this method can result in categories that are either empty or have few observations. In this map, the interval from 22.6 to 30.0 contains only one county, as can be seen from the graph (Figure 13-5). Figure 13-6c is truly a map of quintiles, classes containing 20% of data observations (counties).

Figure 13-6d shows the infant mortality mapped by standard deviations

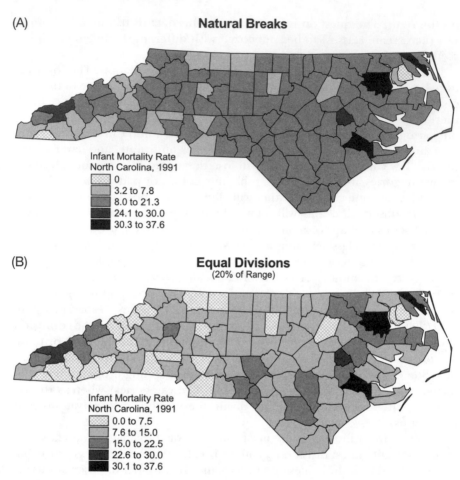

FIGURE 13-6. Choropleth maps of infant mortality in 1991 in North Carolina according to different means of interval determination. (A) Intervals are determine by natural breaks, or change in the slope of accumulating units along frequency distribution. (B) The range of rates is divided into five equal divisions. (C) The number of observations, 100 counties, is divided into five equal groups, or quintiles. (D) Standard deviations from the mean value for infant mortality determine the intervals.

of the data. As the graph indicates, the mean of the data is 11.8, and so the map shows two standard deviations below the mean and four above the mean. Mapping by standard deviations into six categories around a central mean is one of the most objective methods and is ideal for comparison among maps. It can, however, be done automatically, thoughtlessly, inappropriately, and without regard for the distribution of the data being mapped.

These maps of the same data are quite different. Which one is "right"? They all are. For a given data distribution, one method of classifying intervals

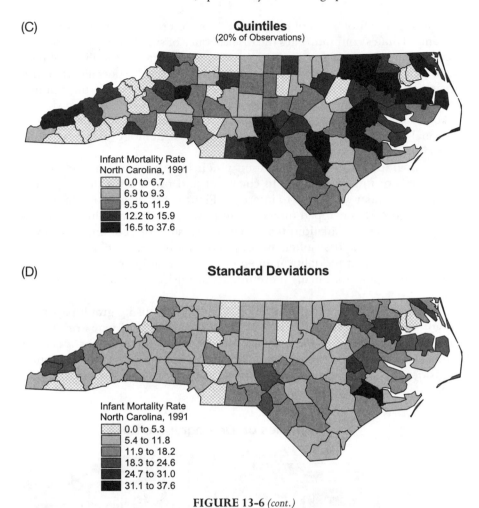

(C)

Quintiles
(20% of Observations)

Infant Mortality Rate
North Carolina, 1991
  0.0 to 6.7
  6.9 to 9.3
  9.5 to 11.9
  12.2 to 15.9
  16.5 to 37.6

(D)

Standard Deviations

Infant Mortality Rate
North Carolina, 1991
  0.0 to 5.3
  5.4 to 11.8
  11.9 to 18.2
  18.3 to 24.6
  24.7 to 31.0
  31.1 to 37.6

FIGURE 13-6 *(cont.)*

may produce results more easy to interpret than another. It can almost be
said, however, that the pattern is in the mind of the cartographer. The map
maker can try to be objective and to derive all the pattern information possible for research, or the map maker can communicate a point strongly for
public education or polemic distortion. Often health professionals who are
rigorous with their statistics and critical of careless interpretation will simply
accept a mapped pattern as given.

Demographic Base Maps

Sometimes better understanding can be achieved by analyzing a distribution
in a less conventional way. We are all accustomed to seeing maps representing *area* on the earth, but in fact human disease occurs in *people*. It is children

that get measles, not acres of corn or trees or desert. A county-level map of the United States communicates the disease rates of small numbers of people over large areas west of the Mississippi and crams the rates of millions of people in places on the East Coast into fractions of an inch. Especially when the disease or health service concern is targeted at a subgroup of the population—whether by age and life stage, ethnicity, or behavioral activity—it makes better sense to construct a map in which the size of the units is proportional to population instead of land area. Such demographic base maps are a kind of cartogram.

Demographic base maps are used much less than they should be because they are time-consuming to construct and often difficult for people who are unfamiliar with them to interpret. Figure 13-7 shows the infant mortality of Figure 13-6 mapped on a demographic base. Because high rates often apply to small populations that are less accessible or economically developed, a population base often portrays conditions very differently. On a global map of infant mortality mapped on a demographic base of births, for example, it is clear that many more infants are dying in South Asia than in Africa.

These maps are best constructed by hand, usually using graph paper, although physically modeling with small blocks of some kind may work better when there are many units. A square is designated to represent a certain number of people, and then the number of squares necessary to represent a unit is determined. Computer algorithms exist to construct cartograms, that

Quintiles on Demographic Base

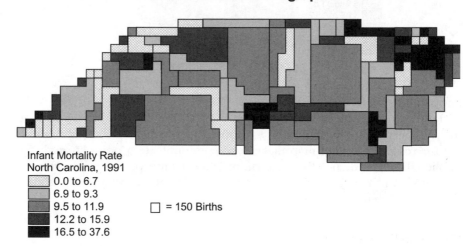

Infant Mortality Rate
North Carolina, 1991
▨ 0.0 to 6.7
▨ 6.9 to 9.3
▨ 9.5 to 11.9   □ = 150 Births
■ 12.2 to 15.9
■ 16.5 to 37.6

FIGURE 13-7. Demographic base map of infant mortality in North Carolina, 1991. Quintiles of data are mapped on a cartogram of county size proportional to county births.

is, to create units proportional to amounts of something. It is especially important, however, in constructing demographic base maps on which health or service concerns will be interpreted by lay people to maintain both *contiguity* and *direction.* If units are to be recognizable as known locations (such as counties), they must touch the units they really do touch and be in the proper directions relative to each other. This context is difficult to maintain when large areas with small populations must be stretched around small areas with large populations, and is still best done by the human eye. Students have constructed demographic base maps to serve later employment and research needs, such as bases for mapping WIC (women, infant, and child) enrollment for supplementary nutrition, infants needing vaccination, and coverage of target population by Meals-on-Wheels.

Without contiguity and direction, demographic cartograms can be sophisticated and portray enormous amounts of information but be unintelligible to health officials and others who should use them. In his landmark national atlas of disease mortality in Britain, Howe (1970) used graduated squares to map disease categories over population size, tilted the squares to show rural or urban classifications, and used solid or dotted line borders to show whether statistical significance had been reached. Broad patterns were sometimes evident, but people found it difficult to interpret unidentifiable squares free-floating in area and his maps' great potential was largely lost. Figure 13-8 illustrates such a demographic cartogram.

Probability Mapping

Sometimes what matters is *what* is mapped rather than how. As discussed in Chapter 12, a denominator problem can result from the relevant subgroups of a population being resident in only small numbers. When incidence rates are low or events not common, the fluctuations inherent in small numbers can be random. Mapping rates or ratios for uncommon cancers, accidents, or other rare events or even for more common events when population subgroups are small can be useless because it can result in serious misdirection. One way around this problem is to step back and realize that the rate of occurrence is not necessarily what is important. Often the researcher really wants to know where something is exceptionally high or low in occurrence.

One way to map less common events is in terms of the probability of their occurrence. Small numbers often follow not a normal distribution but a Poisson distribution. Statistical tables are available that allow a given set of small numbers to be checked to see whether any given number is larger or smaller than could occur by chance. The overall rate is used to generate the numbers predicted for each area and the two distributions are compared. Probabilities from normal distributions can be mapped, too, but other means discussed earlier are available to analyze and portray their spatial distributions. Figure 13-9 illustrates the pattern of strokes in Savannah,

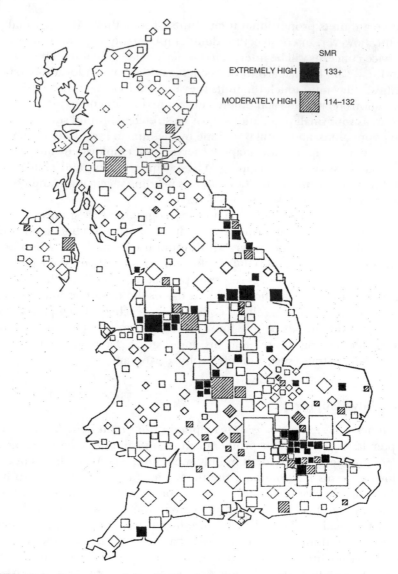

FIGURE 13-8. Cartogram of the distribution of pneumonia mortality in the United Kingdom, 1959–1963. From Howe (1972, p. 237). Copyright 1972 by G. M. Howe. Reprinted by permission.

Georgia. Strokes among white males ages 45–64 are not very common. Furthermore, in any given census tracts the number of people in that demographic category varies greatly. Some census tracts have no white males of that age at all. The map portrays the distribution of strokes that are, according to the statistical probability of their occurring, exceptionally high or low.

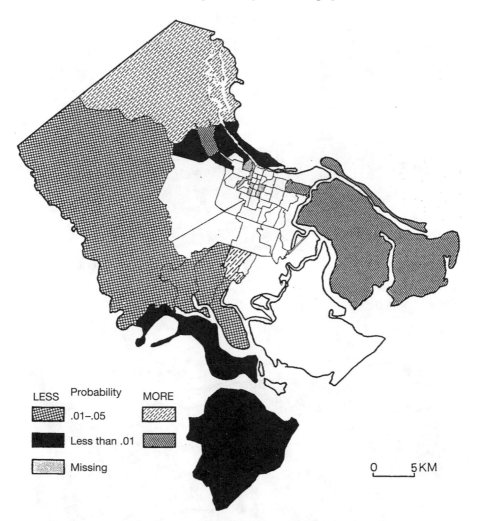

FIGURE 13-9. The probability of the number of strokes for white males ages 45–64 occurring more or less than could occur by chance in each of 54 census tracts. "Missing" refers to tracts without a white male population in the age category that could be used to generate expected deaths.

Trend Surface Mapping

The geographic distribution of health-related phenomena may sometimes be examined through *trend surface analysis*. This form of analysis essentially is regression over space. That is, when a data "surface" exists that has a set of X and Y coordinates for location in space and a Z axis of data values which, like elevation, create a surface of highs and lows, one can use one of several computational programs to carry out a least-squares regression of the data values

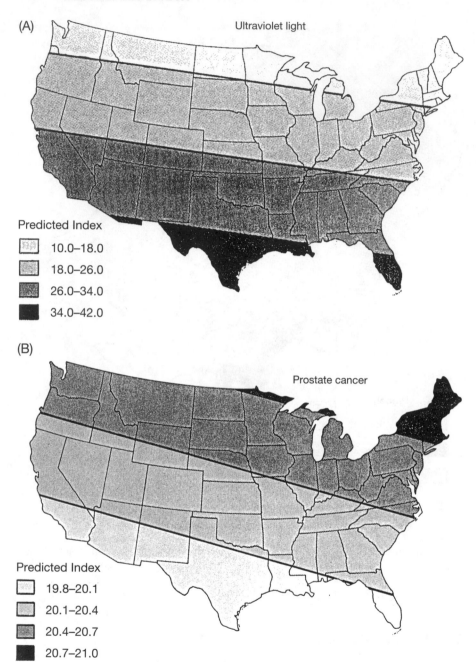

FIGURE 13-10. Maps of trend surface analysis of ultraviolet light as protective of prostate cancer. (A) Linear trend surface by county observations of ultraviolet light measured by the epidemiological index. (B) Linear trend surface by county observations of prostate cancer mortality for white males, aggregated from 1970–1979. From Hanchette (1988). Used with permission.

against the coordinate values that denote distance from the 0,0 point of origin. This technique generalizes patterns by filtering local anomalies from the map. This tends to give a clearer picture of the broader regional trend. Trend surface, a regression procedure, is most appropriate for data that are continuous over space or can be validly interpolated to be so. The simplest trend surface is a plane, the "first order" or linear regression. Just as quadratic equations can move from straight regression line approximations of a data distribution to increasingly better-fitting, curvilinear relations, so it is possible to add warps to the regression surface which more closely fit the local dips and rises in values through the addition of new terms in the regression equation. It is also possible to obtain and map *residuals*, measures of the difference between the actual values at individual data points and those predicted by the fitted trend surface. The examination of such residuals can suggest additional variables that might influence the data distribution but were not adequately incorporated.

In a suggestive study, Hanchette (1988) examined a research question about ultraviolet light as a possible protective factor, through vitamin D production, for prostate cancer. A choropleth county-level map of prostate cancer in the United States suggested vague patterns but nothing that could be clearly identified in the variation of the more than 3000 spatial observations. Figure 13-10 shows the county data in a trend surface of white male mortality that is almost the mirror image of ultraviolet light. The "epidemiological index" used for denoting the ultraviolet light is simply an index based on latitude and altitude and days of cloud cover that has been developed and used primarily with regard to skin cancer. The fifth-order map is included to show the more subtle and adapted surface that can be fitted. How many orders can there be to the quadratic surface? Plotting the explanation derived from successive orders or regressions will show when it levels out and little additional information is gained from another order of analysis. The fifth-order regression achieved an "explanation" of 7.2% of the pattern of prostate cancer (R^2 of .072, compared to R^2 of .02 for the first-order surface; an additional sixth-order surface did not change the R^2 value at all). Although the R^2 of only .072 would indicate only weak explanation and might be laughed at in economic geography, in medicine that small percentage explained could become many deaths prevented. One next step is laboratory studies that can illuminate the biochemical processes involved.

Trend surface analysis should be used with care. It is not suited to analyzing every distribution. It is best addressed to surfaces of continuous data, such as rainfall or altitude or sunlight, and is inappropriate to address discrete point data unless there are enough points to approximate a continuous surface. Thus, it is reasonable to assume that if a dense set of rain gauges measures rainfall, between a gauge registering 1 inch and a gauge measuring 2 inches is a place where 1.5 inches probably fell. It is *not* reasonable to assume that if a city census tract had a population 60% literate and the population of the next county was 95% literate, a census tract located between these two areal, political units would have a literacy rate of 75%. Surfaces fitted to an uneven geographic distribution of sparse data points may not be reliable and are often little more than analogy. Nevertheless, the capacity of this method of spatial analysis to generalize trend over large areas and remove local anomalies is powerful and greatly underutilized in health research.

Computer Mapping

Beginning in the late 1960s, a series of computer mapping programs were developed that promised to automate mapping procedures and allow maps to be rapidly updated, as well as analyzed with such procedures as trend surface analysis. The secret to adapting mapping to computers was assignment of location on an *X* axis and *Y* axis, coordinates of a unique and precise location in space, to every point and line segment symbolizing reality. Latitude and longitude have been used for this purpose for centuries, and these coordinate systems continued to be used. In addition, a variety of local coordinate systems also found favor (e.g., state plane, federal codes, and local road maps). The assignment of location to data was done by *digitizing* and the information was then said to be *geocoded*. Geocoding basically involved putting a map that had borders around areas (census tracts, farm fields), or individual point location (cases, houses, smokestacks), or lines (transport routes), and so on, on a table that had hundreds of wires per inch under its top (a "digitizer"). A hand-held (mouse-like) device with cross hairs could trace the lines or mark the points and, by completing the circuit to the underlying wires, locate coordinates on a grid. Today, much information can be "scanned" onto a grid and converted for digital storage. As this technology developed, census boundaries were digitized so that all the information associated with census tracts could be given location on a map. Other spatial information, such as roads or fields on an air photo, could also be traced over and digitized. There was a lot of "upfront" time and effort in geocoding data sets, but once established as base maps new information could be assigned, such as population change or revised property evaluations or location of cases in an epidemic, and things could be mapped repetitively or easily updated. The future seemed to lie in automation of mapping for planning and other needs, especially as boundary files became increasingly commercially available for common areal features. Powerful programs were developed such as Openshaw et al.'s (1987) GAM (geographic analysis machine) for monitoring point data and detecting clusters of cancer cases or following epidemic outbreaks of infection. The analytical procedures in these mapping programs, however, were limited, especially the ability of the mapping systems to manage large sets of data and to interact or overlay the data sets. The future really lay in the technological transformation of mapping and spatial data management to a new order of being, geographical information systems.

GEOGRAPHIC INFORMATION SYSTEMS

A *geographic information system* is an integrated set of tools and methodologies for collecting, storing, retrieving, analyzing, and displaying spatial as well as nonspatial (attribute) information or data. Its power lies in the ability to manage the spatial and attribute data together for analysis or display. A basic concept is that a common, central data stack is created and spatially referenced (geocoded) which may be used by different people for a variety of purposes. Some systems are user-friendly, work on personal computers, but are limited in capacity and power. Other systems require months of specialized training and experience to handle, run on expensive hardware with large capacities, and universally provoke awe at what they can do in "zooming," overlaying, manipulating, animating, and portraying in a galaxy of color. People sometimes confuse GIS with a specific program. What SAS and SPSS and other software systems are to statistical analysis, ARC/INFO and MapInfo and other software systems are to GIS, a system for support of spatial analysis.

There are several sources from which GIS developed. One was the development of computer cartography discussed earlier, with its evolving capacity for digitizing and geocoding a variety of data and for using Fortran and PASCAL and other computer languages to measure distance and manipulate objects in space. Perhaps the most important source has been the technologies developed in remote sensing and methodologies for analysis of remotely sensed data. Satellites have provided an enormous amount of data, especially American LANDSAT and ERDAS as well as European (SPOT) and Soviet sensing of earth from space. Photography and digital data in multiple bands of the electromagnetic spectrum can be used to differentiate types of land cover and usage or trace pollution in waterways; infrared heat sensing can differentiate thermal plumes in water and air (and thus surface conditions and cover); radio waves can penetrate and record surface declinations in the seas. These and other continuous and repetitive scans of information about the surface of the earth transmitted in digital form to telecommunications satellites, ground receivers, and computer networks overwhelmed existing methods of storage, management, processing, and usage in analysis. Programs sponsored by NASA and the U.S. Geological Survey (USGS) developed models of environmental analysis to integrate this remotely sensed data with biophysical data characterizing soils, topography, climate and the like. Third, needs in urban planning demanded methods for network analysis of transportation, sewage, water, emergency response, and other movements over space. Starting with the 1980 census, metropolitan census information became available in geocoded form in the DIME (dual—for spatial and nonspatial attribute—independent map encoding) files. With the growing capacity, the 1990 census TIGER files (Topologically Integrated Geographic Encoding and Referencing) not only geocoded most census information but integrated it with the digitized, geocoded information of the USGS (1:100,000 base scale) on transportation routes, water bodies and streams. The promising capacity of the TIGER files (in Canada the Area Master File of geocoded street networks, boundaries, and census information covers more than 300 municipalities and more than half of the Canadian population) has in turn encouraged the geocoding of information for data collected from health surveys and cancer registries and the reporting by the National Center for Health Statistics of hospital admissions and discharges. All the signs are that this particular snowball has just started down the slope.

The two fundamental approaches to representing space in a GIS are the *raster* and *vector* models. The vector model represents landscape features (known as cartographic features) as points, lines, and areas through X, Y coordinates. Thus, a line may represent a road, and a connected series of lines may enclose a polygon that is a city block or a field. Every position on the map has a unique coordinate value. The vector model has advantages of a compact structure that efficiently represents spatial relationships and lends itself to network analysis and clear, aesthetic graphics (output maps). The complex data structure, however, makes it difficult to overlay different surfaces on each other. Overlaying plats of property ownership on a surface of urban roads or water pipes, for example, would usually create "slivers," tiny bits of area where the lines on the surfaces do not precisely coincide from data layer to data layer, These slivers themselves become tiny polygons, artifacts encoded into the GIS. Furthermore, representing great spatial variability quickly becomes cumbersome in a vector model. In contrast, a raster model represents space as subdivided by a continuous surface of cells, as if covered with a grid. The location of each object is defined by the row and column position of the cells it occupies. The spatial units are the cells, each with a unique location. Because each cell can have a different digital value (e.g., a line, or scan, of cells across the ground might encode reflectance 1,1,1,1,3,5,2,2,2,4) and cells can be very small, just feet across, they can represent an enormous complexity of spatial variability; and they are easily overlaid on each other as surfaces. A raster surface of vegetation cover could be overlaid on a raster surface of soil with perfect spatial coincidence and tremendous detail encoded. Satellite images of earth are obviously digitally transmitted, stored, and analyzed as rasters. The data structure is not very compact, and it takes a lot of memory storage. Importantly, the simple raster data structure contains little information on topological relationships, only implicitly defining them, whereas the vector model defines topology explicitly.

Topology is the spatial linkage between geographic features. Whether taking one road or another is the shortest distance to a hospital, whether odd-numbered houses on a street get allocated to one census tract and the even-numbered houses on the other side of the street to another, or whether most encephalitis cases are clustered in an area adjacent to a swamp are matters calculated through topology. Line segments (arcs) and nodes (points) at the intersection of two or more arcs being uniquely located in geocoded space, direction, distance relationships, and the enclosure of polygons for which attribute data exists can be calculated, overlain, and interrelated The following section explains the power in this and illustrates the application of a GIS.

A Simplified Summary of How a GIS Is Constructed

A GIS is a system of spatial data management, a system extending from data encoding to display. This means more than locating points, lines, and areas uniquely and displaying them through computer cartography. It means the ability to handle attributes of the relationships between objects and thus to support complex analysis. It means analysis can attempt predictions as a function of the relationships between attributes and thus can attempt simulations and modeling of possible scenarios. It means the mode of operation potentially can be interactive and integrative.

The following discussion uses Figure 13-11 (also Table 13-2), a map of the imaginary town of Search, as its reference. The location of the lake and its shore, the ground cover of Stamp Forest and Fonaroff Swamp, much of the road system, and the altitude of Haggett Eminence would be determined from satellite digital transmissions of raster data and predigitized geographic coverages from the USGS (Digital Line Graph data and Digital Elevation Models). These would be processed, using a GIS, to differentiate the ground cover, calculate the isolines of elevation, and locate the major roads. One geocoded census boundary (from TIGER files) has been included, and encloses the shaded area. Additional overlays of boundaries and areas can be created as additional files. For example, boundaries of state or congressional representative districts can be drawn on the same coordinate system (or one that can be transformed to it) and then digitized and overlain. The location of the hospital has been digitized as well as smelters and smokestacks, as have cases of an unknown disease. The inset of census block 103 shows how this was done, according to the vector model.

Block 103 is bounded by four streets. Each of the corners is treated as a *node*. The first node, the corner of Howe and Shannon Streets, has a precise location in space which the grid determines is 2.0 on the X axis and 8.0 on the Y axis. The node at the corner of Howe and Hunter defines the other end of the line segment (which will have its own arc identification number), and has its own location in space at $X = 3$, $Y = 8$. If one continues "chaining" from node 2 to 3, node 3 to 4, and node 4 back to 1, a polygon that is block number 103 will be defined. This specific locational information for the nodes, line segments (or arcs), and polygons, however, also comes associated with certain topological attributes. The software "knows" that polygon 102 is across the line segment from polygon 103. If house numbers have been associated with that line segment, say odd numbers 5 through 21 on the left and even numbers 8 through 16 on the right, then the home addresses of cases in the cancer registry can be allocated to the separate blocks. Furthermore, if line segment Hunter from Prothero to

(A)

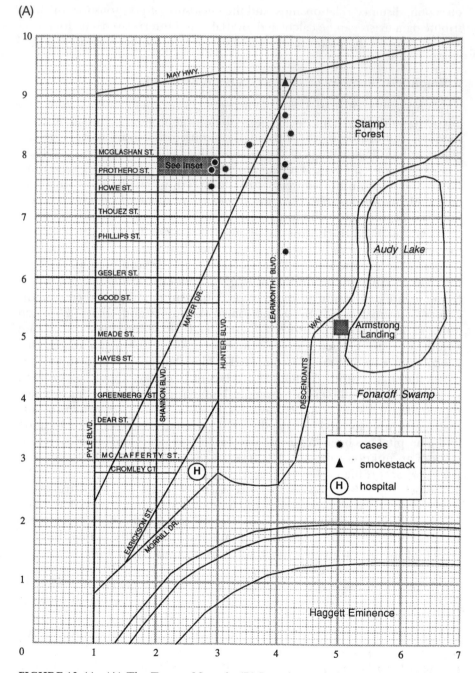

FIGURE 13-11. (A) The Town of Search. (B) Locations relative to tracts and blocks.

(B)

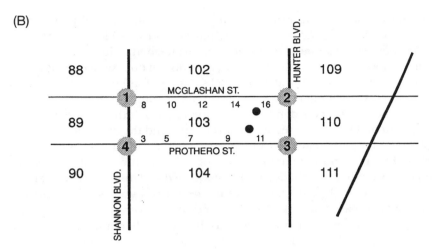

FIGURE 13-11. (*cont.*)

McGlashan is blocked by a reported fallen tree, the GIS could be used to determine the minimum route (distance along line segments) necessary to route an ambulance around the blockage to the hospital.

Separate files are created of attributes associated with these points, lines, and areas (polygons), and it is the job of the GIS to manage and interrelate all these. Thus, there are files that give each line segment its context of other line segments and polygons, so that the ambulance could be routed. Whether the polygons are census tracts or portions of marketing areas or congressional districts, all the attributes the researcher desires and can specify are linked to it. Block 103, for example, is a part of a census tract. Individual household data are not released, but information for the block might include median family income, numbers of single female-headed households, numbers of white children ages 5–9, room density, age of housing, percentage of households with air conditioning, proportion of the population graduated from high school, and numbers speaking Spanish at home. Some information may be confidential at the block level, especially by age/sex/age

TABLE 13-2. Topology of Block 103 of the Town of Search

From node	Coordinate		To node	Coordinate		Polygon to	
	X	Y		X	Y	Right	Left
1	2.0	8.0	2	3.0	8.0	103	102
2	3.0	8.0	3	3.0	7.7	103	110
3	3.0	7.7	4	2.0	7.7	103	104
4	2.0	7.7	1	2.0	8.0	103	89

subdivisions of the population which can get very small (and so inappropriate to use for mapping incidence rates), but because the block is part of a tract, the data for the larger census tract can be attached to it.

Knowing where the smelter is located, the GIS can do distance searches to the cases that have been allocated to blocks. Or "buffers" of specified width could be established along roads and cases in them counted. If the municipal water pipelines have been digitized, age, material, or other characteristics could be matched to the line segments of the pipes and the movement and sitting of water along the segments and at various distances to houses could be modeled. If there is more than one source of water for the people of Search, the separate water delivery sheds could be geocoded and then overlain as areas and the population (by age) and cases in the various watersheds could be counted and compared for risk. People attending the hospital for related reasons could be allocated by their addresses to the blocks where they live, isolines could be constructed of the proportion of people in blocks attending the hospital, and service areas with different distance decay functions could thus be determined. Individuals could be interviewed, and from their responses about where they shopped, visited, exercised, and worked, for example, activity areas could be determined (Vignette 13-2) and could be geocoded as separate surfaces to be overlain on the map of Search. By this point, one can imagine a stack of surfaces, with topography, land use, roads, census tracts and all the associated attributes of education, income, age of housing, case locations, hospital and factories, air pollution, water sources and pipe flow, activity areas, and more. One of the powers of a GIS is not only to stack but to overlay and select and combine these surfaces and create new objects—such as a region of those blocks wherein numbers of Asian women between 20 and 40 live in houses on blocks of predominantly 50-year-old housing with lead soldered pipes and a certain municipal water source downwind within 1 mile from a smokestack at a distance from the hospital where its medical services are underutilized. Then special screening could be instituted to test these people at risk. These blocks could be printed out as a map and workers sent to them.

An Example: Lead Database Evaluation

This ability of a GIS to use overlays to create new objects through combination and deletion (described earlier) can be a powerful analytical tool for disease etiology or service locational selection. This example illustrates the use of GIS modeling of lead database and exposure risk by Hanchette (1996). There are numerous environmental sources and pathways for lead to systemically poison people, but the most important are those absorbed by ingestion. People, especially children, ingest lead from flakes and dust of old paint, in soil contaminated by old automobile or industrial emissions, or from water through lead-soldered pipes or lead-glazed dishware.

As discussed earlier, spatial patterns vary at different scales, and a child's exposure is an individual one, an exposure to microscale risks buffered by nutritional status and parental and personal behavior. Patterns of lead exposure need to be analyzed at a more macroscale for population screening and intervention in public health risks. Aggregate data on environmental sources of lead in soil and dust are not available, however, and thus surrogate measures must be used to define risk factors. Figures 13-12 and 13-13 illustrate GIS modeling of lead database and exposure risk using a technique known as *suitability* mapping from its development in land use planning and facility siting.

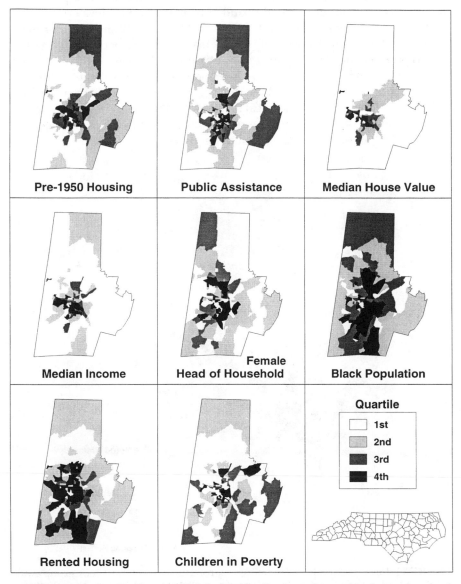

FIGURE 13-12. Lead poisoning risk factors for Durham County block groups, classified by quartiles. From Hanchette (1988). Used with permission.

"Lead poisoning risk potential" was modeled for census block groups across the state of North Carolina, although only the area in Durham County is shown here (Hanchette, 1995). Risk factors known from the literature, such as pre-1950 houses (which have lead-based paint), are mapped as a series of primary maps. Attributes in each primary map are ranked or scaled on the same system to produce a series of derived maps. These derived maps are then overlaid, and a mathematical relation (such as summing the derived values on all the layers) is used to determine a final suitability (risk potential) map. Obviously, a lot of knowledge and care must go into developing accurate values and selecting important variables. Figure 13-12 shows the primary maps of quartile values for each of eight census variables. Derived values were used to produce the map of *comparative* risk potential in Figure 13-13. The addresses of children whose blood was screened for lead were matched to the road network, and the location of those whose blood levels exceeded 10 ug/dl are overlaid. Various statistical means were then used to asses the sensitivity and power of prediction. The methodology and results have met with great demand among state public health agencies.

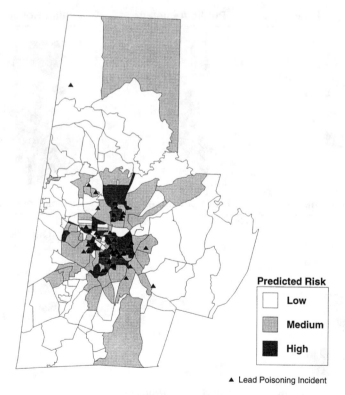

FIGURE 13-13. Predicted lead poisoning risk for Durham County block groups with overlay of lead poisoning cases. From Hanchette (1988). Used with permission.

A SUMMARY EXAMPLE: SPATIAL ANALYSIS OF CVD IN SAVANNAH

The southeast coast of the United States is a region of enigmatically high hypertension, stroke, and cardiovascular disease (CVD). This was not known when rates for CVD were given only at the state level but became evident when they were mapped at county level in the 1970s (Mason, McKay, Hoover, Blot, Franmeni, 1975; 1976). The usual risk factors at the individual level, such as being overweight, consuming salt, lacking exercise, smoking cigarettes, having high cholesterol, working at a stressful job, and so on, undoubtedly apply, but they do not explain the regionalization of the disease rates; that is, they do not covary at the same scale as the disease. A variety of hypotheses have incriminated everything from low selenium in the coastal soil to unknown water factors (CVD varies with water hardness in dozens of countries at the national and international scale) to the dust and ocean air people breath. It is unclear how people who get their food from a national marketing system and most of their water from an underground acquifer shared across much of the South are supposed to be exposed to such factors as a coastal, regional risk (i.e., they do not covary at the same scale). The connections of large metropolitan populations in the Enigma Area to any environmental factors is even less obvious. This section briefly describes the author's attempt to develop some new hypotheses about environmental risk factors by developing new methodological approaches to the question.

The metropolitan area of Savannah, which is located on the coast of Georgia and separated from other urban areas, was chosen as the study site. First, disease and related patterns were mapped. Death certificates were used to develop a probability map of strokes (Figure 13-9) and records of blood pressure measured by nurses with the Community Cardiovascular Center for all high school seniors in the city, aggregated over a 5-year period from 1978 to 1982 to stabilize small numbers and relate them to a census count of data, were mapped. After earlier statistical studies, a factor analysis of measures usually associated with CVD in the literature, such as education, income, age of housing, plumbing, room density, race, employment classification, and so on, was used to identify the components of factors important for several dimensions of the problem and to score their importance for each tract. These were then used in a discriminant analysis to predict the classification of each tract for whites and blacks in terms of blood pressure and strokes. The results of this work were a set of tracts which were well or poorly predicted for high or low strokes or blood pressure for whites and blacks. From these, 10 tracts were selected to represent those where the socioeconomic modeling overpredicted, underpredicted, or well-predicted the CVD outcome. In each of these 10 tracts, two clusters of 10 households were selected and 6 weeks were spent interviewing. Individual data were collected on dietary factors such as frying and salt, exercise behavior, smoking and drinking, and weight and blood pressure. Twenty-four-hour recall of mobility enabled different uses of space and time exposure

(A)

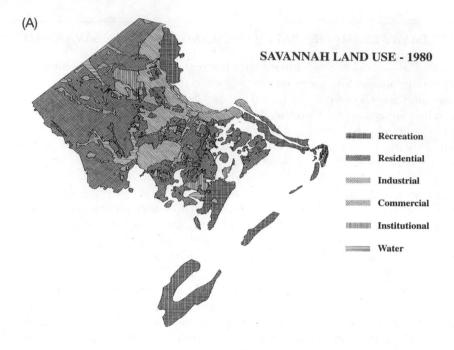

SAVANNAH LAND USE - 1980

▦ Recreation

▨ Residential

▧ Industrial

▩ Commercial

▥ Institutional

▤ Water

(B)

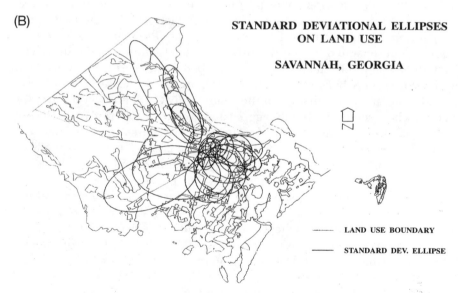

**STANDARD DEVIATIONAL ELLIPSES
ON LAND USE**

SAVANNAH, GEORGIA

------ LAND USE BOUNDARY

——— STANDARD DEV. ELLIPSE

FIGURE 13-14. (A) Land use in Savannah, Georgia, used to create new, combined categories. (B) Standard deviational ellipses of activity areas overlaid.

to be measured and analyzed. Use of health facilities and blood pressure screening and other service dimensions were investigated. Finally, standard questions about activities and locations allowed activity areas to be delimited using standard elliptical cells (Vignette 10-1). At the same time, land-use maps were updated from field observation and industries listed with the Chamber of Commerce were located and classified by type and size of employment.

Figure 13-14A shows the land use of Savannah. The blood pressure of high school seniors was allocated to the census tract in which their home address fell and a map of blood pressure by tract was laid over the land use, creating categories such as commercial-high blood pressure and commercial-low blood pressure, industrial high blood pressure, and so on. One of the findings was that the usual racial difference in blood pressure that has been repeatedly found when residences are classified only as urban, suburban, or rural disappeared when the teenagers were classified according to the land use where they lived (i.e., blood pressure for whites and blacks living in a tract classified as 80% industrial did not differ significantly).

The activity areas, the parts of the territory of Savannah within which people circulated, for the 20 clusters were mapped as a surface of exposure zones and overlaid on census tracts and on land use. Figure 13-14B shows how differently the people experienced the city of Savannah. When these activity areas were overlaid on the census tracts, the proportional areas within the ellipses could be summarized. Figure 13-15 shows the land use that was

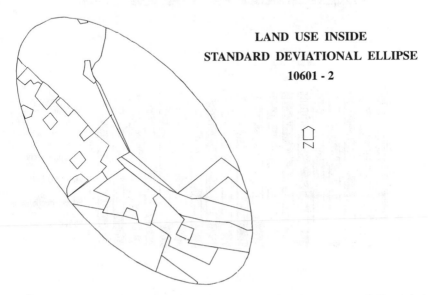

LAND USE INSIDE STANDARD DEVIATIONAL ELLIPSE 10601 - 2

FIGURE 13-15. Activity area of cluster 2, census tract 10601 in Savannah, Georgia cut out of overall land use coverage and showing proportions of various categories of landuse to which people are exposed through circulation within the metropolitan area.

"cut out" of the land-use map by the overlay of the activity area for people in cluster 2 or tract 10601. These are the environments to which the people there are actually exposed as they move around daily, not just what happens to be where their house is located. Finally, Figure 13-16 shows the variation among the clusters in the proportions of different land use or the conditions represented by census data—here, percentage of the population below the poverty line—that the respondents encountered in their daily lives.

Referring the information obtained from summarizing this spatial analysis back to the patterns of blood pressure and stroke mortality, several kinds of things can be said. For example, the average income within activity areas for people living in tracts where the blood pressure was underpredicted was

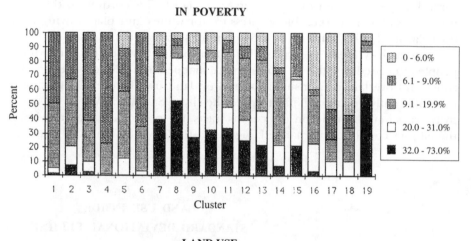

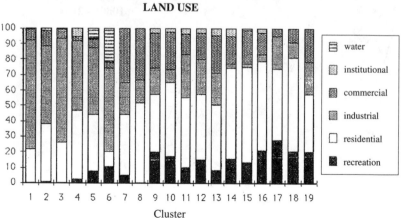

FIGURE 13-16. Bar graphs illustrating the proportion of the activity area of each cluster of interviewed households which is composed of different land uses or census attributes, such as percentage of households below the poverty line.

$11,620; well-predicted, $13,940; and overpredicted, $9,490. The proportion of land use under industry where blood pressure was predicted well or overpredicted by the socioeconomic associations was 24 or 25%, but where blood pressure was underpredicted it was 41.4%. Using the GIS capacity, distances can be measured from the interview clusters or activity area edges to types and sizes of industries overlaid from another surface. These methodologies, like all in this chapter, are still being developed.

CONCLUSION

Geographical methodology has been revolutionized by the information available and the speed and complexity with which it can be manipulated in GIS. Software has been developed to make GIS available on a point-and-click basis in windows and menus. Uses are spreading rapidly into a variety of disciplines, including epidemiology (Croner, 1998; Vine, Degnan, & Hanchette, 1997). It is being picked up internationally by the World Health Organization and others for surveillance of vectored diseases (Pope et al., 1994; Washino & Wood, 1994). Annual GIS and public health conferences are bringing government epidemiologists and statistical analysts (Centers for Disease Control; National Center for Health Statistics), academics, and applied analysts in planning and health services together across disciplines. There are a few careful presentations of concepts and reviews of usage (Clark et al., 1996). The present state is one of euphoria over possibilities.

Caveats are being voiced, however (Vine et al., Matthews, 1990). The proper uses and controls of this technology have not yet been faced, worked through, and academically institutionalized. Remember the problems of analyzing associations across scale and the fallacious and confounding results that can result for causal analysis? There are common sources of error at every stage of using a GIS: data collection (precision, sensing, observation, reporting, responding), data input (geocoding and inaccuracies of digitizing, address matching and incompleteness of coverage), data storage (insufficient processing, space, management), data manipulation (inappropriate class intervals, boundary errors, slivers and artifacts of overlay), data output (scaling inaccuracies, resolution, medium fading or instability), and incomplete understanding or use of results. Remember the issue of variance changing at different scales and the methodological troubles and opportunities of associations covarying over various scales? Then think of the map of the town of Search. The vegetation and other land use was captured in raster format at a resolution of meters by a camera in a satellite. The roads, pipes, and power lines were surveyed by engineering crews to an accuracy of centimeters. The population and other socioeconomic attributes were counted at the individual level but released at an aggregate scale of tracts which covered thousands of meters as their finest resolution. The activity areas were mathematically derived from answers to individual questions and then aggregated to populations determined by the research question. Health service data were accessed from central files at the hospital, and hence already selected as demand rather than need, and then allocated to incompletely matched address locations and converted to usage rates with denominators from census counts themselves incomplete and outdated. When all these different scales and inherent statistical errors are put together into one analysis of pattern association, it is difficult to be certain that truth can be found. Yet, there probably are spatial insights where previously there were none.

On top of all this, the body of knowledge and much of the wisdom of experience accumulated over centuries in cartography is in danger of being ignored, if not totally lost. In particular, all that has been learned about pattern comprehension and the hazards of distortion by poor categorization and sloppy abstraction is being over ridden by the sheer capacity of the hardware and the ignorance of the software writers to make any numbers of categories and colors available and default intervals convenient for the unthinking user.

And yet, the euphoria is real. Health researchers need to proceed with due care, with appreciation of the complexities of scale, but the potentials *are* revolutionary.

REFERENCES

Berghaus, H. (1852). *Physikalischer atlas*. Gotha: J. Perthes.

Burrough & McDonnell (1998). *Principles of geographic information systems*. Oxford: Oxford University Press.

Clarke, K. C. (1997). *Getting started with GIS*. Upper Saddle Road, NJ: Prentice Hall.

Clarke, K. C., McLafferty, S. L., & Tempalski, B. J. (1996). On epidemiology and geographic information systems: a review and discussion of future directions. *Emerging Infectious Diseases, 2*, 85–92.

Cleek, R. K. (1979). Cancer and the environment: The effect of scale. *Social Science and Medicine, 13D*, 241–247.

Cliff, A. D., & Haggett, P. (1988). *Atlas of disease distributions: Analytic approaches to epidemiological data*. New York: Blackwell.

Croner, C. M. (1998). Public health geographic information systems, 1994–1997 [Working paper series, no. 23]. Bethesda, MD: National Center for Health Statistics.

Davis, D. E. (1999). *GIS for everyone*. Redlands, CA: ESRI Press.

Gilbert, E. W. (1958, June). "Pioneer maps of health and disease in England. " *The Geographical Journal, 124*, 172–183.

Haggett, P. (1976). Hybridizing alternative models of an epidemic diffusion process. *Economic Geography, 52*, 136–146.

Hanchette, C. L. (1988). *Geographical patterns of prostate cancer mortality: An investigation of the relationship between prostate cancer and ultraviolet light*. Master's thesis, Department of Geography, University of North Carolina at Chapel Hill.

Hanchette, C. L. (1995.) A predictive model of lead poisoning risk in North Carolina:

Validation and evaluation. In *Proceedings of the International Symposium on Computer Mapping in Epidemiology and Environmental Health,* Tampa, Florida.

Hanchette, C. L. (1996). Lead poisoning risk factors for Durham County block groups. Personal communication of material not used in doctoral dissertation.

Hanchette, C. L., Meyer B., & Atkinson, D. (1993). *Lead database evaluation and GIS modelling project* (Report submitted to National Institute of Environmental Health Sciences, Office of Disease Prevention and Exposure Research [PR-242592]. Raleigh: State Center for Health and Environmental Statistics, North Carolina Department of Environment, Health, and Natural Resources.

Hohl, P., & Mayo, B. (1997). *ArcView GIS exercise book* (2nd ed.). Santa Fe, NM: On-Word Press.

Howe, G. M. (1970). *National atlas of disease mortality in the United Kingdom* (2nd ed.). London: Nelson.

Howe, G. M. (1972). *Man, environment, and disease in Britain.* New York: Barnes & Noble.

Hunter, J. M., & Meade, M. S. (1971). Population models in the high school. *Journal of Geography, 70,* 95–105.

King, P. E. (1979). Problems of spatial analysis in geographical epidemiology. *Social Science and Medicine, 13D,* 249–252.

Mason, T. J., McKay, F. W., Hoover, R., Blot, W. J., & Fraumeni, J. F., Jr. (1975). *Atlas of cancer mortality for U.S. counties: 1950–1969.* Washington, DC: U.S. Department of Health, Education, and Welfare, Epidemiology Branch, National Cancer Institute.

Mason, T. J., McKay, F. W., Hoover, R., Blot, W. J., & Fraumeni, J. F., Jr. (1976). *Atlas of cancer mortality among U.S. nonwhites: 1950–69.* Washington, DC: U.S. Department of Health, Education, and Welfare, Epidemiology Branch, National Cancer Institute.

Matthews, S. A. (1990). Epidemiology using a GIS: The need for caution. *Computer, Environment and Planning, 17,* 213–221.

May, J. M. (1950). Map of the world distribution of poliomyelitis. *Geographical Review, 40,* 646–648.

May, J. M. (1951a). Map of the world distribution of cholera. *Geographical Review, 41,* 272.

May, J. M. (1951b). Map of the world distribution of malaria vectors. *Geographical Review, 41,* 638–639.

May, J. M. (1952a). Map of the world distribution of helminthiases. *Geographical Review, 42,* 98–101.

May, J. M. (1952b). Map of the world distribution of dengue and yellow fever. *Geographical Review, 42,* 282–286.

May, J. M. (1952c). Map of the world distribution of plague. *Geographical Review, 42,* 628–630.

May, J. M. (1953a). Map of the world distribution of leprosy. *Geographical Review, 43.*

May, J. M. (1953b). The mapping of human starvation. *Geographical Review, 43,* 253–255.

May, J. M. (1954a). Maps of the world distribution of rickettsial diseases. *Geographical Review, 44,* 133–136.

May, J. M. (1954b). Map of the world distribution of some viral encephalitides. *Geographical Review, 44,* 408–410.

May, J. M. (1954c). Map of the world distribution of leishmaniasis. *Geographical Review, 44,* 583–584.

May, J. M. (1958). *Ecology of human disease.*

Mayer, J. D. (1981). Problems of spatial analysis in geographical epidemiology. *Social Science and Medicine, 13D,* 249–252.

Mayer, J. D. (1983). The role of spatial analysis and geographic data in detection of disease causation. *Social Science and Medicine, 17,* 1213–1221.

Meade, M. S. (1979). Cardiovascular mortality in the southeastern United States: The coastal plain enigma. *Social Science and Medicine, 13D,* 257–265.

Meade, M. S. (1983). Cardiovascular disease in Savannah, Georgia. In N. D. Mc-Glashan & J. R. Blunden (Eds.), *Geographical aspects of health* (pp. 175–196). London: Academic Press.

Monmonier, M. (1993). *Mapping it out: Expository cartography for the humanities and social sciences.* Chicago: Chicago University Press.

Monmonier, M. (1997). *Cartographies of danger: Mapping hazards in America.* Chicago: University of Chicago Press.

National Center for Health Statistics. (1997). *Atlas of United States mortality.* Washington, DC: U.S. Government Printing Office.

Openshaw, S. (1996). A view on the GIS crisis in geography. In J. Agnew, D. N. Livingstone, & A. Rogers (Eds.), *Human geography: An essential anthology* (pp. 675–685). Oxford: Blackwell.

Openshaw, S., Charlton, M., Wymer, C., & Craft, A. (1987). A mark 1 geographical analysis machine for the automated analysis of point data sets. *International Journal Geographical Information Systems, 1,* 335–358.

Pope, K. O., Rejmankova, E., Savage, H. M., Arredondo-Jimenez, J. I., Rodriguez, M. H., & Roberts, D. R. (1994). Remote sensing of tropical wetlands for malaria control in Chiapas, Mexico. *Ecological Applications, 4,* 81–90.

Rodenwaldt, E., & Jusatz, H. J. (Eds.). (1952–1961). *Welt-Seuchen atlas* (Vols. 1–3). Hamburg: Falk.

Rushton, G. (1998) *Improving public health through geographic information systems: An instructional guide to major systems.* Department of Geography, University of Iowa, Iowa City, Iowa.

Shisematsu, I. (1981). *National atlas of major disease mortalities in Japan,* Tokyo: Japan Health Promotion Federation.

Snow, J. (1855). *On the mode of communication of cholera.* London:

Vine, M., Degnan, D., & Hanchette, C. (1997). Geographic information systems: Their use in environmental epidemiologic research. *Environmental Health Perspectives, 105,* 598–605.

Washino, R. K., & Wood, B. J. (1994). Application of remote sensing to arthropod vector surveillance and control. *American Journal Tropical Medicine and Hygiene, 50* (6 Suppl.), 134–144.

Ziegenfus, R. C., & Gesler, W. M. (1984). Geographical patterns of heart disease in the northeastern United States. *Social Science and Medicine, 18,* 63–72.

FURTHER READING

Abler, R. E. (1993). Everything in its place: GPS, GIS, and geography in the 1990s. *Professional Geographer, 45,* 131–139.

Armstrong, R. W. (1973). Tracing exposure to specific environments in medical geography. *Geographic Analysis, 5,* 122–132.

Bailey, T. C., & Gatrell, A. C. (1995). *Interactive Spatial Data Analysis*. Longman Scientific and Technical. New York: Wiley.

Bennett, R. J. (1979). *Spatial time series*. London: Press.

Cliff, A. D., & Ord, J. K. (1973). *Spatial autocorrelation*. London: Pion.

DeMers, M. N. (1997). *Fundamentals of geographic information systems*. New York: Wiley.

Dobson, J. D. (1993). A rationale for the National Center for Geographic Information and Analysis. *Professional Geographer, 45,* 207–215.

Dobson, J. E., Armstrong, M. P., Cromley, R. G., Goodchild, M. F., Marble,D. F., Peuquet, D. J., Monmonier, M., Pickles, J., Posey, A. S., & Sheppard, E. (1993). "Automated geography" in 1993. *Professional Geographer, 45,* 431–461.

Fotheringham, S., & Rogerson, P. (1994). *Spatial Analysis and GIS* . London: Taylor & Francis

Gesler, W. M. (1986). The uses of spatial analysis in medical geography: A review. *Social Science and Medicine, 23,* 963–973.

Giggs, J. A. (1983). Schizophrenia and ecological structure in Nottingham. In N. D. McGlashan & J. R. Blunden (Eds.), *Geographical aspects of health* (pp. 197–222). London: Academic Press.

Haggett, P. (1990). *The geographer's art*. London: Basil Blackwell.

Heywood, I. (1990). Geographic information systems in the social sciences. *Environment and Planning A, 22,* 849–854.

Lam, N. S., & Quattrochi, D. A. (1992). On the issues of scale, resolution, and fractal analysis in the mapping sciences. *Professional Geographer, 44,* 88–98.

Marble, D. F., Calkins, H. W., & Peuquet, D. J. (1984). *Basic readings in geographic information systems*. Williamsville, NY: SPAD Systems.

Marshall, R. (1991). A review of methods for the statistical analysis of spatial patterns of disease. *Journal Royal Statistical Society, 154,* 421–41.

Meade, M. S. (1980). An interactive framework for geochemistry and cardiovascular disease. In M. S. Meade (Ed.), *Conceptual and methodological issues in medical geography* (pp. 194–221). Chapel Hill: University of North Carolina, Department of Geography.

Odland, J. (1988). *Spatial autocorrelation* [Scientific Geography series, vol. 9, ed., G. I. Thrall]. Newbury Park, CA: Sage.

Ord, K., & A. Getis. (1995). Local spatial autocorrelation statistics: distributional issues and an application. *Geographic Analysis, 24,* 286–306.

Ricketts, T. C., Savitz, L. A., Gesler, W. M., & Osborne, D. N. (1994). *Geographic methods for health services research*. New York: University Press of America.

Robinson, V. B. (1978). Modeling spatial variations in heart disease mortality: Implications of the variable subset selection process. *Social Science and Medicine, 12D,* 165–172.

Scholten, H. J., & Stillwell, J. (Eds.). (1990). *Geographical information systems for urban and regional planning*. Dordrecht: Kluwer Academic.

U.S. Environmental Protection Agency. (1986). *The United States cancer mortality rates and trends 1950–1979:* Vol. 4. *Atlas*. Washington, DC: U.S. Government Printing Office.

Walter, S. D. (1992). The analysis of regional patterns in health data. II. the power to detect environmental effects. *American Journal of Epidemliology, 136,* 742–759.

Wood, D. (1992). *The power of maps*. New York: Guilford Press.

Yuill, R. S. (1971). The standard deviation ellipse: An updated tool for spatial description. *Geografiska Annaler, 53B,* 28–39.

VIGNETTE 13-1.   Spatial Autocorrelation

Spatial autocorrelation is often discussed among geographers because it can be a serious hindrance to their work, but it can also be used as an analytical tool. Spatial autocorrelation means that observations from places next to each other are influenced by each other, in the same way that the real estate value of one piece of property affects that of the property around it. If one city block is poor and black, the adjacent one is probably similar; if one county is affluent and has low unemployment, the adjacent county is probably better off than average as well. One important problem with spatial autocorrelation is that the assumption of independent observations, required for most statistical procedures such as linear regression and correlation, may be wrong.

It is perhaps easiest to explain spatial autocorrelation by mapping a dichotomous (nominal data) variable, one that is either present or absent in each spatial unit of a study area. Consider Vignette 13-1, Figure 1, which diagrams three situations in which a certain disease is either present (black) or absent (white) in each of 16 square units. In the first situation, there is positive spatial autocorrelation: black and white units are grouped together. Perhaps the illness is quite contagious in the black part of the study area but has come up against some type of physical or human barrier in the white area. The second situation illustrates negative autocorrelation; adjacent units are dissimilar. In the third diagram, a random pattern of black and white units indicates no autocorrelation, either positive or negative.

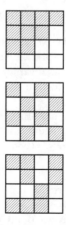

VIGNETTE 13-1, FIGURE 1. Spatial autocorrelation. Three types of spatial autocorrelation with a dichotomous variable are illustrated.

There are two important things to consider in measuring autocorrelation: whether units are adjoining ("have a join") and what the value of a variable or phenomenon is in each unit. One can say that there is a join if units have a common nonzero boundary (rook's case, from chess), a common vertex or point (bishop's case), or either of these (queen's case). In the figure, the unit values were simple presence or absence of a phenomenon.

How can one tell, statistically, whether there is autocorrelation in a particular situation? Basically, one counts the number of black–white (BW), black–black (BB), and white–white (WW) joins and compares these with the number of joins that would be expected if the black and white units were distributed randomly. In the third diagram of Vignette Figure 13-1a, there are 6 BB joins, 4 WW joins, and 14 BW joins (rook's case). The appropriate formulas using this joint count can be found in texts that deal with autocorrelation. If there are significantly more BB or WW joins than expected, there is positive autocorrelation, and if significantly more BW joins than expected there is negative autocorrelation.

Unit values need not only represent absence or presence of a disease; they could also represent high and low disease rates. In addition, more than two nominal data categories can be considered and the analysis taken from the "two-color" to the "k-color" case. Furthermore, definitions of a join can be altered in innovative ways. For example, Haggett (1976) in a study of measles diffusion in England (discussed in Chapter 8) defined joins in seven ways, based on different types of paths along which the disease might be diffusing (e.g., along journey-to-work routes). If a certain path type indicated positive spatial autocorrelation, that particular path type could be important in the spread of measles, and, indeed, Haggett identified the importance of different pathways at different stages of the epidemic.

Spatial autocorrelation techniques have been used in a constructive manner to determine links between spatial patterns and causal processes (see Chapter 8). In particular, the techniques can help identify connections between disease rates and environmental and socioeconomic factors. Disease rates, which are interval data, have been most commonly used.

Thirteen counties from central and southern New Jersey were selected to illustrate how to use spatial autocorrelations. The first step is to construct a 13-by-13 join matrix (rook's case) that consists of 0's if two counties do not have a nonzero boundary and 1's if they do (Vignette 13-1, Figure 2). Note that a county does not join itself.

To examine the heart disease rates for spatial autocorrelation, Moran's I statistic, which is used for interval data, can be calculated. If units with similar rates (high or low) tend to be next to each other, the I statistic will be relatively large (positive autocorrelation); if the opposite is the case, the I statistic will be relatively small (negative autocorrelation). The I statistic can be tested for a significance as a standard normal deviate (Z-score) after determining the mean and variance of its distribution. (Appropriate formulas can be found in books dealing with this subject.) If the calculated Z-score for a particular value of Moran's I is significant-

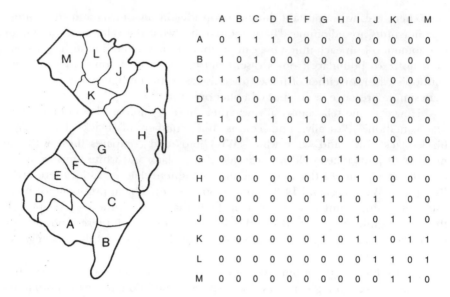

	A	B	C	D	E	F	G	H	I	J	K	L	M
A	0	1	1	1	0	0	0	0	0	0	0	0	0
B	1	0	1	0	0	0	0	0	0	0	0	0	0
C	1	1	0	0	1	1	1	0	0	0	0	0	0
D	1	0	0	0	1	0	0	0	0	0	0	0	0
E	1	0	1	1	0	1	0	0	0	0	0	0	0
F	0	0	1	0	1	0	1	0	0	0	0	0	0
G	0	0	1	0	0	1	0	1	1	0	1	0	0
H	0	0	0	0	0	0	1	0	1	0	0	0	0
I	0	0	0	0	0	0	1	1	0	1	1	0	0
J	0	0	0	0	0	0	0	0	1	0	1	1	0
K	0	0	0	0	0	0	1	0	1	1	0	1	1
L	0	0	0	0	0	0	0	0	0	1	1	0	1
M	0	0	0	0	0	0	0	0	0	0	1	1	0

VIGNETTE 13-1, FIGURE 2. The join matrix for lag 1, neighbors, for a 13-county area in southern New Jersey.

ly positive, then one can say that a particular heart disease rate showed clustering at the level of adjoining counties.

The original join matrix can be modified or refined to reflect two factors simultaneously, the proportion of the boundary of one county that is common to another county and the distance between county centers if there is a nonzero boundary. These modifications can be thought of as adding weights to the simple binary scheme of the original join matrix.

The original join matrix could be modified to reflect a particular potential risk factor. For example, one could assign a join matrix value of 1 if two counties were the same degree urban and within a certain maximum distance of each other. If the value of Moran's I were to increase following this modification, the risk factor might be of importance.

The next stage in the analysis is to produce a spatial correlogram that is a rough indication of the areal extent of disease clustering. The original join matrix is modified to include 1's only if two counties are neighbors of neighbors; for example, county A's neighbors of neighbors are county F and county G. The new matrix can be tested for spatial autocorrelation. If it is significantly positive, one can say that clustering is manifest at a larger scale than the original adjoining county scale. This process can be continued to neighbors of neighbors of neighbors, and so on (the general rule is to carry out approximately $n/4$ steps where n is the number of units of observation). The result is a series of Z-scores for I statistics, which can be plotted as a spatial correlogram. The Z-scores from the original binary matrix are called the first lag and succeeding Z-scores are second, third, and fourth lags, and so on.

Vignette 13-1, Figure 3 shows spatial correlograms for white male and female acute ischemic heart disease for two time periods for a 49-county area surrounding New York City and Philadelphia. For all four sets of rates, there is significant positive spatial autocorrelation at the 99% level for the first lag and significant positive spatial autocorrelation at the 95% level for the second lag; on succeeding lags significant positive autocorrelation is no longer evident. At some lags there is significant negative autocorrelation, indicating that at these scales, adjoining groups of counties have dissimilar rates. It seems that for whites, acute ischemic

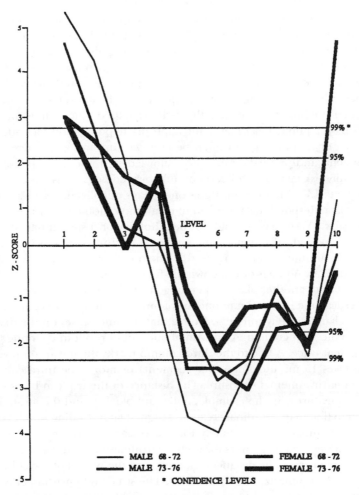

VIGNETTE 13-1, FIGURE 3. Spatial correlograms for whites with acute ischemic heart disease in the New York/Philadelphia metropolitan area, 1968–1972 and 1973–1976.

rates cluster up to the neighbor of neighbor scale, a fairly large area within the 49-county area. Still there are groups of counties within the area that have dissimilar rates, as maps of acute ischemic heart disease rates attest (Ziegenfus & Gesler, 1984).

VIGNETTE 13-2. Microspatial Exposure Analysis

Detailed mobility information is essential for study of exposure to specific environments. For example, knowledge of water contact behavior is critical to understanding the incidence of schistosomiasis. Knowing about exposure to orchard mosquitoes in the evening or stream mosquitoes in the morning helps to identify hazards from specific vectored diseases. Often the environment must be carefully described. The home at night, for example, affects health differently depending on whether the house is screened, the beds are netted, the room is smoke-filled, and so on. At a public health level, the appropriate population for education, intervention, or monitoring can often be targeted through knowledge of critical environments and population mobility. Knowledge of microspatial mobility may help identify risk factors for diseases of unknown etiology.

Vignette 13-2, Figure 1 illustrates one means of collecting such microspatial mobility data. Respondents are asked to recall their mobility over a 24-hour period, yesterday. "Yesterday" should not be a holiday or a special day of the week. The day is marked off in equal time segments by three columns of dots (in the figure a 15-minute segment is used). The interviewer talks the respondent through the day. A line is drawn down the first column of dots until the first trip, to the yard or to another place, depending on the scale being analyzed. The shift of the vertical line from column one to column two and back to column one represents a change in environment. Notice that the line passes on the diagonal to the dot in the next column. A horizontal line would result in counting the same time segment twice. A line to the third column marks the means of travel. When the trip takes 15 minutes (one time segment) or more, the third column dots represent environmental exposure. The distance of the trip can be noted in appropriate measures (in the example, miles and blocks), and the location can be specified so that map coordinates can be assigned later. Coding requires that one specify environments appropriately for the research purpose. The number of dots that the vertical line covers for each environment provides an easy summary. The number of trips, the distances traveled, and the means of travel by purpose are also easily summarized from the form. The scale and environments involved in another interview might specify particular fields, water holes, marketplaces, rooms within a factory, or districts within a city.

Aggregating the responses to mobility interviews permits assessment of dif-

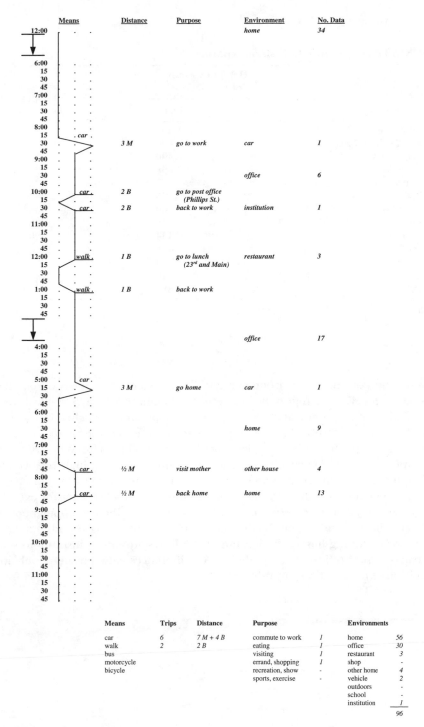

Means			Distance	Purpose	Environment	No. Data
12:00					home	34
6:00						
15						
30						
45						
7:00						
15						
30						
45						
8:00						
15	. car .					
30			3 M	go to work	car	1
45						
9:00						
15						
30					office	6
45						
10:00	. car .		2 B	go to post office (Phillips St.)		
15						
30	. car .		2 B	back to work	institution	1
45						
11:00						
15						
30						
45						
12:00	. walk .		1 B	go to lunch (23rd and Main)	restaurant	3
15						
30						
45						
1:00	. walk .		1 B	back to work		
15						
30						
45						
					office	17
4:00						
15						
30						
45						
5:00	. car .					
15			3 M	go home	car	1
30						
45						
6:00						
15						
30					home	9
45						
7:00						
15						
30						
45	. car .		½ M	visit mother	other house	4
8:00						
15						
30	. car .		½ M	back home	home	13
45						
9:00						
15						
30						
45						
10:00						
15						
30						
45						
11:00						
15						
30						
45						

Means	Trips	Distance	Purpose		Environments	
car	6	7 M + 4 B	commute to work	1	home	56
walk	2	2 B	eating	1	office	30
bus			visiting	1	restaurant	3
motorcycle			errand, shopping	1	shop	-
bicycle			recreation, show	-	other home	4
			sports, exercise	-	vehicle	2
					outdoors	-
					school	-
					institution	1
						96

VIGNETTE 13-2, FIGURE 1. Mobility recall form. Diagonal lines between the first two columns of dots show change of habitat, while the third column is used to indicate the means of transportation, which may itself become a habitat exposure.

483

VIGNETTE 13-2, TABLE 1. Risk of Exposure

Environment	Dots of exposure of population[a]		Control population relative risk
	Sick	Healthy	
Total home	1,613	1,498	1.08
Home 7 A.M. to 7 P.M.	260	196	1.3
Office	86	490	.18
Factory	518	58	8.9
Restaurant	28	86	.33
Shop	29	55	.53
Other home	86	60	1.43
Vehicles	115	58	1.98
Outdoors	29	144	.20
School	346	403	.86
Institution	5	18	.28
Church	25	10	2.5
Total dots of exposure	2,880	2,880	

[a]Population, 30 sick and 30 healthy individuals.

ferences in exposure to environments and of the extent and means of mobility. Vignette 13-2, Table 1 represents the results obtained from a hypothetical study population with an illness and a healthy control population, matched by age, sex, ethnicity, income level, and other appropriate criteria. Because there are 96 15-minute segments (dots) in a day, each population of 30 has a total of 2,880 dots of exposure to some environment. The sick population has a high relative risk (Chapter 12) for exposure to a factory environment and to vehicles during the commute to work. It is much less exposed to the outdoors (perhaps for exercise or recreation). There are also social differences between the two populations, as reflected in more time spent by the sick population in visiting friends, going to church, and staying home, and less time spent in restaurants or institutions such as banks or post offices. The significance of differences between the population can be assessed statistically by using a t-test.

Concluding Words

This textbook describes the systems, such as biology, ecology, economics, politics, culture, meteorology, demographics, and medicine, whose interactions form the status of human health. Health-related phenomena have a certain distribution, move in certain directions at varying speeds, and affect people's perceptions about their communities and surrounding environments. Medical geographers who examine these spatial processes draw on the concepts and techniques of all the subdisciplines of geography. New diseases emerge from the changed landscape and patterns of settlement of the earth and from disease agents' adaptation to our biomedical solutions that have neglected ecological considerations; population fertility seems to be falling around the world to below replacement levels and populations are aging; recombinant DNA technologies are transforming the genetics of foods and diseases; globalization brings democratization of technology and information, but also the devolution of power and new insecurities about the loss of regional culture and status—as these things and more happen over the next decades, geographers need to bring their focus on scale, space, and a holistic approach to understanding health to the public discourse and to the promotion of health.

The medical geography of health care freely incorporates the concerns and findings from other disciplines about the social, economic, political, and cultural behavior of individuals and systems. In turn, it contributes its geographical perspective to the emergence of a social science of health care. Similarly, epidemiological design and methodology, parasitology, entomology, microbiology, and the anthropology of medical belief, along with many other disciplinary insights, are synthesized and used in explaining the spatial distribution of disease occurrence. Medical geographers over the past 20 years have become better trained in the cognate fields relevant to their specializations, although some of that is being lost in the embrace of only things social. Most medical geographers recognize their medical limitations, and are eager to collaborate with other health professionals and scientists.

We have discussed problems that arise in available medical statistics and in obtaining microarea data. More important is awareness that ignorance of basic and relevant biology can cause research hypotheses even about spatial form to be deficient, and that ignorance of basic sociocultural processes can result in simplistic genetic or environmental explanations. Spatial perspective, knowledge about differences of scale and spatial autocorrelation, and general familiarity with physical and social sciences can result in fresh geographical insights, new hypotheses, and sounder planning and policy.

As we hope this text illustrates, the literature of medical geography is complex and exciting. There is a rich diversity to the research, a hybrid vigor and vibrancy that has derived from the the mixing of many new ideas. Individual medical geographers may feel most comfortable with some segment of the subdiscipline. Some wish to be only theoretically informed, some to explore spatial analysis of diffusion in a positivist manner, some to focus on microlevel integration and qualitative understanding. Most still pursue the ancient geographical concerns: integrating all the phenomena at a point in space in order to understand the nature of place and understanding and explaining the distribution of varied phenomena over space.

Employment opportunities for health geographers are abundant but usually only for those with a minimum master's degree in that field (although competence in GIS can qualify for some applied geography jobs with a baccalaureate). Besides academic positions, medical geographers with recent graduate degrees from North Carolina alone are now directing Family Health International family planning and AIDS intervention efforts in East Africa, working with the Centers for Disease Control, the Research Triangle Institute, the North Carolina state center for environmental health, the Carter Center's Global 2000 effort to eradicate guinea worm in West Africa, and numerous hospital and regional health care planning organizations. The term "spatial epidemiology" is appearing more often both in the geographic and public health literature. This usually translates to the application of GIS to disease and health problems. Students who are interested in this field should pursue training in GIS and mathematics/statistics. One of the best Internet sites today for following this field and making contacts is the Public Health GIS Users Groups, which is maintained by medical geographer Charles Croner of the National Center for Health Statistics. Dr. Croner publishers an online newsletter monthly at *GIS-GEOG@LISTSERV.CDC.GOV.*

Medical geography as a well-defined subdiscipline of geography has existed for only a few decades. During that time it has grown from a few individuals producing sometimes excellent work to a substantial and varied body of research effort. As it has matured, it has become more introspective and critical. The intellectual ties of geographical perspective link together different projects, data sources, techniques, scales, hypotheses, and general paradigms to contribute a different voice to understanding. Medical geography has reached the point as an emerging body of literature that students and other medical geographers and health researchers generally can expect to draw on it before intiating a research project. It has reached the point where a text such as this, drawing from the work of dozens of individuals and hundreds of publications, can be written. The perspectives are basic to addressing the broader health questions of the role of social institutions, the consequences of environmental management or misuse, and the impact of sociocultural roles and perception which are too frequently ignored.

Index

About the Authors

Melinda S. Meade, PhD, a medical geographer, is currently a professor of geography at the University of North Carolina at Chapel Hill. She is also an adjunct professor of epidemiology, a member of the ecology curriculum committee, and a fellow of the Carolina Population Center. In addition to the first edition of *Medical Geography,* she has published journal articles on the disease ecology of tropical Asia and the United States. She is a member of the Association of American Geographers, and other geographical, public health, and population associations.

Robert J. Earickson, PhD, a medical geographer, is currently an associate professor of geography at the University of Maryland, Baltimore County. He has written the books *Geographic Measurement and Quantitative Analysis* and *The Spatial Behavior of Hospital Patients,* as well as articles on urban health problems. He is a member of the Association of American Geographers and is also Senior Editor of the Geography of Disease, Health, and Development section of the journal *Social Science & Medicine.*